Pocket Guide to
Diagnostic
Tests
- - - - - - - - - - - - - - - - - - - -

sixth edition

Diana Nicoll, [
Clinical Profess
Department of L
University of Cal
Associate Dean
University of Cali
Chief of Staff and Chief, Laboratory Medicine Service
Veterans Affairs Medical Center, San Francisco

Chuanyi Mark Lu, MD
Associate Professor of Laboratory Medicine
University of California, San Francisco
Chief, Hematology and Hematopathology
Director, Molecular Diagnostics
Laboratory Medicine Service
Veterans Affairs Medical Center, San Francisco

Michael Pignone, MD, MPH
Professor of Medicine
Chief, Division of General Internal Medicine
Department of Medicine
University of North Carolina, Chapel Hill

Stephen J. McPhee, MD
Professor of Medicine, Emeritus
Division of General Internal Medicine
Department of Medicine
University of California, San Francisco

With Associate Authors

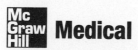 **Medical**

New York Chicago San Francisco Lisbon London Madrid Mexico City
Milan New Delhi San Juan Seoul Singapore Sydney Toronto

The **McGraw·Hill** Companies

Pocket Guide to Diagnostic Tests, Sixth Edition

5 6 7 8 9 0   DOC/DOC   17 16

ISBN 978-0-07-176625-8
MHID 0-07-176625-1
ISSN 1061-3463

This book was set in Times Roman by Cenveo Publisher Services
The editors were Christine Diedrich and Robert Pancotti.
The production supervisor was Catherine H. Saggese.
Project management was provided by Sandhya Gola, Cenveo Publisher Services.
The cover designer was Elizabeth Pisacreta.
RR Donnelley was printer and binder.

This book was printed on acid-free paper.

Contents

Associate Authors

Barbara Haller, MD, PhD
Associate Clinical Professor of Laboratory Medicine
Chief of Microbiology
San Francisco General Hospital & Trauma Center, San Francisco
Microbiology: Test Selection

Fred M. Kusumoto, MD
Associate Professor of Medicine
Department of Medicine
Division of Cardiovascular Diseases
Director of Electrophysiology and Pacing
Mayo Clinic Jacksonville, Florida
Basic Electrocardiography and Echocardiography

Benjamin M. Yeh, MD
Associate Professor of Radiology
Department of Radiology
University of California, San Francisco
Diagnostic Imaging: Test Selection and Interpretation

Phil Tiso
UCSF Principal Editor
Division of General Internal Medicine
Department of Medicine
University of California, San Francisco

Preface

Purpose

The *Pocket Guide to Diagnostic Tests, sixth edition,* is intended to serve as a pocket reference manual for medical, nursing, and other health professional students, house officers, and practicing physicians and nurses. It is a quick reference guide to the selection and interpretation of commonly used diagnostic tests, including laboratory procedures in the clinical setting, laboratory tests (chemistry, hematology, immunology, microbiology, pharmacogenetic, and molecular and genetic testing), diagnostic imaging tests (plain radiography, CT, MRI, and ultrasonography), electrocardiography, echocardiography, and the use of tests in differential diagnosis, helpful algorithms, and nomograms and reference material.

This book enables readers to understand commonly used diagnostic tests and diagnostic approaches to common disease states.

Outstanding Features

- Over 450 tests presented in a concise, consistent, and readable format.
- Full coverage of more than two dozen new laboratory tests.
- Expanded content regarding molecular and genetic tests, including pharmacogenetic tests.
- New section on basic echocardiography.
- Updated and additional microbiologic coverage of emerging (new) and reemerging pathogens and infectious agents.
- Fields covered: internal medicine, pediatrics, surgery, neurology, and obstetrics and gynecology.
- Costs and risks of various procedures and tests.
- Full literature citations with PubMed (PMID) numbers included for each reference.
- An index for quick reference on the back cover.

Organization

This pocket reference manual is not intended to include all diagnostic tests or disease states. The authors have selected the tests and diseases that are most common and relevant to the general practice of medicine.

The *Guide* is divided into 10 sections:
1. Diagnostic Testing and Medical Decision Making
2. Point-of-Care Testing and Provider-Performed Microscopy
3. Common Laboratory Tests: Selection and Interpretation
4. Therapeutic Drug Monitoring and Pharmacogenetic Testing
5. Microbiology: Test Selection
6. Diagnostic Imaging: Test Selection and Interpretation
7. Basic Electrocardiography and Echocardiography
8. Diagnostic Tests in Differential Diagnosis
9. Diagnostic Algorithms
10. Nomograms and Reference Material

New to This Edition

1. More than two dozen new or substantially revised clinical laboratory test entries, including: urine albumin, beta-hCG, CCP antibody, celiac disease serology, serum C-telopeptide and urine N-telopeptide, dehydroepiandrosterone, estradiol, glucagon, hepatitis E, intrinsic factor blocking antibody, urine iodine, islet cell antibody, kappa and lambda light chains, osteocalcin, pancreatic elastase, Quantiferon TB, somatostatin, and thyroid stimulating immunoglobulin.
2. Microbiologic tests for emerging (new) and reemerging pathogens and infectious agents.
3. More than two dozen new or substantially revised tables and algorithms concerning diagnostic approaches to: amenorrhea or oligomenorrhea; ascites and ascitic fluid profiles in various disease states; autoantibodies; molecular diagnostic testing in various genetic diseases; common serologic test patterns in hepatitis B virus infection; hemochromatosis; hyperaldosteronism; female infertility; classification and immunophenotyping of leukemias and lymphomas; severity index for acute pancreatitis; pulmonary embolism, including the revised Geneva Score for pulmonary embolism probability assessment, including a prognostic model (PESI Score) and risk stratification; clinical and laboratory diagnosis in untreated patients with syphilis; genetics and laboratory characteristics of thalassemia syndromes; summary of blood component therapy in transfusion; and diagnostic evaluation of valvular heart disease.

Intended Audience

Medical students will find the concise summary of diagnostic laboratory, microbiologic, and imaging studies, and of electrocardiography and echocardiography in this pocket-sized book of great help during clinical ward rotations.

Busy house officers, physician's assistants, nurse practitioners, and physicians will find the clear organization and current literature references useful in devising proper patient management.

Nurses and other health practitioners will find the format and scope of the *Guide* valuable for understanding the use of laboratory tests in patient management.

Acknowledgments

The editors acknowledge the invaluable editorial contributions of William M. Detmer, MD, and Tony M. Chou, MD, to the first three editions of this book.

In addition, the late G. Thomas Evans, Jr., MD, contributed the electrocardiography section of Chapter 7 for the second and third editions. In the fourth, fifth, and this sixth edition, this section has been revised by Fred M. Kusumoto, MD.

We thank Jane Jang, BS, MT (ASCP) SM, for her revision of the microbiology chapter in the fifth edition. In this sixth edition, the chapter has been substantially revised by Barbara Haller, MD, PhD.

We thank our associate authors for their contributions to this book and are grateful to the many clinicians, residents, and students who have made useful suggestions.

We welcome comments and recommendations from our readers for future editions.

Diana Nicoll, MD, PhD, MPA
Chuanyi Mark Lu, MD
Michael Pignone, MD, MPH
Stephen J. McPhee, MD

1

Diagnostic Testing and Medical Decision Making

Diana Nicoll, MD, PhD, MPA, Michael Pignone, MD, MPH, and
Chuanyi Mark Lu, MD

The clinician's main task is to make reasoned decisions about patient care despite incomplete clinical information and uncertainty about clinical outcomes. Although data elicited from the history and physical examination are often sufficient for making a diagnosis or for guiding therapy, more information may be required. In these situations, clinicians often turn to diagnostic tests for help.

BENEFITS, COSTS, AND RISKS

When used appropriately, diagnostic tests can be of great assistance to the clinician. Tests can be helpful for **screening,** ie, to identify risk factors for disease and to detect occult disease in asymptomatic persons. Identification of risk factors may allow early intervention to prevent disease occurrence, and early detection of occult disease may reduce disease morbidity and mortality through early treatment. Blood pressure measurement is recommended for preventive care of asymptomatic low risk adults. Screening for breast, cervix, and colon cancer is also recommended, whereas screening for prostate cancer and lung cancer remains controversial. Optimal screening tests should meet the criteria listed in Table 1–1.

Tests can also be helpful for **diagnosis,** ie, to help establish or exclude the presence of disease in symptomatic persons. Some tests assist in early diagnosis after onset of symptoms and signs; others assist in developing a differential diagnosis; others help determine the stage or activity of disease.

Tests can be helpful in **patient management:** (1) to evaluate the severity of disease, (2) to estimate prognosis, (3) to monitor the course of disease (progression, stability, or resolution), (4) to detect disease recurrence, and (5) to select drugs and adjust therapy.

**TABLE 1–1. CRITERIA FOR USE OF
SCREENING PROCEDURES.**

Characteristics of population
1. Sufficiently high prevalence of disease.
2. Likely to be compliant with subsequent tests
   and treatments.

Characteristics of disease
1. Significant morbidity and mortality.
2. Effective and acceptable treatment available.
3. Presymptomatic period detectable.
4. Improved outcome from early treatment.

Characteristics of test
1. Good sensitivity and specificity.
2. Low cost and risk.
3. Confirmatory test available and practical.

When ordering diagnostic tests, clinicians should weigh the potential benefits against the potential costs and adverse effects. Some tests carry a risk of morbidity or mortality—eg, cerebral angiogram leads to stroke in 0.5% of cases. The potential discomfort associated with tests such as colonoscopy may deter some patients from completing a diagnostic work-up. The result of a diagnostic test may mandate additional testing or frequent follow-up, and the patient may incur significant cost, risk, and discomfort during follow-up procedures.

Furthermore, a false-positive test may lead to incorrect diagnosis or further unnecessary testing. Classifying a healthy patient as diseased based on a falsely positive diagnostic test can cause psychological distress and may lead to risks from unnecessary or inappropriate therapy. A screening test may identify disease that would not otherwise have been recognized and that would not have affected the patient. For example, early-stage prostate cancer detected by prostate-specific antigen (PSA) screening in a 76-year-old man with known congestive heart failure will probably not become symptomatic during his lifetime, and aggressive treatment may result in net harm.

The costs of diagnostic testing must also be understood and considered. Total costs may be high, or cost-effectiveness may be unfavorable. Even relatively inexpensive tests may have poor cost-effectiveness if they produce very small health benefits.

Factors adversely affecting cost-effectiveness include ordering a panel of tests when one test would suffice, ordering a test more frequently than necessary, and ordering tests for medical record documentation only. The operative question for test ordering is, "Will the test result affect patient management?" If the answer is no, then the test is not justified. Unnecessary tests generate unnecessary labor, reagent, and equipment costs and lead to high health care expenditures.

Molecular and genetic testing is becoming more readily available, but its cost-effectiveness and health outcome benefits need to be carefully examined. Diagnostic genetic testing based on symptoms (eg, testing for fragile X in a boy with mental retardation) differs from predictive genetic testing (eg, evaluating a healthy person with a family history of Huntington disease) and from predisposition genetic testing, which may indicate relative susceptibility to certain conditions or response to certain drug treatment (eg, *BRCA-1* or *HER-2* testing for breast cancer). The outcome benefits of many new pharmacogenetic tests have not yet been established by prospective clinical studies; eg, there is insufficient evidence that genotypic testing for warfarin dosing leads to outcomes that are superior to those using conventional dosing algorithms, in terms of reduction of out-of-range INRs. Other testing (eg, testing for inherited causes of thrombophilia, such as factor V Leiden, prothrombin mutation, etc) has only limited value for treating patients, since knowing whether a patient has inherited thrombophilia generally does not change the intensity or duration of anticoagulation treatment. Carrier testing (eg, for cystic fibrosis) and prenatal fetal testing (eg, for Down syndrome) often require counseling of patients so that there is adequate understanding of the clinical, social, ethical, and sometimes legal impact of the results.

Clinicians order and interpret large numbers of laboratory tests every day, and the complexity of these tests continues to increase. The large and growing test menu has introduced challenges for clinicians in selecting the correct laboratory test and correctly interpreting the test results. Errors in test selection and test result interpretation are common but often difficult to detect. Using evidence-based testing algorithms that provide guidance for test selection in specific disorders and expert-driven test interpretation (eg, reports and interpretative comments generated by clinical pathologists) can help decrease such errors and improve the timeliness and accuracy of diagnosis.

PERFORMANCE OF DIAGNOSTIC TESTS

Test Preparation

Factors affecting both the patient and the specimen are important. The most crucial element in a properly conducted laboratory test is an appropriate specimen.

Patient Preparation

Preparation of the patient is important for certain tests—eg, a fasting state is needed for optimal glucose and triglyceride measurements; posture and sodium intake should be strictly controlled when measuring renin and aldosterone levels; and strenuous exercise should be avoided before taking samples for creatine kinase determinations, since vigorous muscle activity can lead to falsely abnormal results.

Specimen Collection

Careful attention must be paid to patient identification and specimen labeling—eg, two patient identifiers (full name and birth date, or full name and unique institutional identifier, eg, Social Security Number) must be used. Knowing when the specimen was collected may be important. For instance, aminoglycoside levels cannot be interpreted appropriately without knowing whether the specimen was drawn just before ("trough" level) or after ("peak" level) drug administration. Drug levels cannot be interpreted if they are drawn during the drug's distribution phase (eg, digoxin levels drawn during the first 6 hours after an oral dose). Substances that have a circadian variation (eg, cortisol) can be interpreted only in the context of the time of day the sample was drawn.

During specimen collection, other principles should be remembered. Specimens should not be drawn above an intravenous line, because this may contaminate the sample with intravenous fluid and drug (eg, heparin). Excessive tourniquet time leads to hemoconcentration and an increased concentration of protein-bound substances such as calcium. Lysis of cells during collection of a blood specimen results in spuriously increased serum levels of substances concentrated in cells (eg, lactate dehydrogenase and potassium). Certain test specimens may require special handling or storage (eg, specimens for blood gas and serum cryoglobulin). Delay in delivery of specimens to the laboratory can result in ongoing cellular metabolism and therefore spurious results for some studies (eg, low serum glucose).

TEST CHARACTERISTICS

Table 1–2 lists the general characteristics of useful diagnostic tests. Most of the principles detailed below can be applied not only to laboratory and radiologic tests but also to elements of the history and physical examination.

TABLE 1–2. PROPERTIES OF USEFUL DIAGNOSTIC TESTS.

1. Test methodology has been described in detail so that it can be accurately and reliably reproduced.
2. Test accuracy and precision have been determined.
3. The reference interval has been established appropriately.
4. Sensitivity and specificity have been reliably established by comparison with a gold standard. The evaluation has used a range of patients, including those who have different but commonly confused disorders and those with a spectrum of mild and severe, treated and untreated diseases. The patient selection process has been adequately described so that results will not be generalized inappropriately.
5. Independent contribution to overall performance of a test panel has been confirmed if a test is advocated as part of a panel of tests.

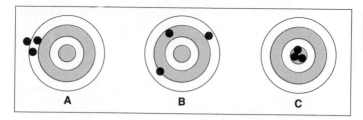

Figure 1–1. Relationship between accuracy and precision in diagnostic tests. The center of the target represents the true value of the substance being tested. **(A)** A diagnostic test that is precise but inaccurate; repeated measurements yield very similar results, but all results are far from the true value. **(B)** A test that is imprecise and inaccurate; repeated measurements yield widely different results, and the results are far from the true value. **(C)** An ideal test that is both precise and accurate.

An understanding of these characteristics is very helpful to the clinician when ordering and interpreting diagnostic tests.

Accuracy

The accuracy of a laboratory test is its correspondence with the true value. A test is deemed inaccurate when the result differs from the true value even though the results may be reproducible (Figure 1–1A), this represents **systematic error** (or bias). For example, serum creatinine is commonly measured by a kinetic Jaffe method, which has a systematic error as large as 0.23 mg/dL when compared with the gold standard gas chromatography-isotope dilution mass spectrometry method. In the clinical laboratory, accuracy of tests is maximized by calibrating laboratory equipment with reference material and by participation in external proficiency testing programs.

Precision

Test precision is a measure of a test's reproducibility when repeated on the same sample. If the same specimen is analyzed many times, some variation in results (random error) is expected; this variability is expressed as a **coefficient of variation** (CV: the standard deviation divided by the mean, often expressed as a percentage). For example, when the laboratory reports a CV of 5% for serum creatinine and accepts results within ± 2 standard deviations, it denotes that, for a sample with serum creatinine of 1.0 mg/dL, the laboratory may report the result as anywhere from 0.90 to 1.10 mg/dL on repeated measurements from the same sample.

An imprecise test is one that yields widely varying results on repeated measurements (Figure 1–1B). The precision of diagnostic tests, which is monitored in clinical laboratories by using control material, must be good enough to distinguish clinically relevant changes in a patient's status from the analytic variability (imprecision) of the test. For instance, the manual peripheral white blood cell differential count may not be precise enough to detect important changes in the distribution of cell types, because it is calculated by subjective evaluation of a small sample (eg, 100 cells). Repeated measurements by different technicians on the same sample result in widely differing results. Automated differential counts are more precise because they are obtained from machines that use objective physical characteristics to classify a much larger sample (eg, 10,000 cells).

An ideal test is both precise and accurate (Figure 1–1C).

Reference Interval

Some diagnostic tests are reported as positive or negative, but many are reported quantitatively. Use of reference intervals is a technique for interpreting quantitative results. Reference intervals are often method- and laboratory-specific. In practice, they often represent test results found in 95% of a small population presumed to be healthy; by definition, then, 5% of healthy patients will have an abnormal test result (Figure 1–2). Slightly abnormal results should be interpreted critically—they may be either truly abnormal or falsely abnormal. Statistically, the probability that a healthy person will have 2 separate test results within the reference interval is

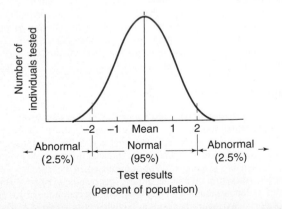

Figure 1–2. The reference interval is usually defined as within 2 SD of the mean test result (shown as −2 and 2) in a small population of healthy volunteers. Note that in this example, test results are normally distributed; however, many biologic substances have distributions that are skewed.

TABLE 1–3. RELATIONSHIP BETWEEN NUMBER OF TESTS AND PROBABILITY OF ONE OR MORE ABNORMAL RESULTS IN A HEALTHY PERSON.

Number of Tests	Probability of One or More Abnormal Results (%)
1	5
6	26
12	46
20	64

$(0.95 \times 0.95)\%$, ie, 90.25%; for 5 separate tests, it is 77.4%; for 10 tests, 59.9%; and for 20 tests, 35.8%. The larger the number of tests ordered, the greater the probability that one or more of the test results will fall outside the reference intervals (Table 1–3). Conversely, values within the reference interval may not rule out the actual presence of disease, since the reference interval does not establish the distribution of results in patients with disease.

It is important to consider also whether published reference intervals are appropriate for the particular patient being evaluated, since some intervals depend on age, sex, weight, diet, time of day, activity status, posture, or even season. Biologic variability occurs among individuals as well as within the same individual. For instance, serum estrogen levels in women vary from day to day, depending on the menstrual cycle; serum cortisol shows diurnal variation, being highest in the morning and decreasing later in the day; and vitamin D shows seasonal variation with lower values in winter.

Interfering Factors

The results of diagnostic tests can be altered by external factors, such as ingestion of drugs; and internal factors, such as abnormal physiologic states. These factors contribute to the biologic variability and must be considered in the interpretation of test results.

External interferences can affect test results *in vivo* or *in vitro*. *In vivo*, alcohol increases γ-glutamyl transpeptidase, and diuretics can affect sodium and potassium concentrations. Cigarette smoking can induce hepatic enzymes and thus reduce levels of substances such as theophylline that are metabolized by the liver. *In vitro*, cephalosporins may produce spurious serum creatinine levels due to interference with a common laboratory method of analysis.

Internal interferences result from abnormal physiologic states interfering with the test measurement. For example, patients with gross lipemia may have spuriously low serum sodium levels if the test methodology includes a step in which serum is diluted before sodium is measured, and patients with endogenous antibodies (eg, human anti-mouse antibodies) may have falsely high or low results in automated immunoassays. Because of the potential for test interference, clinicians should be wary of unexpected test results and should investigate reasons other than disease that may explain abnormal results, including pre-analytical and analytical laboratory error.

Sensitivity and Specificity

Clinicians should use measures of test performance such as sensitivity and specificity to judge the quality of a diagnostic test for a particular disease.

Test **sensitivity** is the ability of a test to detect disease and is expressed as the percentage of patients with disease in whom the test is positive. Thus, a test that is 90% sensitive gives positive results in 90% of diseased patients and negative results in 10% of diseased patients (false negatives). Generally, a test with high sensitivity is useful to exclude a diagnosis because a highly sensitive test renders fewer results that are falsely negative. To exclude infection with the virus that causes AIDS, for instance, a clinician might choose a highly sensitive test, such as the HIV antibody test or antigen/antibody combination test.

A test's **specificity** is the ability to detect absence of disease and is expressed as the percentage of patients without disease in whom the test is negative. Thus, a test that is 90% specific gives negative results in 90% of patients without disease and positive results in 10% of patients without disease (false positives). A test with high specificity is useful to confirm a diagnosis, because a highly specific test has fewer results that are falsely positive. For instance, to make the diagnosis of gouty arthritis, a clinician might choose a highly specific test, such as the presence of negatively birefringent needle-shaped crystals within leukocytes on microscopic evaluation of joint fluid.

To determine test sensitivity and specificity for a particular disease, the test must be compared against an independent "gold standard" test or established standard diagnostic criteria that define the true disease state of the patient. For instance, the sensitivity and specificity of rapid antigen detection testing in diagnosing group A β-hemolytic streptococcal pharyngitis are obtained by comparing the results of rapid antigen testing with the gold standard test, throat swab culture. Application of the gold standard test to patients with positive rapid antigen tests establishes specificity. Failure to apply the gold standard test to patients with negative rapid antigen tests will result in an overestimation of sensitivity, since false negatives will not be identified. However, for many disease states (eg, pancreatitis), an independent gold standard test either does not exist or is very difficult or expensive to apply—and in such cases reliable estimates of test sensitivity and specificity are sometimes difficult to obtain.

Sensitivity and specificity can also be affected by the population from which these values are derived. For instance, many diagnostic tests are evaluated first using patients who have severe disease and control groups who are young and well. Compared with the general population, these study groups will have more results that are truly positive (because patients have more advanced disease) and more results that are truly negative (because the control group is healthy). Thus, test sensitivity and specificity will be higher than would be expected in the general population, where more of a spectrum of health and disease is found. Clinicians should be aware of this **spectrum bias** when generalizing published test results to their own practice. To minimize spectrum bias, the control group should include individuals who have diseases related to the disease in question, but who lack this principal disease. For example, to establish the sensitivity and specificity of the anti-cyclic citrullinated peptide test for rheumatoid arthritis, the control group should include patients with rheumatic diseases other than rheumatoid arthritis. Other biases, including spectrum composition, population recruitment, absent or inappropriate reference standard, and verification bias, are discussed in the references.

It is important to remember that the reported sensitivity and specificity of a test depend on the analyte level (threshold) used to distinguish a normal from an abnormal test result. If the threshold is lowered, sensitivity is increased at the expense of decreased specificity. If the threshold is raised, sensitivity is decreased while specificity is increased (Figure 1–3).

Figure 1–4 shows how test sensitivity and specificity can be calculated using test results from patients previously classified by the gold standard test as diseased or nondiseased.

The performance of two different tests can be compared by plotting the receiver operator characteristic (ROC) curves at various reference interval cutoff values. The resulting curves, obtained by plotting sensitivity against

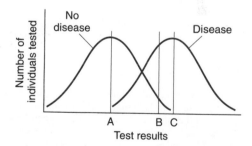

Figure 1–3. Hypothetical distribution of test results for healthy and diseased individuals. The position of the "cutoff point" between "normal" and "abnormal" (or "negative" and "positive") test results determines the test's sensitivity and specificity. If point A is the cutoff point, the test would have 100% sensitivity but low specificity. If point C is the cutoff point, the test would have 100% specificity but low sensitivity. For many tests, the cutoff point (B) is set at the value of the mean plus 2 SD of test results for healthy individuals. In some situations, the cutoff is altered to enhance either sensitivity or specificity.

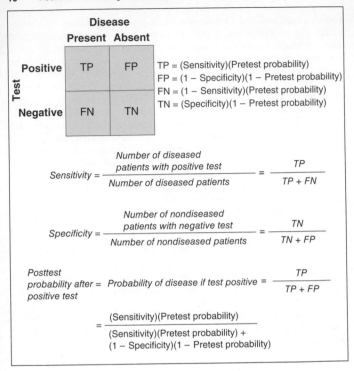

Figure 1–4. Calculation of sensitivity, specificity, and probability of disease after a positive test (posttest probability). TP, true positive; FP, false positive; FN, false negative; TN, true negative.

(1 − specificity) at different cut-off values for each test, often show which test is better; a clearly superior test will have an ROC curve that always lies above and to the left of the inferior test curve, and, in general, the better test will have a larger area under the ROC curve. For instance, Figure 1–5 shows the ROC curves for PSA and prostatic acid phosphatase in the diagnosis of prostate cancer. PSA is a superior test because it has higher sensitivity and specificity for all cutoff values.

Note that, for a given test, the ROC curve also allows one to identify the cutoff value that minimizes both false-positive and false-negative results. This is located at the point closest to the upper-left corner of the

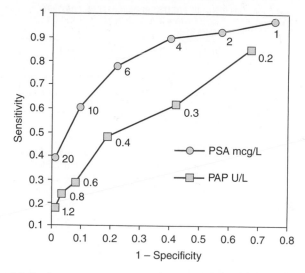

Figure 1–5. Receiver operator characteristic (ROC) curves for prostate-specific antigen (PSA) and prostatic acid phosphatase (PAP) in the diagnosis of prostate cancer. For all cutoff values, PSA has higher sensitivity and specificity; therefore, it is a better test based on these performance characteristics. (*Data from Nicoll CD et al. Routine acid phosphatase testing for screening and monitoring prostate cancer no longer justified.* Clin Chem 1993;39:2540.)

curve. The optimal clinical cutoff value, however, depends on the condition being detected and the relative importance of false-positive versus false-negative results.

USE OF TESTS IN DIAGNOSIS AND MANAGEMENT

The usefulness of a test in a particular clinical situation depends not only on the test's characteristics (eg, sensitivity and specificity) but also on the probability that the patient has the disease before the test result is known (**pretest probability**). The results of a useful test substantially change the probability that the patient has the disease (**posttest probability**). Figure 1–4 shows how posttest probability can be calculated from the known sensitivity and specificity of the test and the estimated pretest probability of disease (or disease prevalence), based on Bayes theorem.

TABLE 1–4. INFLUENCE OF PRETEST PROBABILITY ON POSTTEST PROBABILITY OF DISEASE WHEN A TEST WITH 90% SENSITIVITY AND 90% SPECIFICITY IS USED.

Pretest Probability	Posttest Probability
0.01	0.08
0.50	0.90
0.99	0.999

The pretest probability, or prevalence, of disease has a profound effect on the posttest probability of disease. As demonstrated in Table 1–4, when a test with 90% sensitivity and specificity is used, the posttest probability can vary from 8% to 99%, depending on the pretest probability of disease. Furthermore, as the pretest probability of disease decreases, it becomes more likely that a positive test result represents a false positive.

As an example, suppose the clinician wishes to calculate the posttest probability of prostate cancer using the PSA test and a cutoff value of 4 mcg/L. Using the data shown in Figure 1–5, sensitivity is 90% and specificity is 60%. The clinician estimates the pretest probability of disease given all the evidence and then calculates the posttest probability using the approach shown in Figure 1–4. The pretest probability that an otherwise healthy 50-year-old man has prostate cancer is the prevalence of prostate cancer in that age group (10%) and the posttest probability after a positive test is 20%. Even though the test is positive, there is still an 80% chance that the patient does not have prostate cancer (Figure 1–6A). If the clinician finds a prostate nodule on rectal examination, the pretest probability of prostate cancer rises to 50% and the posttest probability using the same test is 69% (Figure 1–6B). Finally, if the clinician estimates the pretest probability to be 98% based on a prostate nodule, bone pain, and lytic lesions on spine radiographs, the posttest probability using PSA is 99% (Figure 1–6C). This example illustrates that pretest probability has a profound effect on posttest probability and that tests provide more information when the diagnosis is truly uncertain (pretest probability about 50%) than when the diagnosis is either unlikely or nearly certain.

ODDS-LIKELIHOOD RATIOS

Another way to calculate the posttest probability of disease is to use the odds-likelihood (or odds-probability) approach. Sensitivity and specificity are combined into one entity called the likelihood ratio (LR):

$$LR = \frac{\text{Probability of result in diseased persons}}{\text{Probability of result in nondiseased persons}}$$

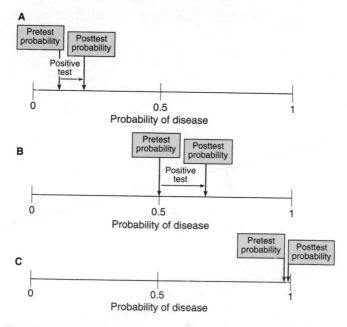

Figure 1–6. Effect of pretest probability and test sensitivity and specificity on the posttest probability of disease. The pretest probability, or prevalence, of the disease has a profound effect on the posttest probability of the disease. Diagnostic tests provide more information when the diagnosis is truly uncertain (pretest probability about 50%, as in Part B) than when the diagnosis is either unlikely (Part A) or nearly certain (Part C).

When test results are dichotomized, every test has two likelihood ratios, one corresponding to a positive test (LR^+) and one corresponding to a negative test (LR^-):

$$LR^+ = \frac{\text{Probability that test is positive in diseased persons}}{\text{Probability that test is positive in nondiseased persons}}$$

$$= \frac{\text{Sensitivity}}{1 - \text{Specificity}}$$

$$LR^- = \frac{\text{Probability that test is negative in diseased persons}}{\text{Probability that test is negative in nondiseased persons}}$$

$$= \frac{1 - \text{Sensitivity}}{\text{Specificity}}$$

TABLE 1–5. LIKELIHOOD RATIOS OF SERUM FERRITIN IN THE DIAGNOSIS OF IRON DEFICIENCY ANEMIA.

Serum Ferritin (mcg/L)	Likelihood Ratios for Iron Deficiency Anemia
≥100	0.08
45–99	0.54
35–44	1.83
25–34	2.54
15–24	8.83
<15	51.85

Adapted from Guyatt G et al: Laboratory diagnosis of iron deficiency anemia. J Gen Intern Med *1992;7(2):145.*

For continuous measures, multiple likelihood ratios can be defined to correspond to ranges or intervals of test results. (See Table 1–5 for an example.)

Likelihood ratios can be calculated using the above formulae. They can also be found in some textbooks, journal articles, and online programs (see Table 1–6 for sample values). Likelihood ratios provide an estimation of whether there will be significant change in pretest to posttest probability of a disease given the test result, and thus can be used to make quick estimates of the usefulness of contemplated diagnostic tests in particular situations. A likelihood ratio of 1 implies that there will be no difference between pretest and posttest probabilities. Likelihood ratios of >10 or <0.1 indicate large, often clinically significant differences. Likelihood ratios between 1 and 2 and between 0.5 and 1 indicate small differences (rarely clinically significant).

The simplest method for calculating posttest probability from pretest probability and likelihood ratios is to use a nomogram (Figure 1–7). The clinician places a straightedge through the points that represent the

TABLE 1–6. EXAMPLES OF LIKELIHOOD RATIOS (LR).

Target Disease	Test	LR+	LR−
Abscess	Abdominal CT scanning	9.5	0.06
Coronary artery disease	Exercise electrocardiogram (1 mm depression)	3.5	0.45
Lung cancer	Chest radiograph	15	0.42
Left ventricular hypertrophy	Echocardiography	18.4	0.08
Myocardial infarction	Troponin I	24	0.01
Prostate cancer	Digital rectal examination	21.3	0.37

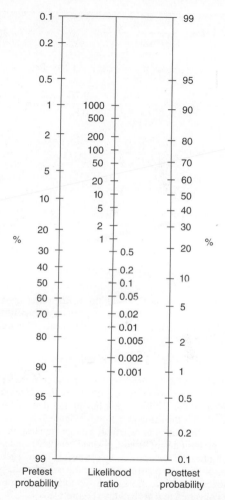

Figure 1–7. Nomogram for determining posttest probability from pretest probability and likelihood ratios. To figure the posttest probability, place a straightedge between the pretest probability and the likelihood ratio for the particular test. The posttest probability will be where the straightedge crosses the posttest probability line. (*Adapted and reproduced, with permission, from Fagan TJ. Nomogram for Bayes theorem. [Letter.] N Engl J Med 1975;293:257.*)

$$\text{Odds} = \frac{\text{Probability}}{1 - \text{Probability}}$$

Example: If probability = 0.75, then

$$\text{Odds} = \frac{0.75}{1 - 0.75} = \frac{0.75}{0.25} = \frac{3}{1} = 3:1$$

$$\text{Probability} = \frac{\text{Odds}}{\text{Odds} + 1}$$

Example: If odds = 3:1, then

$$\text{Probability} = \frac{3/1}{3/1 + 1} = \frac{3}{3 + 1} = 0.75$$

Figure 1–8. Formulae for converting between probability and odds.

pretest probability and the likelihood ratio and then reads the posttest probability where the straightedge crosses the posttest probability line.

A more formal way of calculating posttest probabilities uses the likelihood ratio as follows:

Pretest odds × Likelihood ratio = Posttest odds

To use this formulation, probabilities must be converted to odds, where the odds of having a disease are expressed as the chance of having the disease divided by the chance of not having the disease. For instance, a probability of 0.75 is the same as 3:1 odds (Figure 1–8).

To estimate the potential benefit of a diagnostic test, the clinician first estimates the pretest odds of disease given all available clinical information and then multiplies the pretest odds by the positive and negative likelihood ratios. The results are the **posttest odds,** or the odds that the patient has the disease if the test is positive or negative. To obtain the posttest probability, the odds are converted to a probability (Figure 1–8).

For example, if the clinician believes that the patient has a 60% chance of having a myocardial infarction (pretest odds of 3:2) and the troponin I test is positive (LR$^+$ 24), then the posttest odds of having a myocardial infarction are

$$\frac{3}{2} \times 24 = \frac{72}{2} \text{ or } 36:1 \text{ odds} \left(\frac{36/1}{(36/1) + 1} = \frac{36}{37} = 97\% \text{ probability} \right)$$

If the troponin I test is negative (LR⁻ 0.01), then the posttest odds of having a myocardial infarction are

$$\frac{3}{2} \times 0.01 = \frac{0.03}{2} \text{ odds} \left(\frac{0.03/2}{(0.03/2)+1} = \frac{0.015}{0.015+1} = 1.5\% \text{ probability} \right)$$

Sequential Testing

To this point, the impact of only one test on the probability of disease has been discussed, whereas during most diagnostic work-ups, clinicians obtain clinical information in a sequential fashion. To calculate the posttest odds after three tests, for example, the clinician might estimate the pretest odds and use the appropriate likelihood ratio for each test:

$$\text{Pretest odds} \times LR_1 \times LR_2 \times LR_3 = \text{Posttest odds}$$

When using this approach, however, the clinician should be aware of a major assumption: the chosen tests or findings must be **conditionally independent.** For instance, with liver cell damage, the aspartate aminotransferase (AST) and alanine aminotransferase (ALT) enzymes may be released by the same process and are thus not conditionally independent. If conditionally dependent tests are used in this sequential approach, an inaccurate posttest probability will result.

Threshold Approach to Decision Making

A key aspect of medical decision making is the selection of a treatment threshold, ie, the probability of disease at which treatment is indicated. The treatment threshold is determined by the relative consequences of different actions: treating when the disease is present; not treating when the disease is absent; treating when the disease is actually absent; or failing to treat when the disease is actually present. Figure 1–9 shows a possible way of identifying a treatment threshold by considering the value (utility) of these four possible outcomes.

Use of a diagnostic test is warranted when its result could shift the probability of disease across the treatment threshold. For example, a clinician might decide to treat with antibiotics if the probability of streptococcal pharyngitis in a patient with a sore throat is > 25% (Figure 1–10A).

If, after reviewing evidence from the history and physical examination, the clinician estimates the pretest probability of strep throat to be 15%, then a diagnostic test such as throat culture (LR⁺ 7) would be useful only if a positive test would shift the posttest probability above 25%. Use of the nomogram shown in Figure 1–7 indicates that the posttest probability would be 55% (Figure 1–10B); thus, ordering the test would be justified,

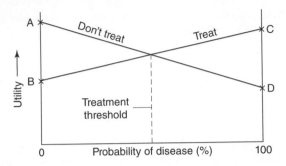

Figure 1–9. The "treat/don't treat" threshold. A, Patient does not have disease and is not treated (highest utility). B, Patient does not have disease and is treated (lower utility than A). C, Patient has disease and is treated (lower utility than A). D, Patient has disease and is not treated (lower utility than C).

since it affects patient management. On the other hand, if the history and physical examination had suggested that the pretest probability of strep throat was 60%, the throat culture (LR− 0.33) would be indicated only if a negative test would lower the posttest probability below 25%. Using the same nomogram, the posttest probability after a negative test would be 33% (Figure 1–10C). Therefore, ordering the throat culture would not be justified because it does not affect patient management.

This approach to decision making is now being applied in the clinical literature.

Decision Analysis

Up to this point, the discussion of diagnostic testing has focused on test characteristics and methods for using these characteristics to calculate the probability of disease in different clinical situations. Although useful, these methods are limited because they do not incorporate the many outcomes that may occur in clinical medicine or the values that patients and clinicians place on those outcomes. To incorporate outcomes and values with characteristics of tests, decision analysis can be used.

Decision analysis is a quantitative evaluation of the outcomes that result from a set of choices in a specific clinical situation. Although it is infrequently used in routine clinical practice, the decision analysis approach can be helpful to address questions relating to clinical decisions that cannot easily be answered through clinical trials.

The basic idea of decision analysis is to model the options in a medical decision, assign probabilities to the alternative actions, assign values (utilities) (eg, survival rates, quality-adjusted life years, or costs) to the various outcomes, and then calculate which decision gives the greatest expected

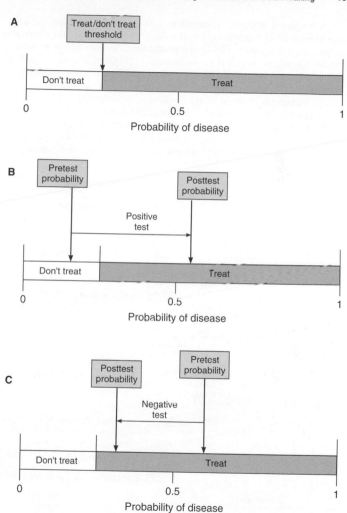

Figure 1–10. Threshold approach applied to test ordering. Diagnostic tests provide more information when the diagnosis is truly uncertain (pretest probability about 50%, as in Part B) than when the diagnosis is either unlikely (Part A) or nearly certain (Part C).

value (expected utility). To complete a decision analysis, the clinician would proceed as follows: (1) Draw a decision tree showing the elements of the medical decision. (2) Assign probabilities to the various branches. (3) Assign values (utilities) to the outcomes. (4) Determine the expected value (expected utility) (the product of probability and value [utility]) of each branch. (5) Select the decision with the highest expected value (expected utility). The results obtained from a decision analysis depend on the accuracy of the data used to estimate the probabilities and values of outcomes.

Figure 1–11 shows a decision tree in which the decision to be made is whether to treat without testing, perform a test and then treat based on the test result, or perform no tests and give no treatment. The clinician begins

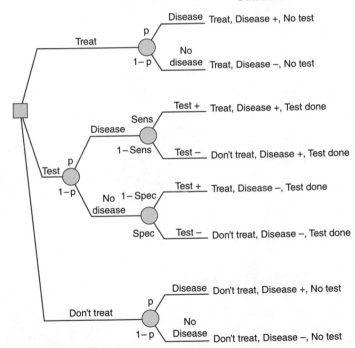

Figure 1–11. Generic tree for a clinical decision where the choices are (1) to treat the patient empirically, (2) to do the test and then treat only if the test is positive, or (3) to withhold therapy. The square node is called a decision node, and the circular nodes are called chance nodes. p, pretest probability of disease; Sens, sensitivity; Spec, specificity.

the analysis by building a decision tree showing the important elements of the decision. Once the tree is built, the clinician assigns probabilities to all the branches. In this case, all the branch probabilities can be calculated from (1) the probability of disease before the test (pretest probability), (2) the chance of a positive test result if the disease is present (sensitivity), and (3) the chance of a negative test result if the disease is absent (specificity). Next, the clinician assigns value (utility) to each of the outcomes.

After the expected value (expected utility) is calculated for each branch of the decision tree, by multiplying the value (utility) of the outcome by the probability of the outcome, the clinician can identify the alternative with the highest expected value (expected utility). When costs are included, it is possible to determine the cost per unit of health gained for one approach compared with an alternative (cost-effectiveness analysis). This information can help evaluate the efficiency of different testing or treatment strategies.

Although time-consuming, decision analysis can help structure complex clinical problems and assist in difficult clinical decisions.

Evidence-Based Medicine

Evidence-based medicine is the care of patients using the best available research evidence to guide clinical decision making. It relies on the identification of methodologically sound evidence, critical appraisal of research studies for both internal validity (freedom from bias) and external validity (applicability and generalizability), and the dissemination of accurate and useful summaries of evidence to inform clinical decision making. Systematic reviews can be used to summarize evidence for dissemination, as can evidence-based synopses of current research. Systematic reviews often use meta-analysis: statistical techniques to combine evidence from different studies to produce a more precise estimate of the effect of an intervention or the accuracy of a test.

Clinical practice guidelines are systematically developed statements intended to assist practitioners in making decisions about health care. Clinical algorithms and practice guidelines are now ubiquitous in medicine, developed by various professional societies or independent expert panels. Diagnostic testing is an integral part of such algorithms and guidelines. Their utility and validity depend on the quality of the evidence that shaped the recommendations, on their being kept current, and on their acceptance and appropriate application by clinicians. Although some clinicians are concerned about the effect of guidelines on professional autonomy and individual decision making, many organizations use compliance with practice guidelines as a measure of quality of care.

Because treatment decisions have not always integrated the best medical knowledge and patient values, there has been growing interest in shared decision making. Shared decision making is a process by which physicians provide patients with evidence-based health information, elicit patient values, and then collaborate to reach a mutually acceptable decision.

Decision aids, tools to help facilitate shared decision making, have been shown in many cases to improve decision making processes and outcomes. In this regard, evidence-based medicine is used to complement, not replace, clinical judgment tailored to individual patients.

Computerized information technology provides clinicians with information from laboratory, imaging, physiologic monitoring systems, and many other sources. Computerized clinical decision support has been increasingly used to develop, implement, and refine computerized protocols for specific processes of care derived from evidence-based practice guidelines. It is important that clinicians use modern information technology to deliver medical care in their practice.

REFERENCES

Benefits, Costs, and Risks

Alonso-Cerezo MC et al. Appropriate utilization of clinical laboratory tests. Clin Chem Lab Med 2009;47:1461. [PMID: 19863300]

Bailey DB et al. Ethical, legal, and social concerns about expanded newborn screening: Fragile X syndrome as a prototype for emerging issues. Pediatrics 2008;121:e693. [PMID: 18310190]

Elder NC et al. Quality and safety in outpatient laboratory testing. Clin Lab Med 2008;28:295. [PMID: 18436072]

Ginsburg GS et al. The long and winding road to warfarin pharmacogenetics testing. J Am Coll Cardiol 2010;55:2813. [PMID: 20579536]

Konstantinopoulos PA et al. Educational and social-ethical issues in the pursuit of molecular medicine. Mol Med 2009;15:60. [PMID: 19043478]

Laposata M et al. "Pre-pre" and "Post-post" analytical error: high-incidence patient safety hazard involving the clinical laboratory. Clin Chem Lab Med 2007;45:712. [PMID: 17579522]

Smith RA et al. Cancer screening in the United States, 2010: a review of current American Cancer Society guidelines and issues in cancer screening. CA Cancer J Clin 2010;60:99. [PMID: 20228384]

Twombly R. Preventive Services Task Force recommends against PSA screening after age 75. J Natl Cancer Inst 2008;100:1571. [PMID: 19001606]

Van Den Bruel A et al. The evaluation of diagnostic tests: evidence on technical and diagnostic accuracy, impact on patient outcome and cost-effectiveness is needed. J Clin Epidemiol 2007;60:1116. [PMID: 17938052]

Performance of Diagnostic Tests

Lippi G et al. Haemolysis: an overview of the leading cause of unsuitable specimens in clinical laboratories. Clin Chem Lab Med 2008;46:764. [PMID: 18601596]

Wagar EA et al. Specimen labeling errors: a Q-probes analysis of 147 clinical laboratories. Arch Pathol Lab Med 2008;132:1617. [PMID: 18834220]

Test Characteristics

Bossuyt X. Clinical performance characteristics of a laboratory test. A practical approach in the autoimmune laboratory. Autoimmun Rev 2009;8:543. [PMID: 19200856]

Christenson RH et al. Evidence-based laboratory medicine—a guide for critical evaluation of in vitro laboratory testing. Ann Clin Biochem 2007;44:111. [PMID: 17362577]

Hicks DG et al. *HER2+* breast cancer: review of biologic relevance and optimal use of diagnostic tools. Am J Clin Pathol 2008;129:263. [PMID: 18208807]

Ismail AA. Interference from endogenous antibodies in automated immuno-assays: what laboratorians need to know. J Clin Pathol 2009;62:673. [PMID: 19638536]

Jung B et al. Clinical laboratory reference intervals in pediatrics: the CALIPER initiative. Clin Biochem 2009;42:1589. [PMID: 19591815]

Smellie WS. What is a significant difference between sequential laboratory results? J Clin Pathol 2008;61:419. [PMID: 17938161]

Use of Tests in Diagnosis and Management

Hargett CW et al. Clinical probability and D-dimer testing: how should we use them in clinical practice. Semin Respir Crit Care Med 2008;29:15. [PMID: 18302083]

Scott IA et al. Cautionary tales in the clinical interpretation of studies of diagnostic tests. Intern Med J 2008;38:120. [PMID: 17645501]

Van Randen A et al. Acute appendicitis: meta-analysis of diagnostic performance of CT and graded compression US related to prevalence of disease. Radiology 2008;249:97. [PMID: 18682583]

Decision Analysis, Evidence-Based Medicine

Aleem IS et al. Clinical decision analysis: incorporating the evidence with patient preferences. Patient Prefer Adherence 2009;3:21. [PMID: 19936141]

Braithwaite RS et al. Influence of alternative thresholds for initiating HIV treatment on quality-adjusted life expectancy: a decision model. Ann Intern Med 2008;148:178. [PMID: 18252681]

Charles C et al. The evidence-based medicine model of clinical practice: scientific teaching or belief-based preaching? J Eval Clin Pract 2011;17:597. [PMID: 21087367]

Elamin MB et al. Accuracy of diagnostic tests for Cushing's syndrome: a systemic review and meta-analysis. J Clin Endocrinol Metab 2008;93:1553. [PMID: 18334594]

Hayes JH et al. Active surveillance compared with initial treatment for men with low-risk prostate cancer: a decision analysis. JAMA 2010;304:2373. [PMID: 21119084]

Lennon S et al. Utility of serum *HER2* extracellular domain assessment in clinical decision making: pooled analysis of four trials of trastuzumab in metastatic breast cancer. J Clin Oncol 2009;27:1685. [PMID: 19255335]

O'Connor AM et al. Do patient decision aids meet effectiveness criteria of the inter-national patient decision aid standards collaboration? A systematic review and meta-analysis. Med Decis Making 2007;27:554. [PMID: 17873255]

Petersen PH et al. 'Likelihood-ratio' and 'odds' applied to monitoring of patients as a supplement to 'reference change value' (RCV). Clin Chem Lab Med 2008;46:157. [PMID: 18076354]

Sucher JF et al. Computerized clinical decision support: a technology to implement and validate evidence based guidelines. J Trauma 2008;64:520. [PMID: 18301226]

2

Point-of-Care Testing and Provider-Performed Microscopy

Chuanyi Mark Lu, MD, and Stephen J. McPhee, MD

This chapter presents information on common point-of-care (POC) tests and provider-performed microscopy (PPM) procedures.

POC testing is defined as medical testing at or near the site of patient care. POC tests are performed outside a central clinical laboratory using portable and hand-held devices and test kits or cartridges. PPM procedures are microscopic examinations performed by a healthcare provider during the course of a patient visit. PPM procedures involve using specimens that are labile and not easily transportable, or for which delay in performing the test could compromise the accuracy of the test result.

POC testing is considered as an integrated part of clinical laboratory service and is under the direction of the central laboratory. Physician interpretation of PPM findings (eg, direct wet mount preparation and KOH preparation) requires appropriate clinical privileges.

In the United States, test results can be used for patient care only when the tests are performed according to the requirements of the Clinical Laboratory Improvement Amendments of 1988 (CLIA '88). These include personnel training and competence assessment before performing any test or procedure, following standard operating procedures and/or manufacturer instructions, performance and documentation of quality control for all tests, and participation in a proficiency testing program, if applicable.

Contents   *Page*

1. OBTAINING AND HANDLING SPECIMENS

Specimens should be collected and handled according to the institution's policies and procedures.
   A. **Safety Considerations**
      General Safety Considerations
         Because all patient specimens are potentially infectious, the following precautions should be observed:
         a. Universal body fluid and needle stick precautions must be observed at all times. Safety needle devices should be used.
         b. Disposable medical gloves, gown, and sometimes mask, goggle, and face shield should be worn when collecting specimens.
         c. Gloves must be changed and hands washed after contact with each patient. Dispose of gloves in an appropriate biohazard waste container.
         d. Care should be taken not to spill or splash blood or other body fluids. Any spills should be cleaned up with freshly made 10% bleach solution.
      Handling and Disposing of Needles and Gloves
         a. Do not resheathe needles.
         b. Discard needles in a sharps container and gloves in a designated biohazard container.
         c. Do not remove a used needle from a syringe by hand. The entire assembly should be discarded as a unit into a designated sharp container.
         d. When obtaining blood cultures, it is unnecessary to change venipuncture needle when filling additional culture bottles.

   B. **Specimen Handling**
      Identification of Specimens
         a. Identify the patient by having the patient state two identifiers (eg, full name plus date of birth or social security number) before obtaining any specimen.
         b. Label each specimen tube or container with the patient's name and unique identification number (eg, medical record number).

Specimen Tubes: Standard specimen tubes that contain a vacuum (called evacuated tubes) are now widely available and are easily identified by the color of the stopper (see also p. 48 in Chapter 3). The following is a general guide:

a. Red-top tubes contain no anticoagulants or preservatives and are used for serum chemistry tests and certain serologic tests.

b. Serum separator tubes (SST) contain material that allows separation of serum and clot by centrifugation and are used for serum chemistry tests.

c. Lavender-top (purple) tubes contain EDTA and are used for hematology tests (eg, blood cell counts, differentials), blood banking (plasma), flow cytometry, and molecular diagnostic tests.

d. Green-top tubes contain heparin and are used for plasma chemistry tests and chromosome analysis.

e. Blue-top tubes contain sodium citrate and are used for coagulation tests.

f. Gray-top tubes contain sodium fluoride and are used for some chemistry tests (eg, glucose or alcohol requiring inhibition of glycolysis) if the specimen cannot be analyzed immediately.

g. Yellow-top tubes contain acid citrate dextrose (ACD) and are used for flow cytometry and HLA typing.

Procedure

Venipuncture is typically performed to obtain blood samples for acid-base and electrolyte studies, metabolic studies, hematologic studies, and coagulation studies. Arterial punctures are performed to obtain blood samples to assess arterial blood gases. Some tests (eg, glucose, rapid HIV test) can be performed on capillary blood obtained by puncturing the fingertip or heel using a lancet device.

a. When collecting multiple blood specimens by venipuncture, follow the recommended order of filling evacuated tubes, ie, blood culture bottles, coagulation tube (blue), non-additive tube (eg, plain red glass tube), SST, heparin tube (green), EDTA tube (lavender/purple), sodium fluoride tube (gray), and ACD tube (yellow). When using a butterfly collection device and drawing blood for a coagulation test, prime the tubing with a discard tube prior to specimen collection.

b. Fill each tube completely. Tilt each tube containing anticoagulant or preservative to mix thoroughly. Do not shake tube. Deliver specimens to the laboratory promptly.

c. For each of the common body fluids, Table 2–1 summarizes commonly requested tests and requirements for specimen handling and provides cross-references to tables and figures elsewhere in this book for help in interpretation of the results.

TABLE 2–1. BODY FLUID TESTS, HANDLING, AND INTERPRETATION.

Body Fluid	Commonly Requested Tests	Specimen Tube and Handling	Interpretation Guide
Arterial blood	pH, Po_2, Pco_2, HCO_3^-	Plastic syringe. Evacuate air bubbles; remove needle; position rubber cap; place sample on ice; deliver immediately.	See acid–base nomogram, Figure 9–1.
Ascitic fluid	Cell count, differential Protein, amylase Gram stain, culture Cytology (if neoplasm suspected)	Lavender top Red top Sterile tube Lavender top	See ascitic fluid profiles, Table 8–5.
Cerebrospinal fluid (collect in sterile and numbered plastic tubes)	Cell count, differential Gram stain, culture Protein, glucose, LDH VDRL or other studies (oligoclonal bands, IgG index) Cytology (if neoplasm suspected)	Tube #1, or #3 if #1 is bloody Tube #2 Tube #3 Tube #3 or #4 Any (#1–#4)	See cerebrospinal fluid profiles, Table 8–8.
Pleural fluid	Cell count, differential Protein, glucose, amylase Gram stain, culture Cytology (if neoplasm suspected)	Lavender top Red top Sterile tube Lavender top	See pleural fluid profiles, Table 8–18.
Synovial fluid	Cell count, differential Gram stain, culture Microscopic examination for crystals Cytology (if neoplasm [villonodular synovitis, metastatic disease] suspected)	Lavender top Sterile tube Green or lavender top Lavender or green top	See synovial fluid profiles, Table 8–4, and Figure 2–4.

Urine (collect in clean and/or sterile plastic tube or container)	Urinalysis
	  Dipstick
	
	  Microscopic examination
	  Gram stain, culture
	
	Cytology (if neoplasm suspected)
		
		Clean tube or container
		Centrifuge tube
		Sterile tube or container
		Clean tube or container
			See Table 8–28.
			See Table 2–3.
			
			See Figure 2–1.

Time to Test

For most accurate results, samples should be tested immediately after collection. Samples are suitable for analysis for a limited time and thus should be tested within the time limits specified by the laboratory's standard operating procedures.

2. COMMONLY USED POINT-OF-CARE TESTS

POC testing is typically performed in a primary care clinic, physician office, emergency room, operating room, or intensive care unit. It is usually performed by non-laboratory personnel. Certain self-testing can also be performed by the patient at home.

Table 2–2 lists the commonly used POC tests, many of which are CLIA waived (waived from regulatory procedures).

Advantages of POC testing include:
   a. Potential to improve patient outcome and/or workflow by having results immediately available for patient management.
   b. Potential to expedite medical decision-making.
   c. Use of portable or hand-held devices, allowing laboratory testing in a variety of locations, sites, and circumstances.
   d. Use of small sample volume (minimizes blood loss to patient).

Disadvantages of POC testing include:
   a. Given the variable training levels and experience of staff performing the tests, quality of test results is difficult to assure.
   b. Competency assessment can be challenging.
   c. Test methods are often different from central laboratory methods and thus can have unique interferences and limitations (eg, interference of POC blood glucose by maltose and xylose).
   d. Results are not necessarily comparable to central laboratory results and may not be approved for all uses that a similar central laboratory test can be used for (eg, waived PT/INR is approved only for monitoring warfarin therapy and thus cannot be used for assessment of bleeding diathesis).
   e. Interfacing results to the electronic patient record may be more difficult.
   f. Per test cost is often significantly higher than the cost of central laboratory testing.

3. PROVIDER-PERFORMED MICROSCOPY PROCEDURES

   A. **Urinalysis (Urine Dipstick and Sediment Examination)**
      Collection and Preparation of Specimen
         a. Obtain a midstream, clean-catch urine specimen in a clean container.

TABLE 2–2. COMMONLY USED POINT-OF-CARE (POC) TESTS.

POC Test Systems	Menu of Tests	Comments
Abbott *i-STAT* System	Chemistry/electrolytes 　Sodium (Na) 　Potassium (K) 　Chloride (Cl) 　Total CO_2 (Tco_2) 　Anion Gap (calculated) 　Ionized calcium (iCa) 　Glucose (Glu) 　Urea nitrogen (BUN) 　Creatinine (Creat) 　Lactate Hematology 　Hematocrit (Hct) 　Hemoglobin (Hgb) Blood gases 　pH 　Pco_2 　Po_2 　HCO_3^- Coagulation 　Activated clotting time (ACT) 　Prothrombin time (PT/INR) Cardiac markers 　Cardiac troponin I (cTnI) 　CK-MB 　BNP (B-type natriuretic 　　peptide)	The *i-STAT* System uses a hand-held device and various single-use test cartridges. Each test cartridge contains chemically sensitive biosensors on a silicon chip that are configured to perform specific tests. To perform a test or a test panel (eg, electrolytes), 2–3 drops whole blood are applied to a cartridge, which is then inserted into the hand-held device. The system is interfaceable to an electronic laboratory information system (LIS), and a wireless device is also available.
Roche CoaguChek Systems (XS, XS Plus, and XS Pro)	Prothrombin time (PT/INR)	Used for monitoring coumadin (warfarin) anticoagulation therapy. The XS system uses a hand-held meter and PT test strip. Test can be performed on fresh capillary (fingerstick) or on nonanticoagulated venous whole blood. The test strip is first inserted into the meter and warmed. After 1 drop of blood is applied to the strip, the result appears on the meter in about 1 minute. The XS Plus system has built-in quality control and data management. The XS Pro system is based on the XS Plus but with an added bar code scanner.

TABLE 2–2. COMMONLY USED POINT-OF-CARE (POC) TESTS. (*CONTINUED*)

POC Test Systems	Menu of Tests	Comments
Roche Accu-Chek Inform System	Blood glucose	The system uses a hand-held meter and reagent test strips and is intended for use in the quantitative determination of glucose levels in whole blood samples. Capillary blood from a fingerstick is typically used. The GDH-PQQ (glucose dehydrogenase pyrroloquinoline quinine) containing test strips cannot distinguish between glucose and certain non-glucose sugars, including maltose, xylose, and galactose. Patients who are receiving therapeutic products containing these non-glucose sugars will have falsely elevated blood glucose results.
Biosite Triage Meter Pro	BNP Cardiac panel (CK-MB, myoglobin, cTnl) D-dimer Drugs of abuse panel	The system is based on sensitive fluorescence immunoassay technology. It uses a portable Triage Meter and various diagnostic devices. It provides quantitative results for blood BNP, cardiac markers, and D-dimer, and qualitative results for urine toxicology screen in about 15 minutes.
POC HIV Test (eg, OraQuick ADVANCE HIV1/2, Uni-Gold Recombigen HIV)	Rapid HIV-1,2 antibody test	These tests are approved for oral fluid, fingerstick, or venipuncture whole blood specimens. Each test provides results within 20 minutes, enabling patients to learn their status in a single visit.
Rapid Strep Test (eg, CLIA waived Inc., Inverness Medical Clearview)	Rapid group A streptococcal antigen test	The test is approved for throat/tonsil swab specimen, and result is generally available in 10–15 minutes. It is used to determine whether a patient has streptococcal pharyngitis. The test is typically used in physicians' offices and emergency rooms.

(continued)

TABLE 2–2. COMMONLY USED POINT-OF-CARE (POC) TESTS. (*CONTINUED*)

POC Test Systems	Menu of Tests	Comments
Reagent strips for urinalysis (eg, Siemens Combistix, Multistix)	Urinalysis, nonautomated	Urine dipsticks (strips) are used to analyze urine specimens for various biochemicals (eg, blood, glucose, protein, bilirubin, nitrite, leukocyte esterase, ketone, etc); and results are available within a few minutes. Results are interpreted using visual comparison of reagent pads to the color chart guide or using a compatible dipstick reader. See Table 2–3 for more details.
Fecal occult blood test (FOBT) (eg, Hemoccult Sensa, HemoSure, Clearview ULTRA, InSure FIT, Polymedco FIT-CHEK)	Rapid FOBT	Test is used for rapid, qualitative detection of human blood (hemoglobin) in feces. It is mainly used for colorectal cancer (CRC) screening in outpatient setting. If guaiac-based FOBT (gFOBT) is used, three specimens on three different days are recommended to improve sensitivity. The fecal immunochemical test (FIT) selectively detects human globin-protein in stool and is specific for colorectal bleeding.
Urine pregnancy test (various over-the-counter FDA-approved, CLIA waived tests are available)	Urine beta-hCG (human chorionic gonadotropin), qualitative	Based on detection of the hormone hCG in urine. In healthy subjects of childbearing age, positive hCG in urine provides an early indication of pregnancy. The detection limit for pregnancy is the day of the first missed period. If negative, recommend repeat testing in 5–7 days if menses have not occurred.
Pulse oximetry	Oxygen saturation of hemoglobin (S_{O_2}) and pulse rate (PR) (finger, ear, foot)	Pulse oximetry allows for noninvasive and continuous monitoring of arterial blood oxygen saturation (Sa_{O_2}). Sa_{O_2} is not directly proportional to oxygen partial pressure (Pa_{O_2}). A relatively small change in Sa_{O_2} (eg, from 94% to 83%) can represent a large change in Pa_{O_2} (eg, from 80 mm Hg to 50 mm Hg). To ensure accurate assessment of oxygenation status, pulse oximetry should be correlated with arterial blood gas analysis, if available. A reduction in peripheral pulsatile blood flow causes inaccurate reading.

b. Examine the specimen while fresh (within 2 hours; do not refrigerate specimen). Otherwise, bacteria may proliferate, casts and crystals may dissolve, and particulate matter may settle out.

c. Place 10 mL in a conical test tube and centrifuge at 2000–3000 rpm for 5 minutes. Do not apply brake at the end of centrifugation to avoid re-suspension of sediment.

d. Invert the tube and drain off the supernatant without dislodging the sediment button. Return the tube to an upright position, and re-suspend the sediment by gently tapping the bottom of the tube.

e. Place a drop of sediment on a glass slide, cover it with a cover-slip, and examine under the microscope; no stain is needed.

Procedural Technique

a. While the urine is being centrifuged, examine the remainder of the specimen by inspection and reagent strip (dipstick) testing.

b. Inspect the specimen for color and clarity. Normally, urine is light yellow (due to urochrome). Intense yellow urine is caused by urine concentration (dehydration) or B vitamin supplements; dark orange urine, by ingestion of the urinary tract analgesic phenazopyridine (Pyridium, others); red urine, by erythrocytes, hemoglobinuria, myoglobinuria, porphyrins, beets, senna, or rifampin therapy; green urine, by *Pseudomonas* infection or iodochlorhydroxyquin or amitriptyline therapy; brown urine, by bilirubinuria or fecal contamination; black urine, by intra-vascular hemolysis, alkaptonuria, melanoma, or methyldopa therapy; and milky white urine, by pus, chyluria, or amorphous crystals (urates or phosphates). Turbidity of urine is caused by pus, red blood cells, or crystals.

c. Reagent strips provide information about specific gravity, pH, protein, glucose, ketones, bilirubin, blood (heme), nitrite, and leukocyte esterase (Table 2–3). Dip a reagent strip in the urine and compare it with the interpretation guide chart on the bottle. Follow the timing instructions carefully. *Note:* Reagent strips cannot be relied on to detect some proteins (eg, globulins, light chains) or reducing sugars (other than glucose). Falsely positive protein results may be obtained with alkaline urine (eg, urine pH > 8.0); sulfosalicylic acid (SSA) test can be used to confirm the presence of protein. Positive bilirubin on a reagent strip should be confirmed by an Ictotest tablet. Substances that cause abnormal urine color may affect the readability of test pads on reagent strips (eg, visible levels of blood or bilirubinuria and drugs containing dyes, nitrofurantoin, or rifampicin).

d. Record and report the results.

Manual Microscopic Urine Sediment Examination

a. Examine the area under the coverslip under low-power (10×) and high-dry (40×) lenses for cells, casts, crystals, and bacteria.

TABLE 2–3. COMPONENTS OF THE URINE DIPSTICK.[1]

Test	Normal Values	Sensitivity	Comments
Specific gravity	1.001–1.035	1.000–1.030[2]	Highly buffered alkaline urine may cause low specific gravity readings. Moderate proteinuria (100–750 mg/dL) may cause high readings. Loss of concentrating or diluting capacity indicates renal dysfunction. If the specific gravity of a random urine specimen is 1.023 or greater, the concentrating ability of the kidneys can be considered normal.
pH	4.6–8.0	5.0–8.5[2]	Excessive urine on strip may cause protein reagent to run over onto pH area, yielding falsely low pH reading. Bacterial growth by certain organisms (eg, proteus) in a specimen may cause a marked alkaline shift (pH > 8), usually because of urea conversion to ammonia.
Protein	Negative <15 mg/dL	15–30 mg/dL albumin	False-positive readings can be caused by highly buffered alkaline urine. Reagent is more sensitive to albumin than other proteins. A negative result does not rule out the presence of globulins, hemoglobin, Bence Jones proteins, or mucoprotein. 1+ = 30 mg/dL 3+ = 300 mg/dL 2+ = 100 mg/dL 4+ = ≥2000 mg/dL
Glucose	Negative <15 mg/dL	75–125 mg/dL	Test is specific for glucose. False-negative results occur with urinary ascorbic acid concentrations ≥ 0 mg/dL and with ketone body levels ≥ 40 mg/dL. Test reagent reactivity also varies with specific gravity and temperature. Trace = 100 mg/dL 1 = 1000 mg/dL ¼ = 250 mg/dL 2 = ≥2000 mg/dL ½ = 500 mg/dL
Ketone	Negative	5–10 mg/dL acetoacetate	Test does not react with acetone or β-hydroxybutyric acid. (Trace) false-positive results may occur with highly pigmented urines or those containing levodopa metabolites or sulfhydryl-containing compounds (eg, Mesna). Trace = 5 mg/dL Moderate = 40 mg/dL Small = 15 mg/dL Large = 80–160 mg/dL

TABLE 2–3. COMPONENTS OF THE URINE DIPSTICK.[1] (*CONTINUED*)

Test	Normal Values	Sensitivity	Comments
Bilirubin	Negative (0.02 mg/dL or less)	0.4–0.8 mg/dL	Positive (conjugated) bilirubin indicates hepatitis. False-negative readings can be caused by ascorbic acid concentrations ≥25 mg/dL. False-positive readings can be caused by metabolites of etodolac. Test is less specific than Ictotest Reagent Tablets. A positive test should be confirmed by Ictotest Reagent Tablets.
Blood	Negative (<0.010 mg/dL hemoglobin or <3 RBC/mcL)[3]	0.015–0.062 mg/dL hemoglobin or 5–20 RBC/mcL	Test is equally sensitive to myoglobin and hemoglobin (including both intact RBC and free hemoglobin). False-positive results can be caused by oxidizing contaminants (hypochloride) and microbial peroxidase (urinary tract infection). Test sensitivity is reduced in urines with high specific gravity, captopril, or heavy proteinuria.
Nitrite	Negative	0.06–0.10 mg/dL nitrite ion	Test depends on the conversion of nitrate (derived from the diet) to nitrite by gram-negative bacteria in urine when their number is >10^5/mcL (≥0.075 mg/dL nitrite ion). Test specific for nitrite. False-negative readings can be caused by ascorbic acid. Test sensitivity is reduced in urines with high specific gravity. A negative result does not rule out significant bacteriuria.
Leukocytes (esterase)	Negative[4]	5–15 WBCs/hpf in clinical urine	Indicator of urinary tract infection. Test detects esterases contained in granulocytic leukocytes. Test sensitivity is reduced in urines with elevated glucose concentrations ≥3 g/dL), or presence of cephalexin, cephalothin, tetracycline, or high concentrations of oxalate.

[1] Package insert, revised 11/05. Bayer Diagnostics Reagent Strips for Urinalysis, Siemens Healthcare Diagnostics.
[2] Analytical measurement range (AMR) of the reagent strips.
[3] Except in menstruating females.
[4] Except in females with vaginitis.

   b. Cells may be red cells, white cells, squamous cells, transitional (bladder) or tubular epithelial cells, or atypical (tumor) cells. Red cells suggest upper or lower urinary tract infections (cystitis, prostatitis, pyelonephritis), glomerulonephritis, collagen vascular disease, trauma, renal calculi, tumors, drug reactions, and structural abnormalities (polycystic kidneys). White cells suggest inflammatory processes such as urinary tract infection (most common), collagen vascular disease (eg, lupus), or interstitial nephritis. Red cell casts are considered pathognomonic of glomerulonephritis; white cell casts, of pyelonephritis; and fatty (lipid) casts, of nephrotic syndrome.

   c. Presence of crystals is often of no clinical significance. Presence of casts, however, is associated with various pathologic conditions. For example, WBC (leukocyte) casts are seen in patients with pyelonephritis and interstitial nephritis; RBC (erythrocyte) casts in acute glomerulonephritis, lupus nephritis, Goodpasture syndrome, and subacute bacterial endocarditis; renal epithelial casts in toxic tubular necrosis; waxy casts in severe chronic renal disease and amyloidosis; and fatty casts in nephrotic syndrome and diabetes mellitus.

Comments

See Table 8–28 for a guide to interpretation of urinalysis; and Figure 2–1 for a guide to microscopic findings in urine.

Note: Fully automated urinalysis systems (either image- or flow cytometry-based) are now available in many clinical laboratories, so manual microscopy examination may not be performed routinely in a central laboratory.

B. Vaginal Fluid Wet-Mount Preparation
Preparation of Smear and Staining Technique
   a. Apply a small amount of vaginal discharge to a glass slide.
   b. Add 2 drops of sterile saline solution.
   c. Place a coverslip over the area to be examined.

Microscopic Examination
   a. Examine under the microscope, using the high-dry (40×) lens and a low light source.
   b. Look for motile trichomonads (undulating protozoa propelled by four flagella). Look for clue cells (vaginal epithelial cells with large numbers of organisms attached to them, obscuring cell borders), which are pathognomonic of *Gardnerella vaginalis*-associated vaginosis.
   c. See Figure 2–2 for an example of a positive wet prep (trichomonads, clue cells) and Table 8–29 for the differential diagnosis of vaginal discharge.

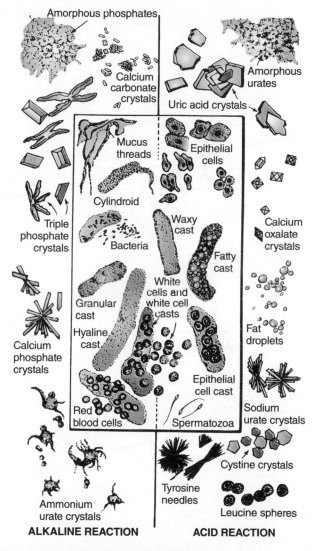

Figure 2–1. Microscopic findings on examination of the urine.

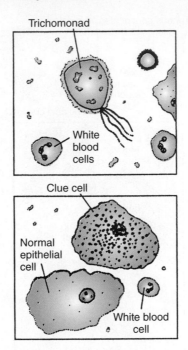

Trichomonad

White blood cells

Clue cell

Normal epithelial cell

White blood cell

Figure 2–2. Wet-mount preparation showing trichomonads, white blood cells, and clue cells.

C. Skin or Vaginal Fluid KOH Preparation
Preparation of Smear and Staining Technique

    a. Obtain a skin specimen by using a scalpel blade to scrape scales from the skin lesion onto a glass slide or to transfer the top of a vesicle to the slide or, place a single drop of vaginal discharge on the slide.

    b. Place 1 or 2 drops of potassium hydroxide (KOH) (15%) on top of the specimen (skin scrapings or vaginal discharge) on the slide. Put a coverslip over the area to be examined.

    d. Allow the KOH prep to sit at room temperature until the material has been cleared. The slide may be warmed to speed the clearing process.

      Note: A fishy amine odor upon addition of KOH to a vaginal discharge is typical of bacterial vaginosis caused by *Gardnerella vaginalis.*

Microscopic Examination

a. Examine the smear under low-power (10×) and high-dry (40×) lenses for mycelial forms. Branched, septate hyphae are typical of dermatophytosis (eg, trichophyton, epidermophyton, microsporum species); branched, septate pseudohyphae with or without budding yeast forms are seen with candidiasis (candida species); and short, curved hyphae plus clumps of spores ("spaghetti and meatballs") are seen with tinea versicolor (*Malassezia furfur*).

b. Record and report any yeast, pseudohyphae, or hyphae, indicating budding and septation.

Comments

See Figure 2–3 for an example of a positive KOH prep.

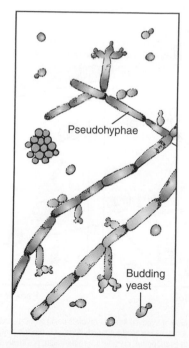

Figure 2–3. KOH preparation showing mycelial forms (pseudohyphae) and budding yeast typical of *Candida albicans*.

D. Synovial Fluid Examination for Crystals
Preparation of Smear Technique
   a. Place a small amount of synovial fluid on a glass slide. No stain is necessary.
   b. Place a coverslip over the area to be examined.

Microscopic Examination
   a. Examine under a polarized light microscope with a red compensator, using the high-dry lens and a moderately bright light source.
   b. Look for needle-shaped, negatively birefringent urate crystals (crystals parallel to the axis of the compensator appear yellow) in gout, or rhomboidal, positively birefringent calcium pyrophosphate crystals (crystals parallel to the axis of the compensator appear blue) in pseudogout.

Comments
See Figure 2–4 for examples of positive synovial fluid examinations for these two types of crystals.

E. Fern Test of Amniotic Fluid
The Fern test, in conjunction with pH determination using pH paper (Nitrazine test), detects the leakage of amniotic fluid from the membrane surrounding the fetus during pregnancy.

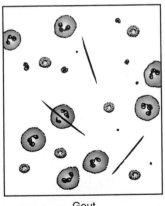
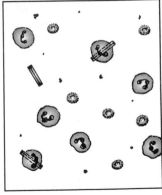

Gout   Pseudogout

Figure 2–4. Examination of synovial fluid for crystals using a compensated, polarized microscope. In gout, crystals are needle shaped, negatively birefringent, and composed of monosodium urate. In pseudogout, crystals are rhomboidal, positively birefringent, and composed of calcium pyrophosphate dihydrate. In both diseases, crystals can be found free-floating or within polymorphonuclear cells.

Preparation of Smear Technique
  a. Collect vaginal secretion from the posterior vaginal fornix with a sterile swab. Do not touch the mucus plug in the cervix.
  b. Immediately rub the swab against a clean glass slide, creating a very thin smear.
  c. Allow slide to dry. Do not cover with a coverslip.

Microscopic Examination
  a. Examine the dried smear under the low-power (10×) lens.
  b. If present, the amniotic fluid crystallizes to form a fern-like pattern (ferning) (Figure 2–5).

Comments
The Fern test should be performed together with the Nitrazine test. If both tests are positive, amniotic membrane rupture has occurred. If the Fern test is positive but the Nitrazine test is negative, there is probable rupture of membrane. If the Fern test is negative but the Nitrazine test is positive, a second specimen should be collected and examined using both tests.

Premature rupture of the membranes may lead to fetal infection and subsequent morbidity. Induction of labor should be evaluated in this situation.

F. Pinworm Tape Test
This test is a method used to diagnose a pinworm infection by microscopic examination of specimens taken from the perianal region to identify *Enterobius vermicularis* eggs or adult female worms, if present.

Procedural Technique
  a. Firmly press the sticky side of a 1-inch strip of transparent adhesive (Cellophane) tape over the right and left perianal folds for a few seconds.
  b. Place the tape on a clean glass slide, sticky side down.
  c. Using a microscope, examine the entire tape for eggs or worms under the low-power (10×) lens. The eggs are oval, elongated, and flattened on one side, with a thick colorless shell. The adult female worms are tiny, white, and threadlike, with a long, pointed tail.
  d. Record and report findings.
  e. See Figure 2–6 for an example of a positive Pinworm tape test.

Comments
Test should be done first thing in the morning before a bowel movement or bath. Note that specimen may also be collected at home with a collection paddle (eg, Becton-Dickinson SWUBE Paddle), and kept in a specimen tube until microscopic examination. Female pinworms deposit eggs sporadically, so test must be done on at least 4 consecutive days to rule out the infection.

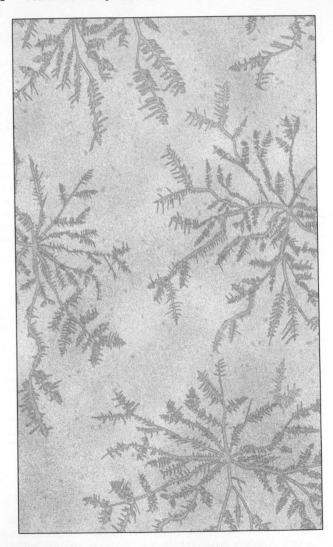

Figure 2–5. Positive Fern test showing crystallized amniotic fluid collected from the posterior vaginal fornix.

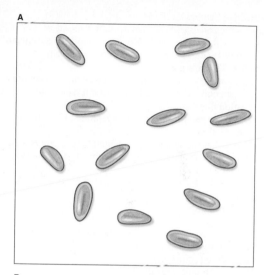

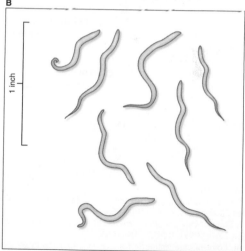

Figure 2–6. Positive Pinworm tape test showing *Enterobius vermicularis* eggs (**A**) and adult female worms (**B**).

G. Qualitative Semen Analysis

Qualitative semen analysis is used to document the success of vasectomy. Semen samples should be examined for presence or absence of motile and/or non-motile sperm at 8–12 weeks post-vasectomy.

Procedural Technique

a. Ask patient to collect the entire ejaculate by masturbation into a clean container labeled with patient name and unique identification number.

b. Keep the specimen at body temperature (37°C) to ensure proper liquefaction.

c. Verify that the semen has liquefied before proceeding with the test. If not liquefied, check specimen at 10-minute intervals until it has liquefied.

d. Place a small drop of liquefied semen on a clean glass slide and add a coverslip.

Microscopic Examination

a. Immediately examine under the high-dry (40×) lens. For presence or absence of sperm, examine several fields before reporting the absence of sperm. If sperm are present, classify them according to their motility (motile versus non-motile) in percentages.

b. Record and report results.

Comments

Semen samples should be collected after an abstinence period of no less than 48 hours and no more than 7 days and maintained at body temperature. Specimen must be examined as soon as possible to ensure maximum accuracy of results. Specimens collected in condoms should be rejected. If sperm are present, the patient should be cautioned to continue temporary contraception and to resubmit a second specimen for re-examination after 4–6 additional weeks.

For evaluation of infertility, full semen analysis should be performed at a central laboratory.

REFERENCES

Point-of-Care Testing

Campbell S et al. HIV testing near the patient: changing the face of HIV testing. Clin Lab Med 2009;29:491. [PMID: 19840682]

Casagranda I. Point-of-care in critical care: the clinician's point of view. Clin Chem Lab Med 2010;48:931. [PMID: 20441464]

Perry DJ et al. Point-of-care testing in haemostasis. Br J Haematol 2010;150:501. [PMID: 20618331]

Rhee AJ et al. Laboratory point-of-care monitoring in the operating room. Curr Opin Anaesthesiol 2010;23:741. [PMID: 20881483]

Urinalysis

Budak YU et al. Comparison of three automated systems for urine chemistry and sediment analysis in routine laboratory practice. Clin Lab 2011;57:47. [PMID: 21391464]

Perazella MA et al. Urine microscopy is associated with severity and worsening of acute kidney injury in hospitalized patients. Clin J Am Soc Nephrol 2010;5:402. [PMID: 20089493]

Tworek JA et al. The rate of manual microscopic examination of urine sediment: a CAP Q-Probes study of 11,243 urinalysis tests from 88 institutions. Arch Pathol Lab Med 2008;132:1868. [PMID: 19061282]

Vaginal Wet-Mount Preparation

Harp DF et al. Trichomoniasis: evaluation to execution. Eur J Obstet Reprod Biol 2011;157:3. [PMID: 21440359]

Roth AM et al. Changing sexually transmitted infection screening protocol will result in improved case finding for *Trichomonas vaginalis* among high-risk female populations. Sex Transm Dis 2011;38:398. [PMID: 21217417]

Synovial Fluid Examination

Pascual E et al. Synovial fluid analysis for crystals. Curr Opin Rheumatol 2011;23.161. [PMID: 21285711]

Vanltallie TB. Gout: epitome of painful arthritis. Metabolism 2010;59(Suppl 1):S32. [PMID: 20837191]

Pinworm Tape Test

Stermer E et al. Pruritus ani: an approach to an itching condition. J Pediatr Gastroenterol Nutr 2009;48:513. [PMID: 19412003]

Semen Analysis, Qualitative

Senanayake E et al. A novel cost-effective approach to post-vasectomy semen analysis. BJU Int 2011;107:1447. [PMID: 21388491]

Sigman M et al. Semen analysis and sperm function assays: what do they mean? Semin Reprod Med 2009;27:115. [PMID: 19247913]

Steward B et al. Diagnostic accuracy of an initial azoospermic reading compared with results of post-centrifugation semen analysis after vasectomy. J Urol 2008;180:2119. [PMID: 18804227]

3

Common Laboratory Tests: Selection and Interpretation

Diana Nicoll, MD, PhD, MPA, Chuanyi Mark Lu, MD, Stephen J. McPhee, MD, and Michael Pignone, MD, MPH

HOW TO USE THIS SECTION

This section contains information about commonly used laboratory tests. It includes most of the blood, urine, and cerebrospinal fluid tests found in this book, with the exception of drug levels and pharmacogenetic tests (see Chapter 4). Entries are in outline format and are arranged alphabetically.

Test/Reference Range/Collection

This first outline listing begins with the common test name, the specimen analyzed, and any test name abbreviation (in parentheses).

Below this, in the first outline listing, is the reference range (also called reference interval) for each test. The first entry is in conventional units, and the second entry (in [brackets]) is in SI units (Système International d'Unités). Any panic values for a particular test are placed here after the word *Panic*. The reference ranges provided are from several large medical centers; consult your own clinical laboratory for those used in your institution.

This outline listing also shows which tube to use for collecting blood and other body fluids, how much the test costs (in relative symbolism; see below), and how to collect the specimen.

The scale used for the cost of each test is:

Approximate Cost	Symbol Used in Tables
$1–20	$
$21–50	$$
$51–100	$$$
>$100	$$$$

Listed below are the common collection tubes and their contents:

Tube Top Color	Tube Contents	Typically Used In
Lavender or Pink	K$_2$EDTA	Complete blood count; blood banking (plasma); molecular testing (cell-based)
Serum separator tube (SST)	Clot activator and serum separator gel	Serum chemistry tests
Red	None	Blood banking (serum)
Blue	Sodium citrate	Coagulation studies
Green	Sodium heparin or lithium heparin	Plasma chemistry tests; chromosome analysis (sodium heparin)
Yellow	Acid citrate dextrose (ACD); sodium polyanethol sulfonate (SPS)	ACD: HLA typing; blood banking (plasma); flow cytometry. SPS: Blood culture (microbiology)
Navy	Trace metal-free	Trace metals (eg, lead, mercury, arsenic)
Gray	Inhibitor of glycolysis (sodium fluoride)	Lactic acid; glucose
Plasma preparation tube (PPT)	K$_2$EDTA and separator gel	Molecular testing (plasma-based), plasma chemistry tests

Physiologic Basis

This outline listing contains physiologic information about the substance being tested. Information on classification and biologic importance, as well as interactions with other biologic substances and processes, is included.

Interpretation

This outline lists clinical conditions that affect the substance being tested. Generally, conditions with higher prevalence are listed first. When the sensitivity of the test for a particular disease is known, that information follows the disease name in parentheses, for example, "rheumatoid arthritis (83%)." Some of the common drugs that can affect the test substance *in vivo* are also included in this outline listing.

Comments

This outline listing sets forth general information pertinent to the use and interpretation of the test and important *in vitro* interferences with the test procedure. Appropriate general references are also listed.

Test Name

The test name is placed as a header to the rest of the outline list to allow for quick referencing.

	ABO Typing		
Test/Range/Collection	**Physiologic Basis**	**Interpretation**	**Comments**
ABO typing, serum or plasma and red cells (ABO) Red or lavender/pink $ Properly identified and labeled blood specimens are critical.	The ABO antigen and antibodies remain the most significant for transfusion practice. The 4 blood groups A, B, O, and AB are determined by the presence of antigens A and B or their absence (O) on a patient's red blood cells. Individuals possess antibodies directed toward the A or B antigen absent from their own red cells. In the US white population, 45% are type O, 40% A, 11% B, 4% AB. In the US Hispanic population, 57% are type O, 30% A, 10% B, 3% AB. In the African American population, 49% are type O, 27% A, 20% B, 4% AB. In the US Asian population, 40% are type O, 28% A, 27% B, 5% AB. In the Native American population, 55% are type O, 35% A, 8% B, 2% AB.	Type O patients can receive type O red cells and type A, B, O, or AB plasma. Type A patients can receive type A or O red cells and type A or AB plasma. Type B patients can receive type B or O red cells and type B or AB plasma. Type AB patients can receive type AB, A, B, or O red cells but only type AB plasma. In an emergency situation, type O red cells and type AB plasma may be given to patients with any ABO blood types.	For both blood donors and recipients, routine ABO typing includes both red cell and serum testing, as checks on each other. Tube testing is as follows: patients red cells are tested with anti-A and anti-B for the presence or absence of agglutination (forward or cell type), and patient's serum or plasma is tested against known A and B cells (reverse or serum/plasma type). *Technical Manual of the American Association of Blood Banks,* 17th ed. American Association of Blood Banks, 2011. Malomgré W et al. Recent and future trends in blood group typing. Anal Bioanal Chem 2009;393:1443. [PMID: 18839152]

Acetaminophen

Test/Range/Collection	Physiologic Basis	Interpretation	Comments
Acetaminophen, serum (Tylenol; others) 10–20 mg/L [66–132 mcmol/L] **Panic:** >50 mg/L Red $$ For suspected overdose, draw 2 samples at least 4 hours apart, at least 4 hours after ingestion. Note time of ingestion, if known. Order test stat.	In overdose, liver and renal toxicity are produced by the hydroxylated metabolite if it is not conjugated with glutathione in the liver.	**Increased in:** Acetaminophen overdose. Interpretation of serum acetaminophen level depends on time since ingestion. Levels drawn <4 hr after ingestion cannot be interpreted, since the drug is still in the absorption and distribution phase. Use nomogram (Figure 10–1) to evaluate possible toxicity. Levels >150 mg/L at 4 hours or >50 mg/L at 12 hours after ingestion suggest toxicity. Nomogram is inaccurate for chronic ingestions.	Do not delay acetylcysteine (Mucomyst) treatment (140 mg/kg orally) if stat levels are unavailable. Chun LJ et al. Acetaminophen hepatotoxicity and acute liver failure. J Clin Gastroenterol 2009;43:342. [PMID: 19169150] Green TJ et al. When do the aminotransferases rise after acute acetaminophen overdose? Clin Toxicol (Phila) 2010;48:787. [PMID: 20969501] Klein-Schwartz W et al. Intravenous acetylcysteine for the treatment of acetaminophen overdose. Expert Opin Pharmacother 2011;12:119. [PMID: 21126198]

Acetoacetate		
Acetoacetate, blood or urine	Acetoacetate, acetone, and β-hydroxybutyrate contribute to ketoacidosis when oxidative hepatic metabolism of fatty acids is impaired.	**Present in:** Diabetic keto-acidosis, alcoholic ketoacidosis, prolonged fasting, starvation, severe carbohydrate restriction with normal fat intake, prolonged exercise.	Nitroprusside test is semiquantitative; it detects aceto-acetate and is sensitive down to 5–10 mg/dL.
0 mg/dL [mcmol/L]			Trace = 5 mg/dL, small = 15 mg/dL, moderate = 40 mg/dL, large = 80 mg/dL [1 mg/dL = 100 mcmol/L].
Red, lavender, or urine container	Proportions in serum vary but are generally 20% acetoacetate, 78% β-hydroxybutyrate, and 2% acetone.		β-Hydroxybutyrate has no ketone group; therefore, it is not detected by the nitroprusside test. Acetone is also not reliably detected by this method because the sensitivity for acetone is poor.
$			Failure of nitroprusside test to detect β-hydroxybutyrate in ketoacidosis may produce a seemingly paradoxical increase in ketones with clini-cal improvement as nondetectable β-hydroxybutyrate is replaced by detectable acetoacetate. Testing for blood β-hydroxybutyrate is clinically more useful in this setting.
Urine sample should be fresh.			Prisco F et al. Blood ketone bodies in patients with recent-onset type 1 diabetes (a multicenter study). Pediatr Diabetes 2006;7:223. [PMID: 16911010] Weber C et al. Prevention of diabetic ketoacidosis and self-monitoring of ketone bodies: an overview. Curr Med Res Opin 2009;25:1197. [PMID: 19327102]

Acetylcholine receptor antibody		
Test/Range/Collection	Physiologic Basis	Interpretation	Comments

Test/Range/Collection	Physiologic Basis	Interpretation	Comments
Acetylcholine receptor antibody, serum Negative SST, red $$	Acetylcholine receptor antibodies are involved in the pathogenesis of myasthenia gravis. Sensitive radioimmunoassay or enzyme-linked immunosorbent assay (ELISA) is available based on inhibition of binding of ^{125}I α-bungarotoxin to the acetylcholine receptor.	**Positive in:** Myasthenia gravis (sensitivity 87–98%, specificity 98–100%)	Antibody levels correlate with severity of autonomic failure. Antibodies can also be associated with other neurologic disorders unrelated to the autonomic nervous system. Leite MI et al. Diagnostic use of autoantibodies in myasthenia gravis. Autoimmunity 2010;43:371. [PMID: 20380582] Meriggioli MN. Myasthenia gravis with anti-acetylcholine receptor antibodies. Front Neurol Neurosci 2009;26:94. [PMID: 19349707] Meriggioli MN et al. Autoimmune myasthenia gravis: emerging clinical and biological heterogeneity. Lancet Neurol 2009;8:475. [PMID: 19375665] Winston N et al. Recent advances in autoimmune autonomic ganglionopathy. Curr Opin Neurol 2010;23:514. [PMID: 20634694]

Activated clotting time		
Activated clotting time, whole blood (ACT) 70–180 sec (method-specific) $$ Obtain blood in a plastic syringe without antico-agulant. Test should be performed immediately at patient's bedside. A clean venipuncture is required. A special vacutainer tube containing activator (eg, celite, kaolin) is also available.	ACT is a point-of-care test used to monitor high-dose heparin as an anticoagulant during cardiac surgery (extracorporeal circulation), angioplasty, and hemodialysis. It is also used to determine the dose of protamine sulfate to reverse the heparin effect on completion of the procedure. ACT is also used to monitor heparin or direct thrombin inhibitor in patients with documented lupus anticoagulant.	**Prolonged in:** Heparin therapy, direct thrombin inhibitor therapy, severe deficiency of clotting factors (except factors VII and XIII), functional platelet disorders. In general, the accepted goal during cardiopulmonary bypass surgery is 400–500 sec. For carotid artery stenting the optimal ACT is 250–300 sec.	ACT is the choice of test when heparin levels are too high (eg, >1.0 U/mL heparin) to allow monitoring with PTT and/or when a rapid result is necessary to monitor treatment. Because different methodologies and a number of variables (eg, platelet count and function, hypothermia, hemodilution, and certain drugs like aprotinin) may affect the ACT, the ACT test is not yet standardized. Reproducibility of prolonged ACTs may be poor. Bosch YP et al. Comparison of ACT point-of-care measurements: repeatability and agreement. Perfusion 2006;21:27. [PMID: 16485696] Perry DJ et al. Point-of-care testing in haemostasis. Br J Haematol 2010;150:501. [PMID: 20618331] Saw J et al. Evaluating the optimal activated clotting time during carotid artery stenting. Am J Cardiol 2006;97:1657. [PMID: 16728233]

	Adrenocorticotropic hormone		
Test/Range/Collection	**Physiologic Basis**	**Interpretation**	**Comments**
Adrenocorticotropic hormone, plasma (ACTH) 9–52 pg/mL [2–11 pmol/L] Lavender, pink $$$$ Separate plasma from cells and freeze ASAP Send promptly to laboratory on ice. ACTH is unstable in plasma, is inactivated at room temperature, and adheres strongly to glass. Avoid all contact with glass.	Pituitary ACTH (release stimulated by hypothalamic corticotropin-releasing factor) stimulates cortisol release from the adrenal gland. There is feedback regulation of the system by cortisol. ACTH is secreted episodically and shows circadian variation, with highest levels at 6:00–8:00 AM; lowest levels at 9:00–10:00 PM.	**Increased in:** Pituitary (40–200 pg/mL) and ectopic (200–71,000 pg/mL) Cushing syndrome, primary adrenal insufficiency (>250 pg/mL), adrenogenital syndrome with impaired cortisol production. **Decreased in:** Adrenal Cushing syndrome (<20 pg/mL), pituitary ACTH (secondary adrenal) insufficiency (<50 pg/mL).	ACTH levels can be interpreted only when measured with cortisol after standardized stimulation or suppression tests (see Adrenocortical insufficiency algorithm, Figure 9–3, and Cushing syndrome algorithm, Figure 9–8). Findling JW et al. Cushing's syndrome: important issues in diagnosis and management. J Clin Endocrinol Metab 2006;91:3746. [PMID: 16868050] Neary N et al. Adrenal insufficiency: etiology, diagnosis and treatment. Curr Opin Endocrinol Diabetes Obes 2010;17:217. [PMID: 20375886] Pecori Giraldi F. Recent challenges in the diagnosis of Cushing's syndrome. Horm Res 2009;71(Suppl 1):123. [PMID: 19153521]

Alanine aminotransferase		
Alanine aminotransferase, serum or plasma (ALT, SGPT, GPT) 0–35 U/L [0–0.58 mckat/L] (laboratory-specific) SST, PPT, green, lavender $	Intracellular enzyme involved in amino acid metabolism. Present in large concentrations in liver, kidney; in smaller amounts, in skeletal muscle and heart. Released with tissue damage, particularly liver injury.	**Increased in:** Acute viral hepatitis (ALT > AST), biliary tract obstruction (cholangitis, choledocholithiasis), alcoholic hepatitis and cirrhosis (AST > ALT), liver abscess, metastatic or primary liver cancer; nonalcoholic steatohepatitis; right heart failure, ischemia or hypoxia, injury to liver ("shock liver"), extensive trauma; drugs that cause cholestasis or hepatotoxicity. **Decreased in:** Pyridoxine (vitamin B_6) deficiency.	ALT is the preferred enzyme for evaluation of liver injury. Screening ALT in low-risk populations has a low (12%) positive predictive value and is not recommended. See Liver function tests (Table 8–14). Fraser A et al. Alanine aminotransferase, gamma-glutamyltransferase, and incident diabetes: the British Women's Heart and Health Study and meta-analysis. Diabetes Care 2009;32:741. [PMID: 19131466] McMahon BJ. The natural history of chronic hepatitis B virus infection. Hepatology 2009;49(5 Suppl):S45. [PMID: 19399792] St George A et al. Effect of a lifestyle intervention in patients with abnormal liver enzymes and metabolic risk factors. J Gastroenterol Hepatol 2009;24:399. [PMID: 19067776]

	Albumin

Test/Range/Collection	Physiologic Basis	Interpretation	Comments
Albumin, serum or plasma 3.4–4.7 g/dL [34–47 g/L] SST, PPT, green $	Major component of plasma proteins; influenced by nutritional state, hepatic function, renal function, and various diseases. Major binding protein. Although there are more than 50 different genetic variants (alloalbumins), only occasionally does a mutation cause abnormal binding (eg, in familial dysalbuminemic hyperthyroxinemia).	**Increased in:** Dehydration, shock, hemoconcentration. **Decreased in:** Decreased hepatic synthesis (chronic liver disease, malnutrition, malabsorption, malignancy, congenital analbuminemia [rare]). Increased losses (nephrotic syndrome, burns, trauma, hemorrhage with fluid replacement, fistulas, enteropathy, acute or chronic glomerulonephritis). Hemodilution (pregnancy, CHF). Drugs: estrogens.	Serum albumin indicates severity in chronic liver disease. Useful in nutritional assessment if there is no impairment in production or increased loss of albumin. Independent risk factor for all-cause mortality in the elderly (age >70) and for complications in hospitalized and post-surgical patients. There is a 10% reduction in serum albumin level in late pregnancy (related to hemodilution). See liver function tests (Table 8–14) and MELD scoring systems for staging cirrhosis (Table 8–9). Ghany MG et al. HALT-C Trial Group. Predicting clinical and histologic outcomes based on standard laboratory tests in advanced chronic hepatitis C. Gastroenterology 2010;138:136. [PMID: 19766643] Hennessey DB et al. Preoperative hypoalbuminemia is an independent risk factor for the development of surgical site infection following gastrointestinal surgery: a multi-institutional study. Ann Surg 2010;252:325. [PMID: 20647925] Pencharz PB. Assessment of protein nutritional status in children. Pediatr Blood Cancer 2008;50(2 Suppl):445.

Albumin		
Albumin, urine <30 mg/24 hr <20 mcg/min (timed collection) $$$$	The normal urinary albumin excretion is less than 30 mg/24 hr. On random spot urine collection, the albumin-to-creatinine ratio (ACR, mcg/mg) should be less than 30. The term microalbuminuria is defined as a subtle increase in the urinary excretion of albumin that cannot be detected by conventional urinalysis. Specifically, the excretion of 30–300 mg albumin per 24 hours or an ACR of 30–300 (mcg/mg) is considered microalbuminuria (urine albumin is high). 300 mg or more of albumin excretion per day or an ACR of 300 or higher indicates gross albuminuria (urine albumin very high or nephrotic) range.	**Increased in:** Diabetes mellitus, diabetic nephropathy.	Microalbuminuria is a useful indicator of early nephropathy in diabetic patients. Urine albumin measurement requires a sensitive immunochemical assay. Urine dipstick analysis is often insensitive to microalbuminuria. Screening for microalbuminuria is often performed by measurement of the ACR in a random spot urine collection (preferred method). Twenty-four-hour or timed urine collections are more burdensome. Comper WD et al. Detection of urinary albumin. Adv Chronic Kidney Dis 2005;12:170. [PMID: 15822052] Miller WG et al. Current issues in measurement and reporting of urinary albumin excretion. Clin Chem 2009;55:24. [PMID: 19028824] Ritz E et al. Renal protection in diabetes: lessons from ONTARGET. Cardiovasc Diabetol 2010;9:60. [PMID: 20920303]

Test/Range/Collection	Physiologic Basis	Interpretation	Comments
Aldosterone, serum	Aldosterone is the major miner-alocorticoid hormone and is a major regulator of extracellular volume and serum potassium concentration. For evaluation of hypoaldosteronism (associated with hyperkalemia), patients should be salt-depleted and upright when specimen is drawn.	**Increased in:** Primary hyperaldosteronism (2/3 from adrenal hyperplasia, 1/3 from adrenal adenomas) may account for 5–10% of hypertension. **Aldosterone/PRA ratio >15** (mL/dL/h) (sensitivity 73–87%, specificity 74–75%) **Decreased in:** Primary or secondary hypoaldosteronism.	Screening for hyperaldosteronism should use simultaneous determination of serum aldosterone and plasma renin activity (PRA) (see Figure 9–12). In primary aldosteronism, plasma aldosterone is usually elevated whereas PRA is low; in secondary hyperaldosteronism, both serum aldosterone and PRA are usually elevated. The aldosterone/PRA ratio is often used for diagnosis of hyperaldosteronism, but the cutoff value has not been well established and the specificity is low. Mulatero P et al. Evaluation of primary aldosteronism. Curr Opin Endocrinol Diabetes Obes 2010;17:188. [PMID: 20389241] Mulatero P et al. Confirmatory tests in the diagnosis of primary aldosteronism. Horm Metab Res 2010;42:406. [PMID: 20119882] Tomaschitz A. Aldosterone to renin ratio—a reliable screening tool for primary aldosteronism? Horm Metab Res 2010;42:382. [PMID: 20251167]
Salt-loaded (120 meq Na+/d for 3–4 days):			
Supine: 3–10 ng/dL			
Upright: 5–30 ng/dL			
Salt-depleted (10 meq Na+/d for 3–4 days):			
Supine: 12–36 ng/dL			
Upright: 17–137 ng/dL			
SST, Red			
$$$$			
Early AM fasting specimen. Separate immediately and freeze.			

Aldosterone, urine		
Aldosterone, urine*	Secretion of aldosterone is controlled by the renin-angiotensin system. Renin (synthesized and stored in juxtaglomerular cells of kidney) is released in response to both decreased perfusion pressure at the juxtaglomerular apparatus and negative sodium balance. Renin then hydrolyzes angiotensinogen to angiotensin I, which is converted to angiotensin II, which then stimulates the adrenal gland to produce aldosterone.	**Increased in:** Primary and secondary hyperaldosteronism, some patients with essential hypertension. **Decreased in:** Primary hypoaldosteronism (eg, 18-hydroxylase deficiency), secondary hypoaldosteronism (hyporeninemic hypoaldosteronism).	Urinary aldosterone is the most sensitive test for primary hyperaldosteronism. Levels >14 mcg/24 hours after 3 days of salt-loading have a 96% sensitivity and 93% specificity for primary hyperaldosteronism: 7% of patients with essential hypertension have urinary aldosterone levels >14 mcg/24 hr after salt-loading. Giacchetti G et al. Analysis of screening and confirmatory tests in the diagnosis of primary aldosteronism: need for a standardized protocol. J Hypertens 2006;24:737. [PMID: 16331803] Rossi GP et al. Primary aldosteronism: cardiovascular, renal and metabolic implications. Trends Endocrinol Metab 2008;19:88. [PMID: 18314347] Tomaschitz A et al. Aldosterone and arterial hypertension. Nat Rev Endocrinol 2010;6:83. [PMID: 20027193]

Salt-loaded (120 meq Na+/d for 3–4 days): 1.5–12.5 mcg/24 hr

Salt-depleted (20 meq Na+/d for 3–4 days): 18–85 mcg/24 hr

[1 mcg/24 hr = 2.77 nmol/d]

Bottle containing boric acid

$$$

*To evaluate hyperaldosteronism, patient is salt-loaded and recumbent. Obtain 24-hour urine for aldosterone (and for sodium to check that sodium excretion is ≥ 250 meq/d). To evaluate hypoaldosteronism, patient is salt-depleted and upright; check patient for hypotension before 24-hour urine is collected.

	Alkaline phosphatase		
Test/Range/Collection	Physiologic Basis	Interpretation	Comments
Alkaline phosphatase, serum or plasma (ALP) 41–133 IU/L [0.7–2.2 mckat/L] (method- and age-dependent) SST, PPT, green $	Alkaline phosphatases are primarily found in liver, bone, intestines, kidney, and placenta. Test is used to detect liver disease and bone disorders.	**Increased in:** Obstructive hepatobiliary disease, bone disease (physiologic bone growth, Paget disease, osteomalacia, osteogenic sarcoma, bone metastases), hyperparathyroidism, rickets, benign familial hyperphosphatasemia, pregnancy (third trimester), GI disease (perforated ulcer or bowel infarct), hepatotoxic drugs. **Decreased in:** Hypophosphatasia.	Alkaline phosphatase performs well in measuring the extent of bone metastases in prostate cancer. Normal in osteoporosis. Alkaline phosphatase isoenzyme separation by electrophoresis or differential heat inactivation is unreliable. Use γ-glutamyl transpeptidase, which increases in hepatobiliary disease but not in bone disease, to infer origin of increased alkaline phosphatase (ie, liver rather than bone). Aragon G et al. When and how to evaluate mildly elevated liver enzymes in apparently healthy patients. Cleve Clin J Med 2010;77:195. [PMID: 20200170] Rajarubendra N et al. Diagnosis of bone metastasis in urological malignancies—an update. Urology 2010;76:782. [PMID: 20346492] Whyte MP. Physiological role of alkaline phosphatase explored in hypophosphatasia. Ann NY Acad Sci 2010;1192:190. [PMID: 20392236]

Amebic serology		
Amebiasis, antibody, serum Negative SST $$	Test for infection with *Entamoeba histolytica* (amebiasis) by detection of IgG antibodies that develop 2–4 weeks after infection. Tissue invasion by the organism may be necessary for antibody production.	**Increased in:** Current or past infection with *E. histolytica*. Amebic abscess (91%), amebic dysentery (84%), asymptomatic cyst carriers (9%), patients with other diseases, and healthy people (2%).	Seroconversion between acute and convalescent sera is considered evidence of recent infection. A positive antibody test can indicate infection even though stool findings are negative. *E. dispar* and *E. moshkovskii* are morphologically indistinguishable from *E. histolytica*. Only *E. histolytica* causes disease in humans. Molecular tests are now available to distinguish between them for research and epidemiologic purposes. Ali K et al. Molecular epidemiology of amebiasis. Infect Genet Evol 2008;8:698. [PMID: 18571478] van Doorn HR et al. Use of rapid dipstick and latex agglutination tests and enzyme-linked immunosorbent assay for serodiagnosis of amebic liver abscess, amebic colitis, and *Entamoeba histolytica* cyst passage. J Clin Microbiol 2005;43:4801. [PMID: 16145144]

	Ammonia		
Test/Range/Collection	**Physiologic Basis**	**Interpretation**	**Comments**
Ammonia, plasma (NH₃) 18–60 mcg/dL [11–35 mcmol/L] Green $$ Separate plasma from cells immediately. Avoid hemolysis. Analyze immediately. Place on ice.	Ammonia is liberated by bacteria in the large intestine or by protein metabolism and is rapidly converted to urea in the liver. In liver disease or portal-systemic shunting, the blood ammonia concentration increases. In acute liver failure, elevation of blood ammonia may cause brain edema; in chronic liver failure, it may be responsible for hepatic encephalopathy.	**Increased in:** Liver failure, hepatic encephalopathy (especially if protein consumption is high or if there is GI bleeding), fulminant hepatic failure, Reye syndrome, portacaval shunting, cirrhosis, urea cycle metabolic defects, urea-splitting urinary tract infection with urinary diversion, and organic acidemias. Drugs: diuretics, acetazolamide, asparaginase, fluorouracil (transient), others. Spuriously increased by any ammonia-containing detergent on laboratory glassware. **Decreased in:** Decreased production by gut bacteria (kanamycin, neomycin). Decreased gut absorption (lactulose).	Plasma ammonia level correlates poorly with degree of hepatic encephalopathy in chronic liver disease. Test not useful in adults with known liver disease. Ammonia toxicity is probably mediated by glutamine, synthesized in excess from ammonia and glutamate. Albrecht J et al. Glutamine as a mediator of ammonia neurotoxicity: a critical appraisal. Biochem Pharmacol 2010;80:1303. [PMID: 20654582] Prakash R et al. Mechanisms, diagnosis and management of hepatic encephalopathy. Nat Rev Gastroenterol Hepatol 2010;7:515. [PMID: 20703237] Wilkinson DJ et al. Ammonia metabolism, the brain and fatigue; revisiting the link. Prog Neurobiol 2010;91:200. [PMID: 20138956]

Amylase		
Amylase, serum or plasma 20–110 U/L [0.33–1.83 mckat/L] (laboratory-specific) SST, PPT $	Amylase hydrolyzes complex carbohydrates. Serum amylase is derived primarily from pancreas and salivary glands and is increased with inflammation or obstruction of these glands. Other tissues have some amylase activity, including ovaries, small and large intestine, and skeletal muscle.	**Increased in:** Acute pancreatitis (70–95%), pancreatic pseudo-cyst, pancreatic duct obstruction (cholecystitis, choledocholithiasis, pancreatic carcinoma, stone, stricture, duct sphincter spasm), bowel obstruction and infarction, mumps, parotitis, diabetic keto-acidosis, penetrating peptic ulcer, peritonitis, ruptured ectopic pregnancy, macroamylasemia. Drugs: azathioprine, hydrochlorothiazide. **Decreased in:** Pancreatic insufficiency, cystic fibrosis. Usually normal or low in chronic pancreatitis.	Macroamylasemia is indicated by high serum but low urine amylase. Serum or plasma lipase is an alternative test for acute pancreatitis. It has clinical sensitivity equivalent to that of amylase but with better specificity. There is no advantage to performing both tests. Amylase isoenzymes are not of practical use because of technical problems. Carroll JK et al. Acute pancreatitis: diagnosis, prognosis, and treatment. Am Fam Physician 2007;75:1513. [PMID: 17555143] Matull WR et al. Biochemical markers of acute pancreatitis. J Clin Pathol 2006;59:340. [PMID: 16567468] Shah AM et al. Acute pancreatitis with normal serum lipase: a case series. JOP 2010;11(4):369. [PMID: 20601812]

	Angiotensin-converting enzyme		
Test/Range/Collection	**Physiologic Basis**	**Interpretation**	**Comments**
Angiotensin-converting enzyme, serum (ACE) 200–590 nkal/L (method-dependent) SST, red $$	ACE is a dipeptidyl carboxypeptidase that converts angiotensin I to the vasopressor, angiotensin II. ACE is normally present in the kidneys and other peripheral tissues. Serum levels in healthy subjects are dependent on polymorphisms in ACE genes. In granulomatous disease, ACE levels increase, derived from epithelioid cells within granulomas.	**Increased in:** Sarcoidosis, hyperthyroidism, acute hepatitis, primary biliary cirrhosis, diabetes mellitus, multiple myeloma, osteoarthritis, amyloidosis, Gaucher disease, pneumoconiosis, histoplasmosis, miliary tuberculosis. Drugs: dexamethasone. **Decreased in:** Renal disease, obstructive pulmonary disease, hypothyroidism.	Test is not useful as a screening test for sarcoidosis (low sensitivity). Specificity is compromised by positive tests in diseases more common than sarcoidosis. Some advocate measurement of ACE to follow disease activity in sarcoidosis. Biller H et al. Gene polymorphisms of ACE and the angiotensin receptor AT2R1 influence serum ACE levels in sarcoidosis. Sarcoidosis Vasc Diffuse Lung Dis 2009;26:139. [PMID: 20560294] Herbort CP et al: members of Scientific Committee of First International Workshop on Ocular Sarcoidosis. International criteria for the diagnosis of ocular sarcoidosis: results of the first International Workshop on Ocular Sarcoidosis (IWOS). Ocul Immunol Inflamm 2009;17:160. [PMID: 19585358]

Antibody screen		
Antibody screen, serum or plasma Red or lavender/pink $ Properly identified and labeled blood specimens are critical.	Detects antibodies to non-ABO red blood cell antigens in recipient's serum or plasma, using reagent red cells selected to possess antigens against which common antibodies can be produced. Further identification of the specificity of any antibody detected (using panels of red cells of known antigenicity) makes it possible to test donor blood for the absence of the corresponding antigen. Primary response to first antigen exposure requires 20–120 days; antibody is largely IgM with a small quantity of IgG. Secondary response requires 1–14 days; antibody is mostly IgG.	**Positive in:** Presence of alloantibody, autoantibodies.	In practice, a type and screen (ABO and Rh grouping and antibody screen) is adequate work-up for patients undergoing operative procedures unlikely to require transfusion. A negative antibody screen implies that a recipient can receive type-specific (ABO-Rh identical) blood with minimal risk. Some antibody activity (eg, anti-Jk^a, anti-E) may become so weak as to be undetectable but increase rapidly after secondary stimulation with the same antigen. *Technical Manual of the American Association of Blood Banks*, 17th ed. American Association of Blood Banks, 2011.

	Antidiuretic hormone		
Test/Range/Collection	**Physiologic Basis**	**Interpretation**	**Comments**
Antidiuretic hormone, plasma (ADH) If serum osmolality <290 mosm/kg H_2O: 2–12 pg/mL If serum osmolality >290 mosm/kg H_2O: <2 pg/mL Lavender, pink $$$$ Draw in two chilled tubes and deliver to lab on ice. Specimen for serum osmolality must be drawn at same time.	Antidiuretic hormone, also known as arginine vasopressin hormone, is a hormone secreted from the posterior pituitary that acts on the distal nephron to conserve water and regulate the tonicity of body fluids. Water deprivation provides both an osmotic and a volume stimulus for ADH release by increasing plasma osmolality and decreasing plasma volume. Water administration lowers plasma osmolality and expands blood volume, inhibiting the release of ADH by the osmo-receptor and the atrial volume receptor mechanisms. Copeptin, the C-terminal part of the AVP precursor peptide, is more stable and may serve a sensitive surrogate marker for ADH release.	**Increased in:** Nephrogenic diabetes insipidus, syndrome of inappropriate antidiuretic hormone (SIADH). Drugs: nico-tine, morphine, chlorpropamide, clofibrate, cyclophosphamide. **Normal relative to plasma osmolality in:** Primary poly-dipsia. **Decreased in:** Central (neurogenic) diabetes insipidus. Drugs: ethanol, phenytoin.	Test very rarely indicated. Measurement of serum and urine osmolality usually suffices. Test not indicated in diagnosis of SIADH. Patients with SIADH show decreased plasma sodium and decreased plasma osmolality, usually with high urine osmolality relative to plasma. These findings in a normovolemic patient with normal thyroid and adrenal function are sufficient to make the diagnosis of SIADH without measuring ADH itself. Fenske W et al. The syndrome of inappropriate secretion of antidiuretic hormone: diagnostic and therapeutic advances. Horm Metab Res 2010;42:691. [PMID: 20607641] Levitchenko EN et al. Nephrogenic syndrome of inappropriate antidiuresis. Nephrol Dial Transplant 2010;25:2839. [PMID: 20543212]

Antiglobulin test, direct

| **Antiglobulin test, direct**, red cells (direct Coombs, DAT)

Negative

Lavender/pink or red

$

Blood anticoagulated with EDTA is used to prevent *in vitro* uptake of complement components. A red top tube may be used, if necessary. | Direct antiglobulin test is used to demonstrate *in vivo* coating of red cells with globulins, in particular IgG and C3d.

DAT is performed with a polyspecific reagent that detects both IgG and C3d. If positive, tests with monospecific reagents (anti-IgG and anti-complement) should be performed to characterize the immune process involved. | **Positive in:** Autoimmune hemolytic anemia, hemolytic disease of the newborn, alloimmune reactions to recently transfused cells, and drug-induced hemolysis. Drugs may induce the formation of antibodies, either against the drug itself or against intrinsic red cell antigens. This may lead to a positive DAT, immune red cell destruction, or both. Some of the antibodies produced appear to be dependent on the presence of the drug (eg, penicillin, quinidine, ceftriaxone), whereas others are independent of the continued presence of the inciting drug (eg, methyldopa, levodopa, procainamide, cephalosporins, fludarabine). | A positive DAT implies *in vivo* red cell coating by immunoglobulins or complement. Such red cell coating may or may not be associated with immune hemolytic anemia.

The DAT can detect a level of 100–500 molecules of IgG per red cell and 400–1100 molecules of C3d per red cell, depending on the reagent and technique used. Positive DATs without clinical manifestations of immune-mediated red cell destruction are reported in the range of 1 in 1000 up to 1 in 14,000 blood donors and 1–15% of hospital patients.

A false-positive DAT is often seen in patients with hypergammaglobulinemia, eg, in some HIV-positive patients.

Technical Manual of the American Association of Blood Banks, 17th ed. American Association of Blood Banks, 2011. |

	Antiglobulin test, indirect

Test/Range/Collection	Physiologic Basis	Interpretation	Comments
Antiglobulin test, indirect, serum or plasma (indirect Coombs) Negative Red or lavender, pink $	Indirect antiglobulin test is used to demonstrate the presence in the patient's serum/plasma of unexpected antibody to ABO and Rh-compatible reagent red blood cells. Patient serum or plasma is incubated *in vitro* with reagent red cells, which are then washed to remove unbound globulins. Agglutination that occurs when antihuman globulin (AHG, Coombs) reagent is added indicates that antibody has bound to a specific antigen present on the red cells.	**Positive in:** Presence of alloantibody or autoantibody. Drugs: methyldopa.	The technique is used in antibody detection and identification, and in the AHG crossmatch prior to transfusion (see Type and crossmatch). *Technical Manual of the American Association of Blood Banks,* 17th ed. American Association of Blood Banks, 2011.

Antistreptolysin O

Antistreptolysin O, serum (ASO)	Detects the presence of antibody to the antigen streptolysin O produced by group A streptococci. Streptococcal antibodies appear about 2 weeks after infection. Titer rises to a peak at 4–6 weeks and may remain elevated for 6 months to 1 year. Test is based on the neutralization of hemolytic activity of streptolysin O toxin by antistreptolysin O antibodies in serum.	**Increased in:** Recent infection with group A β-hemolytic streptococci: scarlet fever, erysipelas, streptococcal pharyngitis/tonsillitis (40–50%), rheumatic fever (80–85%), poststreptococcal glomerulonephritis. Some collagen vascular diseases. Certain serum lipoproteins, bacterial growth products, or oxidized streptolysin O may result in inhibition of hemolysis and thus cause false-positive results.	Standardization of (Todd) units may vary significantly from laboratory to laboratory. ASO titers are not useful in management of acute streptococcal pharyngitis. In patients with rheumatic fever, test may be a more reliable indicator of recent streptococcal infection than throat culture. An increasing titer is more suggestive of acute streptococcal infection than a single elevated level. Even with severe infection, ASO titers rise in only 70–80% of patients. ASO and anti-DNase-B together increase test sensitivity. Normal range increases with age. Hahn RG et al. Evaluation of poststreptococcal illness. Am Fam Physician 2005;71:1949. [PMID: 15926411] Jeng A et al. The role of beta hemolytic streptococci in causing diffuse non-culturable cellulitis: a prospective investigation. Medicine (Baltimore) 2010;89:217. [PMID: 20616661]
0–1 year: <200 IU/mL;			
2–12 years: <240 IU/mL			
13 years or older: <330 IU/mL (laboratory-specific)			
SST			
$$			

Antithrombin

Test/Range/Collection	Physiologic Basis	Interpretation	Comments
Antithrombin (AT), plasma 84–123% (enzymatic activity, qualitative) 80–130% (antigen, quantitative) Blue $$ Transport to lab on ice. Plasma must be separated and frozen in a polypropylene tube within 2 hours.	Antithrombin is a serine protease inhibitor that protects against thrombus formation by inhibiting thrombin and other factors, including IXa, Xa, XIa. It accounts for 70–90% of the anticoagulant activity of human plasma. Its activity is enhanced 1000-fold by heparin. There are two types of assay: functional/enzymatic (activity) and immunologic (antigen). Since the immunologic assay cannot rule out functional AT deficiency, a functional assay should be ordered first. Functional assays test AT activity in inhibiting thrombin or factor Xa. Given an abnormal functional assay, the immunologic test indicates whether there is decreased production of AT (type I deficiency) or intact synthesis of a dysfunctional protein (type II deficiency).	**Decreased in:** Congenital and acquired AT deficiency (nephrotic syndrome, chronic liver disease), oral contraceptive use, chronic disseminated intravascular coagulation (DIC), acute venous thrombosis (consumption), L-asparginase treatment (decreased synthesis) and heparin therapy (consumption).	Congenital or acquired AT deficiency results in a hypercoagulable state, venous thromboembolism, and heparin resistance. Congenital AT deficiency is present in 1:2000–1:3000 people and is autosomal codominant. Heterozygotes have AT levels 20–60% of normal. Evaluation of AT should be considered in patients with venous thrombosis, especially for thrombosis in unusual sites or associated with heparin resistance. Testing should be performed at least 2 months after the thrombotic event, at a time when the patient is not receiving anticoagulants. De Stefano V et al. The risk of recurrent venous thromboembolism in patients with inherited deficiency of natural anticoagulants antithrombin, protein C and protein S. Haematologica 2006;91:695. [PMID: 16670075] Khor B et al. Laboratory tests for antithrombin deficiency. Am J Hematol 2010;85:947. [PMID: 21108326] Rodgers GM. Role of antithrombin concentrate in treatment of hereditary antithrombin deficiency. An update. Thromb Haemost 2009;101:806. [PMID: 19404531]

α_1-Antitrypsin

| α_1-Antitrypsin (α_1-Antiprotease) serum or plasma

110–270 mg/dL

[1.1–2.7 g/L]

SST, red, PPT, lavender, pink

$$ | α_1-Antitrypsin is an α_1 globulin glycoprotein serine protease inhibitor (Pi) whose deficiency leads to excessive protease activity and panacinar emphysema in adults or liver disease in children (seen as ZZ and SZ phenotypes). Cirrhosis of the liver and liver cancer in adults are also associated with the Pi Z phenotype. | **Increased in:** Inflammation, infection, rheumatic disease, malignancy, and pregnancy as an acute-phase reactant.
Decreased in: Congenital α_1-antitrypsin deficiency, nephrotic syndrome. | Smoking is a much more common cause of chronic obstructive pulmonary disease in adults than is α_1-antitrypsin deficiency.
Testing for α_1-antitrypsin deficiency should be done in young patients (<50 year-old with exercise limitation from emphysema), those with emphysema in absence of cigarette smoking, and in presence of familial clustering or basilar predominance of emphysema.
Bals R. Alpha-1-antitrypsin deficiency. Best Pract Res Clin Gastroenterol 2010;24:629. [PMID: 20955965]
Ferrarotti I et al. Laboratory diagnosis of alpha-1-antitrypsin deficiency. Transl Res 2007;150:267. [PMID: 17964515]
Fromer L. Improving diagnosis and management of alpha-1-antitrypsin deficiency in primary care: translating knowledge into action. COPD 2010;7(3):192. [PMID: 20486818]
Kelly E et al. Alpha-1-antitrypsin deficiency. Respir Med 2010 104(6):763. [PMID: 20303723]
Miravitlles M et al. Laboratory testing of individuals with severe alpha-1-antitrypsin deficiency in three European centres. Eur Respir J 2010;35(5):960. [PMID: 20436173]
Pietrangelo A. Inherited metabolic disease of the liver. Curr Opin Gastroenterol 2009;25(3):2094. [PMID: 19342951]
Sandhaus RA. Alpha-1-antitrypsin deficiency: whom to test, whom to treat? Semin Respir Crit Care Med 2010;31:343. [PMID: 20496303] |

Test/Range/Collection	Physiologic Basis	Interpretation	Comments
Arterial blood gases (ABG), whole blood Heparinized syringe $$$ Collect arterial blood in a heparinized syringe, and send to laboratory immediately.	Blood gas measurements provide information about cardiopulmonary (oxygen and carbon dioxide exchange) and metabolic (acid-base) status. When integrated with the history and physical examination, the rapidly available arterial blood gas (ABG) analysis is useful in the resuscitation of the acutely ill or injured patient.	See Carbon Dioxide (p. 90), Oxygen (p. 224), and pH (p. 229).	Panos RJ et al. Exertional desaturation in patients with chronic obstructive pulmonary disease. COPD 2009;6:478. [PMID: 19938972]

Arterial blood gases

Aspartate aminotransferase

| Aspartate aminotransferase, serum or plasma (AST, SGOT, GOT)

0–35 IU/L

[0–0.58 mckat/L] (laboratory-specific)

SST, PPT, green, lavender

$ | Intracellular enzyme involved in amino acid metabolism. Present in large concentrations in liver, skeletal muscle, brain, red cells, and heart. Released into the bloodstream when tissue is damaged, especially in liver injury. | **Increased in:** Acute viral hepatitis (ALT > AST), biliary tract obstruction (cholangitis, choledocholithiasis), alcoholic hepatitis and cirrhosis (AST > ALT), liver abscess, metastatic or primary liver cancer; right heart failure, ischemic or hypoxic injury to liver ("shock liver"), extensive trauma. Drugs that cause cholestasis or hepatotoxicity.

Decreased in: Pyridoxine (vitamin B_6) deficiency. | Test is not indicated for diagnosis of myocardial infarction.
AST/ALT ratio >1 suggests cirrhosis in patients with hepatitis C.
See Liver function tests (Table 8–14).
Giannini EG et al. Liver enzyme alteration: a guide for clinicians. CMAJ 2005;172:367. [PMID: 15684121]
Ozer J et al. The current state of serum biomarkers of hepatotoxicity. Toxicology 2008;245:194. [PMID: 18291570]
Senior JR. Monitoring for hepatotoxicity: what is the predictive value of liver "function" tests? Clin Pharmacol Ther 2009;85:331. [PMID: 19129750] |

	B cell immunoglobulin heavy-chain (IgH) gene rearrangement		
Test/Range/Collection	**Physiologic Basis**	**Interpretation**	**Comments**
B-cell immunoglobulin heavy-chain (IgH) gene rearrangement Whole blood, bone marrow, frozen or paraffin-embedded tissue Lavender $$$$	In general, the percentage of B lymphocytes with identical immunoglobulin heavy-chain gene rearrangements is very low; in malignancies, however, the clonal expansion of one population leads to a large number of cells with identical B-cell immunoglobulin heavy-chain gene rearrangements. B-cell clonality can be assessed by restriction fragment Southern blot hybridization or more commonly polymerase chain reaction (PCR).	**Positive in:** B-cell neoplasms such as lymphoma (monoclonal B-cell proliferation), plasma cell neoplasms.	The diagnostic sensitivity and specificity are heterogeneous and laboratory- and method-specific. Results of the test must always be interpreted in the context of morphologic and other relevant data (eg, flow cytometry) and should not be used alone for a diagnosis of malignancy. The test is primarily for initial diagnosis, but may also be used to detect minimal residual disease. Bagg A et al. Immunoglobulin heavy chain gene analysis in lymphomas: a multi-center study demonstrating the heterogeneity of performance of polymerase chain reaction assays. J Mol Diagn 2002;4:81. [PMID: 11986398] Garcia-Castillo H et al. Detection of clonal immunoglobulin and T-cell receptor gene recombination in hematological malignancies: monitoring minimal residual disease. Cardiovasc Hematol Disord Drug Targets 2009;9:124. [PMID: 19519371]

BCR/ABL, t(9;22) translocation by RT-PCR

| **BCR-ABL, t(9;22) translocation by RT-PCR,** qualitative

Blood

Lavender

$$$$ | Approximately 95% of cases of chronic myelogenous leukemia (CML) have the characteristic t(9;22)(q34;q11) that results in a BCR-ABL gene fusion on the derived chromosome 22 called the Philadelphia (Ph) chromosome. The remaining cases either have a cryptic translocation between 9q34 and 22q11 that cannot be identified by routine cytogenetic analysis, or have variant translocations involving a third or even a fourth chromosome besides 9 and 22.

The BCR-ABL fusion transcript is found in all cases of CML, including those with a cryptic or variant translocation.

A subset of acute lymphoblastic leukemia (ALL) and occasionally acute myelogenous leukemia (AML, mostly CML blast crisis) also have the Ph chromosome, and therefore are positive for BCR-ABL, t(9;22) translocation. | **Positive in:** All CML, a subset of acute lymphoblastic leukemia (ALL), and rare acute myeloid leukemia (eg, CML blast crisis). | This assay can also be used to distinguish between the major and minor transcripts. The major transcript, characterized by the p210 fusion gene product, is typically detected in CML. The minor transcript, characterized by the p190 fusion gene product, is typically detected in ALL. Detection limit of RT-PCR based assays is at least 1 in 100,000 cells.

Small amounts of p190 transcript can be detected in most patients with CML, due to alternative splicing of the BCR gene.

For treatment monitoring, the BCR-ABL, t(9;22) translocation quantitative RT-PCR assay should be used. The quantitative assay may not distinguish between the major and minor BCR-ABL products.

Foroni L et al. Technical aspects and clinical applications of measuring BCR-ABL1 transcripts number in chronic myeloid leukemia. Am J Hematol 2009;84:517. [PMID: 19544476]

Goldman JM et al. BCR-ABL in chronic myelogenous leukemia—how does it work? Acta Haematol 2008;119:212. [PMID: 18566539]

Ross DM et al. Current and emerging tests for the laboratory monitoring of chronic myeloid leukemia and related disorders. Pathology 2008;40:231. [PMID: 18428043] |

	BCR/ABL mutation analysis		
Test/Range/Collection	Physiologic Basis	Interpretation	Comments
BCR-ABL mutation analysis (*BCR-ABL* genotyping) Blood Lavender $$$$	The analysis involves direct DNA sequencing of the PCR-amplified *BCR-ABL* products. The sequence is then compared with an ABL kinase domain reference sequence to identify single or multiple mutations.	**Positive in:** Imatinib-resistant chronic myeloid leukemia; imatinib-resistant Ph-positive precursor B-lymphoblastic leukemia.	The *BCR-ABL* tyrosine kinase inhibitor imatinib is generally effective in Philadelphia chromosome–positive (Ph-positive) leukemias (eg, chronic myeloid leukemia, CML). However, patients may have an inferior response to imatinib, either failing to respond to primary therapy or demonstrating progression (or relapse) after an initial response. Imatinib resistance is mainly due to leukemic subclones with *BCR-ABL* mutation(s) in the ABL kinase domain that interfere with imatinib binding. The *BCR-ABL* mutation analysis can assist physicians in evaluating resistance to imatinib therapy and facilitate appropriate adjustments to treatment (eg, increase in imatinib dosage or switch to other tyrosine kinase inhibitors). Mutations at 17 different amino acid positions within the BCR-ABL kinase domain have been associated with clinical resistance to imatinib. Patients with T315I mutation are also resistant to dasatinib and nilotinib. Bixby D et al. Seeking the causes and solutions to imatinib-resistance in chronic myeloid leukemia. Leukemia 2011;25:7. [PMID: 21102425] Hughes TP et al. Monitoring disease response to tyrosine kinase inhibitor therapy in CML. Hematology Am Soc Hematol Educ Program 2009:477. [PMID: 20008233]

Beta-hCG		
Beta-hCG, quantitative, serum Males and nonpregnant females: undetectable or <5 mIU/mL [IU/L] SST, red $$	Human chorionic gonadotropin (hCG) is a glycoprotein made up of two subunits (α and β). The β-subunit is specific for hCG. hCG is produced by trophoblastic tissue, and its detection in serum or urine is the basis for pregnancy testing. Serum hCG can be detected as early as 24 hours after implantation at a concentration of 5 mIU/mL. During normal pregnancy, serum levels double every 2–3 days and are 50–100 mIU/mL at the time of the first missed menstrual period. Peak levels are reached 60–80 days after the last menstrual period (LMP) (30,000–100,000 mIU/mL), and levels then decrease to a plateau of 5,000–10,000 mIU/mL at about 120 days after LMP and persist until delivery.	**Increased in:** Pregnancy (including ectopic pregnancy), hyperemesis gravidarum, trophoblastic tumors (hydatidiform mole, choriocarcinoma), some germ cell tumors (teratomas; seminoma), ectopic hCG production by other malignancies. **Decreasing over time:** Threatened abortion.	Routine pregnancy testing is done by *qualitative* urine hCG test, or less commonly quantitative serum hCG test. Test is positive (>50 mIU/mL) in most pregnant women at the time of or shortly after the first missed menstrual period. *Quantitative* hCG test detects hCG levels as low as 1.0 mIU/mL. It is preferred for the evaluation of suspected ectopic pregnancy and threatened abortion. In both situations, hCG levels fail to demonstrate the normal early pregnancy increase. Test is also indicated for following the course of trophoblastic and germ cell tumors. Most commercially available hCG tests detect only regular hCG. In patients with malignancies that produce primarily hCG-H, the test should be interpreted with caution. Chung K et al. The use of serial human chorionic gonadotropin levels to establish a viable or a nonviable pregnancy. Semin Reprod Med 2008;26:383. [PMID: 18825606] Cole LA. Human chorionic gonadotropin tests. Expert Rev Mol Diagn 2009;9:721. [PMID: 19817556] Cole LA. Hyperglycosylated hCG, a review. Placenta 2010;31:653. [PMID: 20619452] Nama V et al. Tubal ectopic pregnancy: diagnosis and management. Arch Gynecol Obstet 2009;279:443. [PMID: 18665380]

	Beta-hCG (*continued*)

Test/Range/Collection	Physiologic Basis	Interpretation	Comments
	Regular hCG produced by differentiated syncytotrophoblast cells primarily functions to promote progesterone production and to maintain the myometrial and the vascular supply of the placenta during the first trimester. Hyperglycosylated hCG (hCG-H) is produced by undifferentiated extravillous cytotrophoblast cells and maintains trophoblast invasion as in implantation of pregnancy. Hyperglycosylated hCG and/or free β-subunit are produced by a high proportion of malignant gestational trophoblastic diseases.		

Bilirubin		
Bilirubin, serum or plasma 0.1–1.2 mg/dL [2–21 mcmol/L] Direct (conjugated to glucuronide) bilirubin: 0.1–0.4 mg/dL [<7 mcmol/L]; Indirect (unconjugated) bilirubin: 0.2–0.7 mg/dL [<12 mcmol/L] SST, PPT $$	Bilirubin is the orange-yellow pigment derived from the breakdown of hemoglobin (heme). The majority of bilirubin comes from senescent red cells. It is biotransformed in the liver and excreted in bile and urine. The conjugated form is water-soluble and reacts directly with diazo dyes in the absence of reaction accelerator, and is therefore called direct bilirubin. The unconjugated form is fat-soluble and reacts with diazo dyes only in the presence of accelerator; so it is called indirect. Some conjugated bilirubin is bound to serum albumin, so-called D (delta) bilirubin.	**Increased in:** Acute or chronic hepatitis, cirrhosis, biliary tract obstruction, toxic hepatitis, neonatal jaundice (neonatal hyperbilirubinemia), congenital liver enzyme abnormalities (Dubin-Johnson, Rotor, Gilbert, Crigler-Najjar syndromes), fasting, hemolytic disorders. Hepatotoxic drugs.	Assay of total bilirubin includes conjugated (direct) and unconjugated (indirect) bilirubin. The unconjugated (indirect) form is the difference between total bilirubin (with reaction accelerator) and the direct bilirubin fraction. Delta bilirubin is determined together with conjugated bilirubin. Delta bilirubin (half-life is about 17 days) accounts for relatively slow regression of jaundice. Only conjugated bilirubin appears in the urine, and it is indicative of liver disease and biliary tract obstruction. Hemolysis is associated with increased unconjugated bilirubin. Unbound (free) serum or plasma bilirubin level correlates better than total bilirubin with CNS bilirubin concentrations and bilirubin encephalopathy (kernicterus) in newborn jaundice. Ahlfors CE et al. Unbound (free) bilirubin: improving the paradigm for evaluating neonatal jaundice. Clin Chem 2009;55:1288. [PMID: 19423734] Cohen RS et al. Understanding neonatal jaundice: a perspective on causation. Pediatr Neonatol 2010;51:143. [PMID: 20675237] Fevery J. Bilirubin in clinical practice: a review. Liver Int 2008; 28:592. [PMID: 18433389]

Test/Range/Collection	Physiologic Basis	Interpretation	Comments
Blood urea nitrogen, serum or plasma (BUN) 8–20 mg/dL [2.9–7.1 mmol/L] SST, PPT, green $	Urea is the end product of protein metabolism, which is excreted by the kidney. BUN is directly related to protein intake and nitrogen metabolism and inversely related to the rate of excretion of urea. Urea concentration in glomerular filtrate is the same as in plasma, but its tubular reabsorption is inversely related to the rate of urine formation. Thus, BUN is a less useful measure of glomerular filtration rate than the serum/plasma creatinine (Cr).	**Increased in:** Renal failure (acute or chronic), urinary tract obstruction, dehydration, shock, burns, CHF, GI bleeding, nephrotoxic drugs (eg, gentamicin). **Decreased in:** Hepatic failure, nephrotic syndrome, cachexia (low-protein and high-carbohydrate diets).	Urease assay method is commonly used. Blood BUN/Cr ratio (normally 10:1–20:1) is decreased in acute tubular necrosis, advanced liver disease, low protein intake, and following hemodialysis. Blood BUN/Cr ratio is increased in dehydration, GI bleeding, and increased catabolism. Edelstein CL. Biomarkers of acute kidney injury. Adv Chronic Kidney Dis 2008;15:222. [PMID: 18565474] Waika SS et al. Diagnosis, epidemiology and outcomes of acute kidney injury. Clin J Am Soc Nephrol 2008;3:844. [PMID: 18337550]

Blood urea nitrogen

B-type natriuretic peptide		
B-type natriuretic peptide (BNP), plasma Lavender, pink 0–100 pg/mL [0–347 pmol/L] $$ Point-of-care immunoassays also available.	BNP has biologic effects similar to those of atrial natriuretic peptide (ANP) and is stored mainly in the myocardium of the cardiac ventricles. Blood BNP levels are elevated in hypervolemic states such as congestive heart failure (CHF). BNP is useful for guiding and monitoring heart failure treatment and for predicting prognosis. Clinical applications in the setting of CHF include: to determine the cause of symptoms (eg, dyspnea); to estimate the degree of severity of heart failure; to estimate the risk of disease progression; and to screen for less symptomatic disease in high-risk populations.	**Increased in**: CHF (cutoff concentration, >100 pg/mL yields a sensitivity of 90%, specificity, 73%. BNP <100 pg/mL has a negative predictive value of 90%. BNP >400 pg/mL suggests CHF with specificity exceeding 90%). BNP is also increased in a variety of other cardiac and noncardiac diseases including acute coronary syndrome, left ventricular dysfunction, valvular aortic stenosis, pulmonary embolism, and renal insufficiency.	BNP testing is not a substitute for careful cardiopulmonary evaluation and should not be the sole criterion for admission/discharge of a patient. Although normal levels indicate a low probability of CHF, they do not exclude it or other serious cardiopulmonary disorders. Moderately increased levels are not specific for CHF and can occur with a variety of cardiac and noncardiac diseases. BNP is not recommended for screening for left ventricular dysfunction or hypertrophy in the general population. It is also unnecessary to test BNP in patients with obvious CHF (eg, NYHA class IV). Treatment of CHF has been reported to decrease BNP levels in parallel with clinical improvement. Tests for N-terminal fragment of pro-BNP (NT-pro-BNP) are also available, and diagnostic performance is comparable to that of BNP. The normal reference intervals of pro-BNP are laboratory-dependent and vary with age and sex. Maisel A et al. State of the art: using natriuretic peptide levels in clinical practice. Eur J Heart Fail 2008;10:824. [PMID: 18760965] McCullough PA et al. An evidence-based algorithm for the use of B-type natriuretic testing in acute coronary syndromes. Rev Cardiovasc Med 2010;11(Suppl 2):S51. [PMID: 20700103] Palazzuoli A et al. Natriuretic peptides (BNP and NT-proBNP): measurement and relevance in heart failure. Vasc Health Risk Manag 2010;6:411. [PMID: 20539843] Porapakkham P et al. B-type natriuretic peptide-guided heart failure therapy: a meta-analysis. Arch Intern Med. 2010;170(6):507. [PMID: 20306637]

			***Brucella* antibody**
Test/Range/Collection	**Physiologic Basis**	**Interpretation**	**Comments**
***Brucella* antibodies,** serum Negative SST, red $	Patients with acute brucellosis generally develop an agglutinating antibody titer of >1:160 within 3 weeks. The titer may rise during the acute infection, with relapses, brucellergin skin testing, or use of certain vaccines (see Interpretation). The agglutinin titer usually declines after 3 months or after successful therapy. Low titers may persist for years. Indirect enzyme-linked immunosorbent assay (ELISA) measuring IgM, IgG, and IgA antibodies have higher sensitivity and specificity than the agglutinating antibody test. Routine use of PCR and RT-PCR assays for diagnosis of human brucellosis needs further clinical evaluation.	**Positive in:** *Brucella* infection (except *B. canis*) (97% within 3 weeks of illness); recent brucellergin skin test; infections with *Francisella tularensis*, *Yersinia enterocolitica*, salmonella, Rocky Mountain spotted fever; vaccinations for cholera and tularemia. **Negative in:** *B. canis* infection.	This test detects antibodies against all of the *Brucella* species except *B. canis*. A fourfold or greater rise in titer in separate specimens drawn 1–4 weeks apart is indicative of recent exposure. Since titers can remain high for a prolonged period, they are not suitable for patient follow-up. Specimens testing positive or equivocal for *Brucella* antibodies by ELISA should be confirmed by bacterial agglutination. Final diagnosis depends on isolation of organism by culture. Araj GF. Update on laboratory diagnosis of human brucellosis. Int J Antimicrob Agents 2010;36(Suppl 1):S12. [PMID: 20692128] Franco MP et al. Human brucellosis. Lancet Infect Dis 2007;7:775. [PMID: 18045560]

C-peptide		
C-peptide, serum or plasma 0.8–4.0 ng/mL [mcg/L] (0.26–1.3 nmol/L) SST, PPT, lavender, green $$$ Fasting sample preferred.	C-peptide is an inactive by-product of the cleavage of proinsulin to active insulin. Its presence indicates endogenous release of insulin. The half-life of C-peptide in the blood is about 30 min. C-peptide is largely excreted by the kidney.	**Increased in:** Renal failure, ingestion of oral hypoglycemic drugs, insulinomas, Beta-cell transplants. **Decreased in:** Factitious hypoglycemia due to insulin administration, pancreatectomy, type 1 diabetes mellitus (decreased or undetectable).	Test is most useful to detect factitious insulin injection (increased insulin, decreased C-peptide) or endogenous insulin production in diabetic patients receiving insulin (C-peptide present). A random C-peptide level has reasonable discriminatory power for determining type 1 vs type 2 diabetes. A molar ratio of insulin to C-peptide >1.0 in peripheral venous blood in a hypoglycemic patient is consistent with surreptitious or inadvertent insulin administration but not insulinoma. C-peptide levels of 2 nmol/L or greater suggest insulinoma. Cryer PE et al. Evaluation and management of adult hypoglycemic disorders: an Endocrine Society Clinical Practice Guideline. J Clin Endocrinol Metab 2009;94:709. [PMID: 19088155] Hills CE et al. C-peptide as a therapeutic tool in diabetic nephropathy. Am J Nephrol 2010;31:389. [PMID: 20357430]. Marks V. Murder by insulin: suspected, purported and proven—a review. Drug Test Anal 2009;1:162. [PMID: 20355194]

C-reactive protein, high sensitivity

Test/Range/Collection	Physiologic Basis	Interpretation	Comments
C-reactive protein, high sensitivity (hs-CRP), serum or plasma <1.0 mg/dL (lower 95th percentile) SST, PPT, green $	CRP is an acute-phase reactant protein. Hepatic secretion is stimulated in response to inflammatory cytokines. Unlike other acute-phase proteins, CRP is not affected by hormones. CRP activates the complement system, binds to Fc receptors, and serves as an opsonin for some microorganisms. Rapid, marked increases in CRP occur with inflammation, infection, trauma and tissue necrosis, malignancies, and autoimmune disorders. CRP levels are also valuable in assessing vascular inflammation and cardiovascular risk stratification. CRP level has been shown to be an independent risk factor for atherosclerotic disease. Elevated CRP levels are associated with increased cardiovascular morbidity and mortality in patients with coronary artery disease.	**Increased in:** Inflammatory states, including arteriosclerotic disorders.	CRP is a very sensitive but nonspecific marker of inflammation. A variety of conditions other than arteriosclerosis may cause dramatic increases in CRP levels. CRP levels increase within 2 hours of acute insult (eg, surgery, infection) and should peak and begin decreasing within 48 hours if no other inflammatory event occurs. In patients with rheumatoid arthritis, persistently elevated CRP concentrations are present when the disease is active and usually fall to normal during periods of complete remission. Patients with high hs-CRP concentrations are more likely to develop stroke, myocardial infarction, and severe peripheral vascular disease. hs-CRP results are used to assign risk as follows: <1.0 mg/L lowest tertile, lowest risk; 1.0–3.0 mg/L middle tertile, average risk; >3.0 mg/L highest tertile, highest risk. Noncardiovascular cause should be considered if CRP values are >10 mg/dL with repeat measurements. Bajpai A et al. Should we measure C-reactive protein on earth or just on JUPITER? Clin Cardiol 2010;33:190. [PMID: 20394038] Devaraj S et al. Role of C-reactive protein in contributing to increased cardiovascular risk in metabolic syndrome. Curr Atheroscler Rep. 2010;12:110. [PMID: 20425246] Kaysen GA. Biochemistry and biomarkers of inflamed patients: why look, what to assess. Clin J Am Soc Nephrol 2009;4(Suppl 1):S56. [PMID: 19996007]

C1 esterase inhibitor

C1 esterase inhibitor (C1 INH), serum		Decreased in: Hereditary angioedema (HAE), acquired angioedema.	C1 esterase inhibitor deficiency is an uncommon cause of angioedema. There are three subtypes of HAE. In type 1 (~85%), both antigenic and functional levels are low; in type 2 (~15%), antigenic level is normal but functional level is decreased; in type 3 (rare), the C1-INH levels are normal. In some families, type 3 HAE has been linked to mutations in the Hageman factor.
20–40 mg/dL	C1 esterase inhibitor (C1 INH) is a broad-spectrum protease inhibitor, which controls the first stage of the classic complement pathway and inhibits thrombin, plasmin, activated Hageman factor (factor XIIa) and kallikrein. Deficiency results in spontaneous activation of C1, leading to consumption of C2 and C4. The functional assay involves the measurement of C1 INH antigen is also available.		Acquired angioedema has been attributed to massive consumption of C1 INH (presumably by tumor or lymphoma-related immune complexes) or to anti-C1 INH autoantibody.
(method-dependent)			When clinical suspicion exists, a serum C4 level screens for HAE. Low levels of C4 are present in all cases during an attack. C1 INH levels are not indicated unless either the C4 level is low or there is a very high clinical suspicion of HAE in a patient with normal C4 during an asymptomatic phase between attacks. In acquired C1 INH deficiency, the C1 level is also significantly decreased (often 10% of normal), whereas in HAE the C1 level is normal or only slightly decreased. Frank MM. Complement disorders and hereditary angioedema. J Allergy Clin Immunol 2010;125(Suppl 2):S262. [PMID: 20176263]
SST			Nagy N et al. New insights into hereditary angio-edema: molecular diagnosis and therapy. Australas J Dermatol. 2010;51:157. [PMID: 20695852]
$$			Zuraw BL et al. Pathogenesis and laboratory diagnosis of hereditary angioedema. Allergy Asthma Proc 2009;30:487. [PMID: 19843402]

	Calcitonin		
Test/Range/Collection	Physiologic Basis	Interpretation	Comments
Calcitonin, plasma or serum Males: <8 pg/mL [ng/L] Females: <6 pg/mL [ng/L] Green, SST $$$ Separate serum/plasma from cells ASAP and freeze	Calcitonin is a 32-amino-acid polypeptide hormone secreted by the parafollicular C cells of the thyroid. It decreases osteoclastic bone resorption and lowers serum calcium levels.	**Increased in:** Medullary thyroid carcinoma, Zollinger-Ellison syndrome, pernicious anemia, pregnancy (at term), newborns, carcinoma (breast, lung, pancreas), leukemia, myeloproliferative disorders, chronic renal failure.	Test is useful to diagnose and monitor medullary thyroid carcinoma, although stimulation tests may be necessary (eg, pentagastrin test). Genetic testing (eg, *RET* mutation test) is now available for the diagnosis of multiple endocrine neoplasia type II. (MEN II is the most common familial form of medullary thyroid carcinoma.) Ball DW. Medullary thyroid cancer: therapeutic targets and molecular markers. Curr Opin Oncol 2007;19:18. [PMID: 17133107] Chen H et al. The North American Neuroendocrine Tumor Society consensus guideline for the diagnosis and management of neuroendocrine tumors: pheochromocytoma, paraganglioma, and medullary thyroid cancer. Pancreas 2010;39:775. [PMID: 20664475] Elisei R. Routine serum calcitonin measurement in the evaluation of thyroid nodules. Best Pract Res Clin Endocrinol Metab 2008;22:941. [PMID: 19041824]

Calcium, serum

Calcium, serum or plasma (Ca^{2+})	Serum calcium is the sum of ionized calcium plus complexe calcium and calcium bound to proteins (mostly albumin). Level of ionized calcium is regulated by parathyroid hormone and vitamin D.	**Increased in:** Hyperparathyroidism, malignancies secreting parathyroid hormone-related protein (PTHrP) (especially squamous cell carcinoma of lung and renal cell carcinoma), vitamin D excess, milk-alkali syndrome, multiple myeloma, Paget disease of bone with immobilization, sarcoidosis, other granulomatous disorders, familial hypocalciuria, vitamin A intoxication, thyrotoxicosis, Addison disease. Drugs: antacids (some), calcium salts, chronic diuretic use (eg, thiazides), lithium, others. **Decreased in:** Hypoparathyroidism, vitamin D deficiency, renal insufficiency, pseudohypoparathyroidism, magnesium deficiency, hyperphosphatemia, massive transfusion, hypoalbuminemia.	Need to know serum albumin to interpret calcium level. For every decrease in albumin by 1 mg/dL, calcium should be corrected upward by 0.8 mg/dL. In 10% of patients with malignancies, hypercalcemia is attributable to coexistent hyperparathyroidism, suggesting that serum PTH levels should be measured at initial presentation of all hypercalcemic patients (see Figure 9–13). Carlson D. Parathyroid pathology: hyperparathyroidism and parathyroid tumors. Arch Pathol Lab Med 2010;134:1639. [PMID: 21043817] Habib Z et al. Primary hyperparathyroidism: an update. Curr Opin Endocrinol Diabetes Obes 2010;17:554. [PMID: 20890202] Lietman SA et al. Hypercalcemia in children and adolescents. Curr Opin Pediatr 2010;22:508. [PMID: 20601885]
8.5-10.5 mg/dL			
[2.1-2.6 mmol/L]			
Panic: <6.5 or >13.5 mg/dL			
SST, green			
$			
Prolonged venous stasis during collection causes false increase in serum calcium.			

Calcium, ionized			
Test/Range/Collection	Physiologic Basis	Interpretation	Comments
Calcium, ionized, serum or whole blood

4.4–5.4 mg/dL (at pH 7.4) [1.1–1.3 mmol/L]

Whole blood specimen must be collected anaerobically and anticoagulated with standardized amounts of heparin. Tourniquet application must be brief. Specimen should be analyzed promptly.

SST, green

$$ | Calcium circulates in three forms: as free Ca^{2+} (50–55%), protein-bound to albumin and globulins (40–45%), and as calcium-ligand complexes (5–10%) (with citrate, bicarbonate, lactate, phosphate, and sulfate). Protein binding is highly pH-dependent, and acidosis results in an increased free calcium fraction. Ionized Ca^{2+} is the form that is physiologically active. Ionized calcium is a more accurate reflection of physiologic status than total calcium in patients with altered serum proteins (renal failure, nephrotic syndrome, multiple myeloma, etc), altered concentrations of calcium-binding ligands, and acid-base disturbances. Measurement of ionized calcium is by ion-selective electrodes. Ionized calcium levels vary inversely with pH, about 0.2 mg/dL per 0.1 pH unit change. | **Increased in:** ↓ Blood pH. **Decreased in:** ↑ Blood pH, citrate, EDTA. | Ionized calcium measurements are not needed except in special circumstances, eg, massive blood transfusion, transfusion of whole blood in neonates, liver transplantation, neonatal hypocalcemia, cardiac bypass surgery, and possibly monitoring of patients with secondary hyperparathyroidism from renal failure. Validity of test depends on sample integrity. Ionized calcium normalized to pH 7.4 should be interpreted with caution and along with patient's acid/base status. See diagnostic algorithms for hypercalcemia and hypocalcemia (Figures 9–13 & 9–15). Morton AR et al. Is the calcium correct? Measuring serum calcium in dialysis patients. Semin Dial 2010;23:283. [PMID: 20492582] |

Calcium, urine		
Calcium, urine (U_{Ca}) 100–300 mg/24 hr (for persons with average calcium intake, ie, 600–800 mg/d) [2.5–7.5 mmol/24 hr or 2.3–3.3 mmol/12 hr] Urine bottle containing hydrochloric acid $$$ Collect 24-hour urine or 12-hour overnight urine. Refrigerate during collection.	Ordinarily, there is moderate urinary calcium excretion, the amount depending on dietary calcium, parathyroid hormone (PTH) level, and protein intake. Renal calculi occur much more often in those with hyperparathyroidism than in other hypercalcemic states.	**Increased in:** Hyperparathyroidism, osteolytic bone metastases, myeloma, osteoporosis, vitamin D intoxication, distal RTA, idiopathic hypercalciuria, thyrotoxicosis, Paget disease, Fanconi syndrome, hepatolenticular degeneration, schistosomiasis, sarcoidosis, malignancy (breast, bladder), osteitis deformans, immobilization. Drugs: acetazolamide, calcium salts, cholestyramine, corticosteroids, dihydrotachysterol, initial diuretic use (eg, furosemide), others. **Decreased in:** Hypoparathyroidism, pseudohypoparathyroidism, rickets, osteomalacia, nephrotic syndrome, acute glomerulonephritis, osteoblastic bone metastases, hypothyroidism, celiac disease, steatorrhea, hypocalciuric hypercalcemia, other causes of hypocalcemia. Drugs: aspirin, bicarbonate, chronic diuretic use (eg, thiazides, chlorthalidone), estrogens, indomethacin, lithium, neomycin, oral contraceptives.	Approximately one third of patients with hyperparathyroidism have normal urine calcium excretion. The extent of calcium excretion can be expressed as a urine calcium (U_{Ca})/urine creatinine (U_{Cr}) ratio. Normally, $$\frac{U_{Ca}\ (mg/dL)}{U_{Cr}\ (mg/dL)} < 0.14$$ or $$\frac{U_{Ca}\ (mmol/L)}{U_{Cr}\ (mmol/L)} < 0.40$$ Hypercalciuria is defined as a ratio of >0.20 or >0.57, respectively. Test is useful in the evaluation of renal stones but is not usually needed for the diagnosis of hyperparathyroidism, which can be made using serum calcium (see above) and PTH measurements (see Figure 10–8). It may be useful in hypercalcemic patients to rule out familial hypocalciuric hypercalcemia. In the diagnosis of hypercalciuria, U_{Ca}/U_{Cr} ratios in random single-voided urine specimens correlate well with 24-hour calcium excretions. Srivastava T et al. Diagnosis and management of hypercalciuria in children. Curr Opin Pediatr 2009;21:214. [PMID: 19307900] Stechman MJ et al. Genetic causes of hypercalciuric nephrolithiasis. Pediatr Nephrol 2009;24:2321. [PMID: 18446382] Tasca A et al. Bone disease in patients with primary hypercalciuria and calcium nephrolithiasis. Urology 2009;74:22. [PMID: 19428073]

Test/Range/Collection	Physiologic Basis	Interpretation	Comments
Carbon dioxide, partial pressure (PCO₂), whole blood Arterial: 32–48 mm Hg (4.26–6.38 kPa) Heparinized syringe $$$ Specimen must be collected in heparinized syringe and immediately transported on ice to lab without exposure to air.	The partial pressure of carbon dioxide in arterial blood (PCO_2) provides important information with regard to adequacy of ventilation, and acid–base status.	**Increased in:** Respiratory acidosis: decreased alveolar ventilation (eg, COPD, respiratory depressants), neuromuscular diseases (eg, myasthenia gravis). **Decreased in:** Respiratory alkalosis: hyperventilation (eg, anxiety), sepsis, liver disease, fever, early salicylate poisoning, and excessive artificial ventilation.	See laboratory characteristics of acid–base disturbances (Figure 9–1, Table 8–1). Kraut JA et al. Metabolic acidosis: pathophysiology, diagnosis and management. Nat Rev Nephrol 2010;6:274. [PMID: 20308999] Zhou W et al. Hypercapnia and hypocapnia in neonates. World J Pediatr 2008;4:192. [PMID: 18822927]

Carbon dioxide, partial pressure

Carbon dioxide, (total bicarbonate)		
Carbon dioxide (total bicarbonate), serum or plasma 22–28 meq/L [mmol/L] ***Panic:*** <15 or >40 meq/L [mmol/L] SST, green $	Bicarbonate-carbonic acid buffer is one of the most important buffer systems in maintaining normal body fluid pH. Total carbon dioxide (CO_2) is measured as the sum of bicarbonate (HCO_3^-) concentration and dissolved CO_2 (carbonic acid and dissolved free CO_2). Total CO_2 measurements use either electrode-based or enzymatic methods. Because HCO_3^- makes up 90–95% of the total CO_2 content, total CO_2 is a useful surrogate for HCO_3^- concentration.	**Increased in:** Primary metabolic alkalosis, compensated respiratory acidosis, volume contraction, mineralocorticoid excess, congenital chloridorrhea. Drugs: diuretics (eg, thiazide, furosemide). **Decreased in:** Metabolic acidosis, compensated respiratory alkalosis, Fanconi syndrome, volume overload. Drugs: acetazolamide, outdated tetracycline.	Total CO_2 determination is indicated for all seriously ill patients on admission. Simultaneous measurement of HCO_3, pH, and PCO_2 is required to fully characterize a patient's acid–base status. See Acid–base disturbance (Table 8–1; Figure 9–1). Kraut JA et al. Metabolic acidosis: pathophysiology, diagnosis and management. Nat Rev Nephrol 2010;6:274. [PMID: 20308999]

	Carboxyhemoglobin		
Test/Range/Collection	**Physiologic Basis**	**Interpretation**	**Comments**
Carboxyhemoglobin, whole blood (COHb) <9% [<0.09] Blood gas syringe or green $$ Specimen should be collected before treatment with oxygen is started. Do not remove stopper or cap.	Carbon monoxide (CO) is an odorless and nonirritating gas formed by hydrocarbon combustion. CO binds to hemoglobin with much greater affinity (~240 times) than oxygen, forming carboxyhemoglobin (COHb) and resulting in impaired oxygen transport/delivery and utilization. CO can also precipitate an inflammatory cascade that results in CNS lipid peroxidation and delayed neurologic sequelae.	**Increased in:** Carbon monoxide poisoning, exposure to automobile exhaust, smoke from fires, coal gas, and defective furnaces. Cigarette smokers can have up to 9% carboxyhemoglobin, while nonsmokers have <2%.	Laboratory CO-oximetry is widely available for rapid evaluation of CO poisoning. Toxic effects (headache, dizziness, nausea, confusion, and/or unconsciousness) occur if the COHb level is >10–15%. Levels > 40% may be fatal if not treated immediately with oxygen. PO_2 is usually normal in CO poisoning. Kealey GP. Carbon monoxide toxicity. J Burn Care Res 2009;30(1):146. [PMID: 19060737] Weaver LK. Clinical practice. Carbon monoxide poisoning. N Engl J Med 2009;360:1217.

Carcinoembryonic antigen		
Carcinoembryonic antigen, serum (CEA) <2.5 ng/mL [mcg/L] SST $$	CEA is an oncofetal antigen, a glycoprotein associated with certain malignancies, particularly epithelial tumors (eg, colorectal cancer, pancreatic cancer, etc).	**Increased in:** Colorectal cancer (72%), lung cancer (76%), pancreatic cancer (91%), stomach cancer (61%), cigarette smokers, benign acute (50%) and chronic (90%) liver disease, benign GI disease (peptic ulcer, pancreatitis, colitis). Elevations >20 ng/mL are generally associated with malignancy. For breast cancer recurrence (using 5 ng/mL cutoff), sensitivity is 44.4% and specificity, 95.5%.	**Screening:** Test is not sensitive or specific enough to be useful in cancer screening. CEA levels should be used in conjunction with clinical evaluation and other diagnostic procedures. **Monitoring after surgery:** Test is used to detect recurrence of colorectal cancer after surgery (elevated CEA levels suggest recurrence 3–6 months before other clinical indicators), although such monitoring has not yet been shown to improve survival rates. If monitoring is done, the same assay method must be used consistently to eliminate any method-dependent variability. Holt A et al. Surveillance with serial serum carcinoembryonic levels detect colorectal cancer recurrences in patients who are initial nonsecretors. Am Surg 2010;76:1100. [PMID: 21105619] Tan E et al. Diagnostic precision of carcinoembryonic antigen in the detection of recurrence of colorectal cancer. Surg Oncol 2009;18:15. [PMID: 18619834]

	CD4 cell count	
Test/Range/Collection	**Physiologic Basis**	**Interpretation**	**Comments**
CD4 cell count, absolute, whole blood CD4: 359–1725 cells/mcL (29–61%) Lavender, yellow $$$ For an absolute CD4 count, order T-cell subsets and a CBC with differential.	Lymphocyte identification depends on specific cell surface CD (clusters of differentiation) antigens, which can be detected by flow cytometry analysis using monoclonal antibodies. The CD4 cells (helper T cells) express both CD3 (a pan–T-cell marker) and CD4. The CD8 cells (suppressor T cells) express both CD3 and CD8. CD4 cell levels are a criterion for categorizing HIV-related clinical conditions by CDC's classification system for HIV infection. The measurement of CD4 cell levels has been used to establish decision points for initiating prophylaxis and antiviral therapy and to monitor the efficacy of treatment. It has been recommended that CD4 cell levels be monitored every 3–6 months in all HIV-infected persons.	**Increased in:** Rheumatoid arthritis, type 1 diabetes mellitus, SLE without renal disease, primary biliary cirrhosis, atopic dermatitis, psoriasis, Sézary syndrome, chronic autoimmune hepatitis. **Decreased in:** AIDS/HIV infection, SLE with renal disease, acute cytomegalovirus (CMV) infection, burns, graft-versus-host disease, sunburn, myelodysplastic syndromes, acute lymphoblastic leukemia in remission, recovery from bone marrow transplantation, herpes infection, infectious mononucleosis, measles, ataxia-telangiectasia, vigorous exercise.	During HIV infection, antiviral therapy is often initiated when the absolute CD4 count drops below 500 cells/mcL. When the absolute CD4 count drops below 200 cells/mcL, therapeutic prophylaxis against *Pneumocystis jiroveci* pneumonia (PCP) and other opportunistic infections may be initiated. When the absolute CD4 count drops below 100 cells/mcL, prophylaxis against *Mycobacterium avium* complex is recommended. For longitudinal studies involving serial monitoring, specimen collections should be performed at the same time of day. Cambiano V et al. 'Test-and-treat': the end of the HIV epidemic? Curr Opin Infect Dis 2011;24:19. [PMID: 21157329] Jain V et al. When to start antiretroviral therapy. Curr HIV/AIDS Rep 2010;7:60. [PMID: 20425559] Sabin CA et al. Should HIV therapy be started at a CD4 cell count above 350 cells/microl in asymptomatic HIV-1-infected patients? Curr Opin Infect Dis 2009;22:191. [PMID: 19283914]

Celiac disease, serologic testing

| Celiac disease serologic testing, serum

Negative

SST, red

$$$$ | Celiac disease (gluten-sensitive enteropathy) is associated with a variety of autoantibodies, including tissue transglutaminase (tTG), endomysial, and deamidated gliadin antibodies. Although the IgA isotype of these antibodies usually predominates in celiac disease, individuals may also produce IgG isotypes, particularly those who are IgA deficient. The most sensitive and specific serologic tests are tTG and deamidated gliadin antibodies.

For patients with selective IgA deficiency, serum tTG, gliadin (deamidated), and endomysial autoantibodies of IgG type should be tested. | **Positive in:** Celiac disease (90% cases have 1 or more of the 3 autoantibodies). | Useful for evaluating patients suspected of having celiac disease, including patients with compatible symptoms, those with atypical symptoms, and those at increased risk (family history and/or positivity for DQ2 and/or DQ8). Those with positive laboratory results should then be referred for small intestinal biopsy to confirm the diagnosis.

Genetic susceptibility of celiac disease is related to specific HLA markers, ie, HLA DQ2 and/or DQ8.

Ensari A. Gluten-sensitive enteropathy (celiac disease): controversies in diagnosis and classification. Arch Pathol Lab Med 2010;134:826. [PMID: 20524861]

Green PH et al. Medical progress: Celiac disease. N Engl J Med 2007;357:1731. [PMID: 17960014]

Leffler DA et al. Update on serologic testing in celiac disease. Am J Gastroenterol 2010;105:2520. [PMID: 21131921] |

	Centromere antibody		
Test/Range/Collection	Physiologic Basis	Interpretation	Comments
Centromere antibody, serum (ACA) Negative SST $$	Centromere antibodies (ACA) are antibodies to nuclear proteins, specifically CENP-A, B, and C. The CENP-B is the primary autoantigen and is recognized by all sera that contain ACA. Presence of ACA predicts a favorable prognosis for systemic sclerosis. Both immunofluorescent antibody testing (IFA)- and enzyme-linked immunosorbent assay (ELISA)-based assays are available for ACA detection.	**Positive in:** CREST syndrome (calcinosis, Raynaud phenomenon, esophageal dysmotility, sclerodactyly, and telangiectasia) (80–90%), diffuse scleroderma (5–10%), Raynaud disease (20–30%).	In patients with connective tissue disease, the predictive value of a positive test is >95% for scleroderma or related disease (CREST syndrome, Raynaud disease). Diagnosis of CREST syndrome is made clinically. The presence of detectable ACA may antedate the development of clinical CREST syndrome by several years. ACA is also present in a small percentage of patients with primary biliary cirrhosis, rheumatoid arthritis and systemic lupus erythematosus. (See also Autoantibodies, Table 8–6.) Hamaguchi Y. Autoantibody profiles in systemic sclerosis: predictive value for clinical evaluation and prognosis. J Dermatol 2010;37:42. [PMID: 20175839]

Ceruloplasmin, serum		
Ceruloplasmin, serum or plasma 20–40 mg/dL [200–500 mg/L] (age-dependent) SST, PPT, green (fasting specimen is preferred) $$	Ceruloplasmin, a 120,000–160,000 MW α_2-glycoprotein with oxidase activity synthesized by the liver, is the main (95%) copper-carrying protein in human serum. Any failure during its synthesis whereby copper cannot be incorporated into ceruloplasmin results in secretion of an apoceruloplasmin. The apo form has a short half-life and is rapidly metabolized, leading to reduced serum level of ceruloplasmin.	**Increased in:** Acute and chronic inflammation, pregnancy. Drugs: oral contraceptives, phenytoin. **Decreased in:** Wilson disease (hepatolenticular degeneration) (95%), CNS disease other than Wilson (15%), liver disease other than Wilson (23%), malabsorption (enteropathy), malnutrition, primary biliary cirrhosis, nephrotic syndrome, severe copper deficiency, Menkes disease (X-linked inherited copper deficiency), hereditary aceruloplasminemia.	Serum ceruloplasmin level and slit-lamp examination for Kayser-Fleischer rings are initial recommended tests for diagnosis of Wilson disease. Slit-lamp exam is only 50–60% sensitive in patients without neurologic symptoms. Equivocal cases may need 24-hour urinary copper excretion, liver copper measurement, and/or detection of *ATP7B* gene mutations. Serum/plasma copper level is rarely indicated. Serum/plasma ceruloplasmin for diagnosis of Wilson disease is not reliable in asymptomatic patients. Mak CM et al. Diagnosis of Wilson's disease: a comprehensive review. Crit Rev Clin Lab Sci 2008;45:263. [PMID: 18568852] Nicastro E et al. Re-evaluation of the diagnostic criteria for Wilson disease in children with mild liver disease. Hepatology 2010;52:1948. [PMID: 20967755]

Chloride

Test/Range/Collection	Physiologic Basis	Interpretation	Comments
Chloride, serum or plasma (Cl⁻) 98–107 meq/L [mmol/L] SST, green $	Chloride, the principal inorganic anion of extracellular fluid, is important in maintaining proper body water distribution, osmotic pressure, and normal acid–base balance. If chloride is lost (as HCl or NH₄Cl), alkalosis ensues; if chloride is ingested or retained, acidosis ensues.	**Increased in:** Renal failure, nephrotic syndrome, renal tubular acidosis, dehydration, overtreatment with saline, hyperparathyroidism, diabetes insipidus, metabolic acidosis from diarrhea (loss of HCO_3^-), respiratory alkalosis, hyperadrenocorticism. Drugs: acetazolamide (hyperchloremic acidosis), androgens, hydrochlorothiazide, salicylates (intoxication). **Decreased in:** Vomiting, diarrhea, gastrointestinal suction, renal failure combined with salt deprivation, over-treatment with diuretics, chronic respiratory acidosis, diabetic ketoacidosis, excessive sweating, SIADH, salt-losing nephropathy, acute intermittent porphyria, water intoxication, expansion of extracellular fluid volume, adrenal insufficiency, hyperaldosteronism, metabolic alkalosis. Drugs: chronic laxative or bicarbonate ingestion, corticosteroids, diuretics.	Test is helpful in assessing normal and increased anion gap metabolic acidosis. It is somewhat helpful in distinguishing hypercalcemia due to primary hyperparathyroidism (high serum chloride) from that due to malignancy (normal serum chloride). Yunos NM et al. Bench-to-bedside review: chloride in critical illness. Crit Care 2010;14:226. [PMID: 20663180]

Cholesterol

Cholesterol, serum or plasma Desirable: <200 mg/dL [<5.2 mmol/L] Borderline: 200–239 mg/dL [5.2–6.1 mmol/L] High risk: >240 mg/dL [>6.2 mmol/L] SST, PPT, green $ Fasting specimen is required for LDL-C determination. HDL-C and total cholesterol can be measured with nonfasting specimen.	Cholesterol level is determined by lipid metabolism, which is in turn influenced by heredity, diet, and liver, kidney, thyroid, and other endocrine organ functions. Screening for total cholesterol (TC) may be done with nonfasting specimens, but a complete lipoprotein profile or LDL cholesterol (LDL-C) determination must be performed on fasting specimens. TC, triglyceride (TG), and high-density lipoprotein cholesterol (HDL-C) are directly measured. Although methods have been developed for direct LDL-C measurement, in practice, LDL-C is often indirectly determined by use of the Friedewald equation: $[LDL-C] = [TC] - [HDL-C] - [TG/5]$ Note that this calculation is not valid for specimens having TG >400 mg/dL [>4.52 mmol/L], for patients with type III hyperlipoproteinemia or chylomicronemia, or nonfasting specimens.	**Increased in:** Primary disorders: polygenic hypercholesterolemia, familial hypercholesterolemia (deficiency of LDL receptors), familial combined hyperlipidemia, familial dysbetalipoproteinemia. Secondary disorders: hypothyroidism, uncontrolled diabetes mellitus, nephrotic syndrome, biliary obstruction, anorexia nervosa, hepatocellular carcinoma, Cushing syndrome, acute intermittent porphyria. Drugs: corticosteroids. **Decreased in:** Severe liver disease (acute hepatitis, cirrhosis, malignancy), hyperthyroidism, severe acute or chronic illness, malnutrition, malabsorption (eg, HIV), extensive burns, familial (Gaucher disease, Tangier disease), abetalipoproteinemia, intestinal lymphangiectasia.	Coronary heart disease (CHD) risk depends on the ratio of total cholesterol to HDL cholesterol. The ratio of LDL to HDL cholesterol has similar predictive ability. Treatment decisions should be based on absolute CHD risk. The risk reduction is proportional to the reduction in LDL cholesterol achieved with treatment. The National Cholesterol Education Program (NCEP) expert panel has published clinical recommendations. According to NCEP guidelines, HDL-C <40 mg/dL is a risk factor for coronary heart disease (CHD), and HDL-C ≥60 mg/dL is a "negative" risk factor. In addition, there is a direct relation between LDL-C and the incidence of CHD. Treatment decisions and therapeutic goals are primarily based on LDL-C concentrations. The recommended LDL-C intervention goals are <100 mg/dL for high-risk patients (eg, patients with CHD), <130 mg/dL for moderate-risk patients (≥2 risk factors), and <160 mg/dL for low-risk patients (no or 1 risk factor). See Table 8–12 for risk factor assessment for CHD. Alwaili K et al. High-density lipoproteins and cardiovascular disease: 2010 update. Expert Rev Cardiovasc Ther 2010;8:413. [PMID: 20222819] Baumer JH et al. Hypercholesterolaemia in children guidelines review. Arch Dis Child Educ Pract Ed 2009;94:84. [PMID: 19460897] Viera AJ et al. Global risk of coronary heart disease: assessment and application. Am Fam Physician 2010;82:265. [PMID: 20672791]

Test/Range/Collection	Physiologic Basis	Interpretation	Comments
Clostridium difficile toxins, stool Negative Urine or stool container for collection of diarrheal (unformed) stool $$$ Must be tested within 12 hours of collection because toxin (B) is labile.	*Clostridium difficile*, a motile, gram-positive rod, is the major recognized agent of antibiotic-associated diarrhea, which is toxigenic in origin (see Antibiotic-associated colitis, Chapter 5). There are two toxins (A and B) produced by *C. difficile*, toxin A is an enterotoxin and toxin B is a cytotoxin. Cytotoxicity assay performed in cell culture is used to detect the cytopathic effect of the toxins, whose identity is confirmed by neutralization with specific antitoxins. The assay sensitivity and specificity are 95% and 90%, respectively. However, the assay is expensive and requires 24–48 hours and is thus not clinically practical. Toxin A (more weakly cytopathic in cell culture) is enterotoxic and produces enteric disease. Toxin B (more easily detected in standard cell culture assays) fails to produce intestinal disease.	**Positive in:** Antibiotic-associated diarrhea (15–25%), antibiotic-associated colitis (50–75%), and pseudomembranous colitis (90–100%). About 3% of healthy adults and 10–20% of hospitalized patients have *C. difficile* in their colonic flora. There is also a high carrier rate of *C. difficile* and its toxin in healthy neonates.	Rapid enzyme immunoassay (EIA) (2–4 hour) tests for toxin A or toxins A and B have been used as an alternative to the cytotoxicity assay but are less sensitive and thus suboptimal. New guidelines recommend a two-step testing process, which includes an initial screening of stool samples with a rapid immunoassay for glutamate dehydrogenase (GDH), a common enzyme produced by *C. difficile*. A negative GDH assay effectively rules out infection, while a positive assay requires confirmation with a more specific assay, ie, the cell cytotoxicity assay or toxigenic culture. PCR assay that amplifies the genes responsible for *C. difficile* toxins may ultimately provide a more rapid, sensitive and specific test. Repeat testing during the same episode of diarrhea is of limited value and should be discouraged. Direct visualization with histopathologic examination of pseudomembranes on lower gastrointestinal endoscopy only detects 50–55% of *C. difficile* cases. Cohen SH et al. Clinical practice guidelines for *Clostridium difficile* in adults: 2010 update by the Society for Healthcare Epidemiology of America (SHEA) and the Infectious Diseases Society of America (IDSA). Infect Control Hosp Epidemiol 2010;31:431. [PMID: 20307191] Curry S. *Clostridium difficile*. Clin Lab Med 2010;30(1):329. [PMID: 20513554]

Coccidioides antibodies		
Coccidioides antibodies, serum or CSF Negative SST or red (serum); glass or plastic (CSF) $$	Screens for presence of antibodies to *Coccidioides immitis*. Some centers use the mycelial-phase antigen, coccidioidin, to detect antibody. IgM antibodies appear early in disease in 75% of patients, begin to decrease after week 3, and are rarely seen after 5 months. They may persist in disseminated cases, usually in immunocompromised patients. IgG antibodies appear later in the course of the disease. Meningeal disease may have negative serum IgG and require CSF IgG antibody titers.	**Positive in:** Infection by coccidioides (90%). **Negative in:** Coccidioidin skin testing, many patients with chronic cavitary coccidioides; 5% of meningeal coccidioides is negative by CSF complement fixation (CF) test.	Diagnosis is based on culture and serologic testing. Precipitin (immunodiffusion) and CF tests detect 90% of primary symptomatic cases. Precipitin test (for IgM and IgG antibodies) is most effective in detecting early primary infection or an exacerbation of existing disease. Test is diagnostic but not prognostic. CF test (for IgG antibody) becomes positive later than precipitin test, and titers can be used to assess severity of infection. Titers rise as the disease progresses and decline as the patient improves. ELISA-based test is also available; data suggest good test performance characteristics. Ampel NM. New perspectives on coccidioidomycosis. Proc Am Thorac Soc 2010;7:181. [PMID: 20463246] Parish JM et al. Coccidioidomycosis. Mayo Clin Proc 2008;83:343. [PMID: 18316002]

Test/Range/Collection	Physiologic Basis	Interpretation	Comments
Cold agglutinins, serum <1:32 titer Red, SST $$ Specimen should be kept at 37°C before separation from cells.	Cold agglutinins are IgM (rarely IgG or IgA) autoantibodies that are capable of agglutinating red blood cells (RBCs) at temperature below 35°C (strongly at 4°C, weakly at 24°C, and weakly or not at all at 37°C). Cold agglutinins can be monoclonal or polyclonal, and have been associated with various diseases, particularly infections, neoplasms, and collagen vascular diseases. Cold agglutinins are not necessarily pathologic, and may be detected in asymptomatic individuals during routine blood typing and crossmatching. If the agglutination is not reversible after incubation at 37°C, then the reaction is not due to cold agglutinins.	**Increased in:** Chronic cold agglutinin disease, lymphoproliferative disorders (eg, Waldenström macroglobulinemia, chronic lymphocytic leukemia), autoimmune hemolytic anemia, myeloma, collagen-vascular diseases, *Mycoplasma pneumoniae* pneumonia, infectious mononucleosis, mumps orchitis, cytomegalovirus, listeriosis, tropical diseases (eg, trypanosomiasis, malaria).	Patients with cold agglutinins develop anti-I or anti-i antibodies which are usually of the IgM class and react with adult human RBCs at temperatures below 35°C, resulting in agglutination. In *Mycoplasma* pneumonia, titers of anti-I rise late in the first week or during the second week, are maximal at 3–4 weeks after onset, and then disappear rapidly. A rise in cold agglutinin antibody titer is suggestive of recent mycoplasma infection. Berentsen S. Cold agglutinin-mediated autoimmune hemolytic anemia in Waldenström's macroglobulinemia. Clin Lymphoma Myeloma 2009;9:110. [PMID: 19362990] Mayer B et al. Mixed-type autoimmune hemolytic anemia: differential diagnosis and a critical review of reported cases. Transfusion 2008;48:2229. [PMID: 18564390]

Complement C3		
Complement C3, serum 64–166 mg/dL [640–1660 mg/L] SST $$	The classic and alternative complement pathways converge at the C3 step in the complement cascade. Low levels indicate activation by one or both pathways. Most diseases with immune complexes show decreased C3 levels. Test is usually performed as an immunoassay (by radial immunodiffusion or nephelometry).	**Increased in:** Many inflammatory conditions as an acute-phase reactant, active phase of rheumatic diseases (eg, rheumatoid arthritis, SLE), acute viral hepatitis, myocardial infarction, cancer, diabetes mellitus, pregnancy, sarcoidosis, amyloidosis, thyroiditis. **Decreased by:** Decreased synthesis (protein malnutrition, congenital deficiency, severe liver disease), increased catabolism (immune complex disease, membranoproliferative glomerulonephritis [75%], SLE, Sjögren syndrome, rheumatoid arthritis, DIC, paroxysmal nocturnal hemoglobinuria, autoimmune hemolytic anemia, gram-negative bacteremia), increased loss (burns, gastroenteropathies).	Complement C3 levels may be useful in following the activity of immune complex diseases. The best test to detect inherited deficiencies is CH50 (complement activity assay). Carroll MC. Complement and humoral immunity. Vaccine 2008;26(Suppl 8):128. [PMID: 19388161] Reis E et al. Clinical aspects and molecular basis of primary deficiencies of complement component C3 and its regulatory proteins factor I and factor H. Scand J Immunol 2006;63:155. [PMID: 16499568]

	Complement C4

Test/Range/Collection	Physiologic Basis	Interpretation	Comments
Complement C4, serum 15–45 mg/dL [150–450 mg/dL] SST $$	C4 is a component of the classic complement pathway. Depressed levels usually indicate classic pathway activation. Test is usually performed as an immunoassay and not a functional assay.	**Increased in:** Various malignancies (not clinically useful). **Decreased by:** Decreased synthesis (congenital deficiency), increased catabolism (SLE, rheumatoid arthritis, proliferative glomerulonephritis, hereditary angioedema (HAE)), and increased loss (burns, protein-losing enteropathies).	Low C4 accompanies acute attacks of HAE, and C4 is used as a first-line test for the disease. C1 esterase inhibitor levels are not indicated for the evaluation of HAE unless C4 is low. Congenital C4 deficiency occurs with an SLE-like syndrome. Arason GJ et al. Primary immunodeficiency and autoimmunity: lessons from human diseases. Scand J Immunol 2010;71:317. [PMID: 20500682] Breda L et al. Laboratory tests in the diagnosis and follow-up of pediatric rheumatic diseases: an update. Semin Arthritis Rheum 2010;40:53. [PMID: 19246077] Lipsker D et al. Cutaneous manifestations of complement deficiencies. Lupus 2010;19:1096. [PMID: 20693203]

Complement CH50		
Complement CH50, serum (CH50) 22–40 U/mL (laboratory-specific) Red $$$	The quantitative assay of hemolytic complement activity depends on the ability of the classic complement pathway to induce hemolysis of red cells sensitized with optimal amounts of anti-red cell antibodies. For precise titrations of hemolytic complement, the dilution of serum that lyses 50% of the indicator red cells is determined as the CH50. This arbitrary unit depends on the conditions of the assay and is therefore laboratory-specific.	**Decreased with:** >50–80% deficiency of classic pathway complement components (congenital or acquired deficiencies). **Normal in:** Deficiencies of the alternative pathway complement components.	This is a functional assay of biologic activity. Sensitivity to decreased levels of complement components depends on exactly how the test is performed. It is used to detect congenital and acquired severe deficiency disorders of the classic complement pathway. Botto M et al. Complement in human diseases: lessons from complement deficiencies. Mol Immunol 2009;46:2774. [PMID: 19481265] Chen M et al. The complement system in systemic autoimmune disease. J Autoimmun 2010;34:J276. [PMID: 20005073] Pettigrew HD et al. Clinical significance of complement deficiencies. Ann N Y Acad Sci 2009;1173:108. [PMID: 19758139]

	Complete blood cell count		
Test/Range/Collection	**Physiologic Basis**	**Interpretation**	**Comments**
Complete blood cell count (CBC), blood

Refer to individual test for reference range

Lavender

$ | The CBC consists of a panel of tests that examines whole blood and includes the following: total white blood cell count (WBC, ×10³/mcL) and white blood cell differential (%) (p. 289), red blood cell count (RBC, × 10⁶/mcL) (p. 248), hemoglobin concentration (Hb, g/L) (p. 159), hematocrit (Hct, %) (p. 155), platelet count (Plt, 10³/mcL) (p. 233), red cell indices including mean corpuscular volume (MCV, fL) (p. 207), mean corpuscular hemoglobin (MCH) (p. 206), mean corpuscular hemoglobin concentration (MCHC, g/L) (p. 206), and red cell distribution width (RDW, %).

Several new CBC parameters are being introduced, including nucleated red blood cells, immature granulocytes, immature reticulocyte fraction, immature platelet fraction, red cell fragments as well as new parameters for detection of functional iron deficiency. Automated laboratory hematology analyzers are widely available. The basic principles used for the cell counting and white cell differential are instrument-dependent. | Refer to individual test for detailed information.
Also see Table 8–31 for white cell count and differential. | The CBC provides important information about the types and numbers of cells in the blood, especially red cells, white cells, and platelets. It helps in evaluating symptoms (eg, weakness, fatigue, fever or bruising), diagnosing conditions/diseases (eg, anemia, infection, leukemia, and many other disorders), and determining the stages of a particular disease (eg, leukemia).

Hct, MCH, and MCHC are typically calculated from RBC, Hb, and MCV.

If significantly abnormal CBC values are obtained, a peripheral blood smear should be prepared and examined (eg, red cell morphology, WBC differential, platelet count estimation, identification of immature and malignant cells).

Briggs C. Quality counts: new parameters in blood cell counting. Int J Lab Hematol 2009;31:277. [PMID: 19452619]

Milcic TL. The complete blood count. Neonatal Netw 2010;29:109. [PMID: 20211833] |

Cortisol		
Cortisol, plasma or serum 8:00 AM: 5–20 mcg/dL [140–550 nmol/L] SST, lavender, or green $$	Release of corticotropin-releasing factor (CRF) from the hypothalamus stimulates release of ACTH from the pituitary, which in turn stimulates release of cortisol from the adrenal. Cortisol provides negative feedback to this system. Test measures both free cortisol and cortisol bound to cortisol-binding globulin (CBG). Morning levels are higher than evening levels.	**Increased in:** Cushing syndrome, acute illness, surgery, trauma, septic shock, depression, anxiety, alcoholism, starvation, chronic renal failure, increased CBG (congenita, pregnancy, estrogen therapy). **Decreased in:** Addison disease; decreased CBG (congenital, liver disease, nephrotic syndrome).	Cortisol levels are useful only in the context of standardized suppression or stimulation tests. See Cosyntropin stimulation test and Dexamethasone suppression tests for details. Circadian fluctuations in cortisol levels limit usefulness of single measurements. Analysis of diurnal variation of cortisol is not useful diagnostically. Anagnostis P et al. Clinical review: the pathogenetic role of cortisol in the metabolic syndrome: a hypothesis. J Clin Endocrinol Metab 2009;94:2692. [PMID: 19470627] Newell-Price J. Diagnosis/differential diagnosis of Cushing's syndrome: a review of best practice. Best Pract Res Clin Endocrinol Metab 2009;23(Suppl 1):S5. [PMID: 20129193] Pecori Giraldi F. Recent challenges in the diagnosis of Cushing's syndrome. Horm Res 2009;71(Suppl 1):123. [PMID: 19153521] Satre TJ et al. Clinical inquiries. What's the most practical way to rule out adrenal insufficiency? J Fam Pract 2009;58:281a-b. [PMID: 19442385] Wallace I et al. The diagnosis and investigation of adrenal insufficiency in adults. Ann Clin Biochem 2009;46(Pt 5):351. [PMID: 19675057]

Test/Range/Collection	Physiologic Basis	Interpretation	Comments
Cortisol (urinary free), urine 10–110 mcg/24 hr [30–300 nmol/d] Urine bottle containing boric acid. $$$ Collect 24-hour urine.	Urinary free cortisol measurement is useful in the initial evaluation of suspected Cushing syndrome (see Cushing syndrome algorithm, Figure 9–8).	**Increased in:** Cushing syndrome, acute illness, stress. **Not increased in:** Obesity.	Urinary free cortisol is the initial diagnostic test of choice for Cushing syndrome. Not useful for the diagnosis of adrenal insufficiency. A shorter (12-hour) overnight collection and measurement of the ratio of urine-free cortisol to urine creatinine appears to perform nearly as well as a 24-hour collection for urine-free cortisol. Boscaro M et al. Approach to the patient with possible Cushing's syndrome. J Clin Endocrinol Metab 2009;94:3121. [PMID: 19734443] Carroll TB et al. The diagnosis of Cushing's syndrome. Rev Endocr Metab Disord 2010;11:147. [PMID: 20821267] Newell-Price J. Diagnosis/differential diagnosis of Cushing's syndrome: a review of best practice. Best Pract Res Clin Endocrinol Metab 2009;23(Suppl 1):S5. [PMID: 20129193]

Cosyntropin stimulation test		
Cosyntropin stimulation test, serum or plasma $$$ First draw a cortisol level. Then administer cosyntropin (1 mcg or 250 mcg IV). Draw another cortisol level in 30 minutes.	Cosyntropin (synthetic ACTH preparation) stimulates the adrenal to release cortisol. A normal response is a doubling of basal levels or an increment of 7 mcg/dL (200 nmol/L) to a level above 18 mcg/dL (>504 nmol/L). A poor cortisol response to cosyntropin indicates adrenal insufficiency (see Adrenocortical insufficiency algorithm, Figure 9–3).	**Decreased in:** Adrenal insufficiency, pituitary insufficiency, AIDS.	Test does not distinguish primary from secondary (pituitary) adrenal insufficiency, because in secondary adrenal insufficiency the atrophic adrenal may be unresponsive to cosyntropin. Test may not reliably detect pituitary insufficiency. Metyrapone test may be useful to assess the pituitary-adrenal axis. AIDS patients with adrenal insufficiency may have normal ACTH stimulation tests. Fleseriu M et al. "Relative" adrenal insufficiency in critical illness. Endocr Pract 2009;15:632. [PMID: 19625244] Magnotti M et al. Diagnosing adrenal insufficiency: which test is best—the 1-microg or the 250-microg test? Endocr Pract 2008;14:233. [PMID: 18308665] Sarre TJ et al. Clinical inquiries. What's the most practical way to rule out adrenal insufficiency? J Fam Pract 2009;58:281a-b.[PMID: 19442385]

	Creatine kinase	

Test/Range/Collection	Physiologic Basis	Interpretation	Comments
Creatine kinase, serum or plasma 32–267 IU/L [0.53–4.45 mckat/L] (method-dependent) SST, PPT, green $	Creatine kinase splits creatine phosphate in the presence of ADP to yield creatine and ATP. Skeletal muscle, myocardium, and brain are rich in the enzyme. CK is released by tissue damage.	**Increased in:** Myocardial infarction (MI), myocarditis, muscle trauma, rhabdomyolysis, muscular dystrophy, polymyositis, severe muscular exertion, malignant hyperthermia, hypothyroidism, cerebral infarction, surgery, Reye syndrome, tetanus, generalized convulsions, alcoholism, IM injections, DC countershock. Drugs: clofibrate, HMG-CoA reductase inhibitors.	CK is as sensitive a test as aldolase for muscle damage, so aldolase is not needed for this condition. During an MI, serum CK level rises rapidly (within 3–5 hours); elevation persists for 2–3 days post-MI. Total CK is not specific enough for use in diagnosis of MI, but a normal total CK has a high negative predictive value. A more specific test is needed for diagnosis of MI or acute coronary syndrome (eg, CK-MB, now largely replaced by cardiac troponin I). Brancaccio P et al. Biochemical markers of muscular damage. Clin Chem Lab Med 2010;48:757. [PMID: 20518645] Cervellin G et al. Rhabdomyolysis: historical background, clinical, diagnostic and therapeutic features. Clin Chem Lab Med 2010;48:749. [PMID: 20298139] Ristagno G et al. Biomarkers of myocardial injury after cardiac arrest or myocardial ischemia. Front Biosci (Schol Ed) 2010;2:373. [PMID: 20036954]

Creatine kinase MB

Creatine kinase MB, enzyme activity (CK-MB)	CK consists of three isoenzymes, made up of 2 subunits, M and B.	Increased in: Myocardial infarction, cardiac trauma, certain muscular dystrophies, and	CK-MB is a relatively specific test for MI. It appears in serum approximately 4 hours after infarction, peaks
<16 IU/L	The fraction with the greatest electrophoretic mobility is CK1 (BB), CK2 (MB) is intermediate, and CK3 (MM) moves slowest toward the anode.	polymyositis. Slight persistent elevation reported in a few patients on hemodialysis.	at 12–24 hours, and declines over 48–72 hours. CK-MB mass concentration is a sensitive marker of MI within 4–12 hours after infarction. Because
[<0.27 mckat/L] or <4% of total CK or <7 mcg/L mass units (laboratory-specific)	Skeletal muscle is characterized by isoenzyme MM and brain by isoenzyme BB.		cardiac troponins are now the markers of choice for the diagnosis of acute MI, high sensitivity cardiac troponin I test has largely replaced the conventional CK-MB assay.
SST, PPT, green	Myocardium has approximately 40% MB isoenzyme.		Measurement of CK-MB remains useful in evaluating patients who are already troponin positive and have recurrent chest pain and in follow-up of patients who
$$	Assay techniques include isoenzyme separation by electrophoresis (isoenzyme activity units) or by immunoassay using antibody specific for MB fraction (mass units).		are status post interventional procedures. Estimation of CK-MM and CK-BB is not clinically useful. Use total CK. McLean AS et al. Bench-to-bedside review: the value of cardiac biomarkers in the intensive care patient. Crit Care 2008;12:215. [PMID: 18557993] Saenger AK. A tale of two biomarkers: the use of troponin and CK-MB in contemporary practice. Clin Lab Sci 2010;23:134. [PMID: 20734885]

	Creatinine		
Test/Range/Collection	Physiologic Basis	Interpretation	Comments
Creatinine, serum or plasma (Cr)

0.6–1.2 mg/dL

[50–100 mcmol/L]

SST, PPT, green

$ | Endogenous creatinine is excreted by filtration through the glomerulus and by tubular secretion.
Creatinine clearance is an acceptable clinical measure of glomerular filtration rate (GFR), although it sometimes overestimates GFR (eg, in cirrhosis).
For each 50% reduction in GFR, serum creatinine approximately doubles. | **Increased in:** Acute or chronic renal failure, urinary tract obstruction, nephrotoxic drugs, hypothyroidism.
Decreased in: Reduced muscle mass, cachexia, aging. | In the alkaline picrate method, substances other than Cr (eg, acetoacetate, acetone, β-hydroxybutyrate, α-ketoglutarate, pyruvate, glucose) may give falsely high results. Therefore, patients with diabetic ketoacidosis may have spuriously elevated Cr.
Cephalosporins may spuriously increase or decrease Cr measurement.
Increased bilirubin may spuriously decrease Cr.
Chronic renal insufficiency may be underrecognized. Age, male sex, and black race are predictors of kidney disease.
Serum creatinine levels frequently do not reflect decreased renal function because creatinine production rate is decreased with reduced lean body mass. Increased intravascular volume and increased volume of distribution associated with anasarca may also mask decreased renal function by reducing serum creatinine levels.
See glomerular filtration rate, estimated (eGFR).
Fliser D. Assessment of renal function in elderly patients. Curr Opin Nephrol Hypertens 2008;17:604. [PMID: 18941354]
Pottel H et al. On the relationship between glomerular filtration rate and serum creatinine in children. Pediatr Nephrol 2010;25:927. [PMID: 20012996]
Wu I et al. Screening for kidney diseases: older measures versus novel biomarkers. Clin J Am Soc Nephrol 2008;3:1895. [PMID: 18922990] |

Creatinine clearance			
Creatinine clearance (Cl_{Cr}) Adults: 90–130 mL/min/1.73 m² BSA $$$ Collect carefully timed 24-hour urine and simultaneous serum/plasma creatinine sample. Record patient's weight and height.	Widely used test of glomerular filtration rate. Theoretically reliable, but often compromised by incomplete urine collection. Creatinine clearance is calculated from measurement of urine creatinine (U_{Cr} [mg/dL]), plasma/serum creatinine (P_{Cr} [mg/dL]), and urine flow rate (V [mL/min]) according to the formula: $$Cl_{Cr}\,(mL/min) = \frac{U_{Cr} \times V}{P_{Cr}}$$ where $$V\,(mL/min) = \frac{24\text{-hour urine volume (mL)}}{1440\ (min/24h)}$$ Creatinine clearance is often "corrected" for body surface area (BSA [m²]) according to the formula: $$Cl_{Cr}\ (corrected) = \frac{Cl_{Cr}\ (uncorrected)}{BSA} \times 1.73$$	**Increased in:** High cardiac output, exercise, acromegaly, diabetes mellitus (early stage), infections, hypothyroidism. **Decreased in:** Acute or chronic renal failure, decreased renal blood flow (shock, hemorrhage, dehydration, CHF). Drugs: nephrotoxic drugs.	Serum Cr may, in practice, be a more reliable indicator of renal function than 24-hour Cl_{Cr} unless urine collection is carefully monitored. An 8-hour collection provides results similar to those obtained with a 24-hour collection. Cl_{Cr} will overestimate glomerular filtration rate to the extent that Cr is secreted by the renal tubules (eg, in cirrhosis). Cl_{Cr} can be estimated from the serum creatinine using the following formula: $$Cl_{Cr}\,(mL/min) = \frac{(140 - Age) \times Wt\ (kg)}{72 \times P_{Cr}}$$ Serial decline in Cl_{Cr} is the most reliable indicator of progressive renal dysfunction. Also see GFR, estimated (eGFR). Fliser D. Assessment of renal function in elderly patients. Curr Opin Nephrol Hypertens 2008;17:604. [PMID: 18941354] Stevens LA et al. Measured GFR as a confirmatory test for estimated GFR. J Am Soc Nephrol 2009;20:2305. [PMID: 19833901] White CA et al. Performance of creatinine-based estimates of GFR in kidney transplant recipients: a systematic review. Am J Kidney Dis 2008;51:1005. [PMID: 18455847]

	Cryoglobulins		
Test/Range/Collection	**Physiologic Basis**	**Interpretation**	**Comments**
Cryoglobulins, serum Negative SST $ Patients should be fasting and blood sample must be drawn in a pre-warmed vacutainer tube, kept at 37°C and immediately transported to the laboratory.	Cryoglobulins are immuno-globulins (IgG, IgM, IgA, or light chains) that precipitate on exposure to the cold. The sample is stored at 4°C and examined daily for the presence or absence of cryoglobulins over a period of 3–5 days. Type I cryoglobulins (25%) are monoclonal immunoglobulins, most commonly IgM, occasionally IgG, and rarely IgA or Bence Jones protein. Type II (25%) are mixed cryoglobulins with a monoclonal component (usually IgM but occasionally IgG or IgA) that complexes with polyclonal normal IgG in the cryoprecipitate. Type III (50%) are mixed poly-clonal cryoglobulins (IgM and IgG).	**Positive in:** Immunoproliferative disorders (multiple myeloma, Waldenström macroglobu-linemia, chronic lymphocytic leukemia, lymphoma), collagen vascular disease (SLE, poly-arteritis nodosa, rheumatoid arthritis, Sjögren syndrome), hemolytic anemia, infections (eg, HCV, HIV), glomerulonephritis, chronic liver disease. The term "essential mixed cryoglobuli-nemia" (a vasculitic syndrome) is used to refer to patients with no primary disease other than Sjögren syndrome; other cases are classified as secondary mixed cryoglobulinemia.	All types of cryoglobulins may cause cold-induced symptoms, including Raynaud phenomenon, vascular purpura, and urticaria. Patients with type I cryoglobulinemia usually suffer from underlying disease (eg, multiple myeloma). Patients with type II and III cryoglobulinemia often have immune complex disease, with vascular purpura, bleeding tendencies, arthritis, and nephritis. Typing of cryoglobulins by electrophoresis is not nec-essary for diagnosis or clinical management. About 50% of essential mixed cryoglobulinemia patients have evidence of hepatitis C infection. Cacoub P et al. Hepatitis C virus infection induced vasculitis. Clin Rev Allergy Immunol 2008;35:30. [PMID: 18196478] Sargur R et al. Cryoglobulin evaluation: best practice? Ann Clin Biochem 2010;47(Pt 1):8. [PMID: 20040797]

Cryptococcal antigen		
Cryptococcal antigen, serum or CSF Negative SST (serum) or glass or plastic tube (CSF) $$	The capsular polysaccharide of *Cryptococcus neoformans* potentiates opportunistic infections by the yeast. The cryptococcal antigen test used is often a latex agglutination test.	**Increased in:** Cryptococcal infection.	False-positive and false-negative results have been reported. False positives due to rheumatoid factor can be reduced by pretreatment of serum using pronase before testing. Sensitivity and specificity of serum cryptococcal antigen titer for cryptococcal meningitis are 91% and 83%, respectively. Ninety-six percent of cryptococcal infections occur in AIDS patients. Sloan D et al. Treatment of acute cryptococcal meningitis in HIV infected adults, with an emphasis on resource-limited settings. Cochrane Database Syst Rev 2008:CD005647. [PMID: 18843697]

	C-telopeptide, beta-cross-linked		
Test/Range/Collection	Physiologic Basis	Interpretation	Comments
C-telopeptide, beta-cross-linked (Beta-CTx), serum Adult male: 60–850 pg/mL Adult female: premenopausal 60–650 pg/mL; postmenopausal 104–1010 pg/mL (age- and laboratory-specific). SST, red $$$$	During bone resorption, osteoclasts secrete a mixture of proteases that degrade the type I collagen fibrils into fragments including C-terminal telopeptide (CTx). One of the fragments is beta-CTx, which is released into blood and is considered a specific marker for increased bone resorption.	**Increased in:** Osteoporosis, osteopenia, osteomalacia, rickets, Paget disease, hyperparathyroidism, and hyperthyroidism.	Test aids in the diagnosis of medical conditions associated with increased bone turnover, but cannot replace bone mineral density to diagnose osteoporosis. Test may be useful for monitoring antiresorptive treatment in postmenopausal women treated for osteoporosis and individuals diagnosed with osteopenia. Reduced renal function may lead to reduced urinary excretion of beta-CTx and consequent increase in the serum beta-CTx concentration. Also see N-telopeptide, cross-linked (p. 218). Civitelli R et al. Bone turnover markers: understanding their value in clinical trials and clinical practice. Osteoporos Int 2009;20:843. [PMID: 19190842] Delmas PD et al. The use of biochemical markers of bone turnover in osteoporosis. Committee of Scientific Advisors of the International Osteoporosis Foundation. Osteoporos Int 2000;11:S2. [PMID: 11193237] Garnero P. Biomarkers for osteoporosis management: utility in diagnosis, fracture risk prediction and therapy monitoring. Mol Diagn Ther 2008;12:157. [PMID: 18510379]

Cyclic citrullinated protein antibody		
Cyclic citrullinated protein antibody (anti-CCP), serum Negative SST, red $$$$	Post-translational deamination of arginine residues by peptidyl arginine deaminase (citrullination) during inflammation results in production of antigenic epitope. Antibodies to citrullinated proteins (particularly filaggrin) are frequently elevated in rheumatoid arthritis (RA).	**Increased in:** RA (sensitivity 70–80%).	Specificity of anti-CCP (90–95%) for RA is higher than that of rheumatoid factor. Pincus T et al. Laboratory tests to assess patients with rheumatoid arthritis: advantages and limitations. Rheum Dis Clin North Am 2009;35:731. [PMID: 19962677] Raptopoulou A et al. Anti-citrulline antibodies in the diagnosis and prognosis of rheumatoid arthritis: evolving concepts. Crit Rev Clin Lab Sci 2007;44:339. [PMID: 17558653] Whiting PF et al. Systematic review: accuracy of anti-citrullinated peptide antibodies for diagnosing rheumatoid arthritis. Ann Intern Med 2010;152:456. [PMID: 20368651]

Cytomegalovirus antibody			
Test/Range/Collection	Physiologic Basis	Interpretation	Comments
Cytomegalovirus antibody, serum (CMV) Negative SST $$$	Detects the presence of antibody to CMV, either IgG or IgM. CMV infection is usually acquired during childhood or early adulthood. By age 20–40 years, 40–90% of the population has CMV antibodies.	**Increased in:** Previous or active CMV infection. False-positive CMV IgM tests occur when rheumatoid factor or infectious mononucleosis is present.	Serial specimens exhibiting a greater than fourfold titer rise suggest a recent infection. Active CMV infection must be documented by viral isolation. Useful for screening of potential organ donors and recipients. Universal prophylaxis reduces infection in transplant recipients. Detection of CMV IgM antibody in the serum of a newborn usually indicates congenital infection. Detection of CMV IgG antibody is not diagnostic, because maternal CMV IgG antibody passed via the placenta can persist in newborn's serum for 6 months. CMV seronegative blood components are more efficacious than leukocyte-reduced blood components in preventing transfusion-acquired CMV infection. Hyde TB et al. Cytomegalovirus seroconversion rates and risk factors: implications for congenital CMV. Rev Med Virol 2010;20:311. [PMID: 20645278] Kalil AC et al. Meta-analysis: the efficacy of strategies to prevent organ disease by cytomegalovirus in solid organ transplant recipients. Ann Intern Med 2005;143:870. [PMID: 16365468]

D-dimer		
D-dimer, plasma

Negative

Blue

$$ | D-dimer is one of the terminal fibrin degradation products. The presence of D-dimers indicates that a fibrin clot was formed and subsequently degraded by plasmin. Essentially, D-dimer is elevated whenever the coagulation system has been activated, followed by fibrinolysis. | **Increased in:** Deep vein thrombosis (DVT), venous thromboembolism (VTE), pulmonary embolism (PE), disseminated intravascular coagulation (DIC), arterial thromboembolism, pregnancy (especially postpartum period), malignancy, surgery, thrombolytic therapy. | D-dimer assay is a very sensitive test for DIC, DVT and VTE or PE. The D-dimer can be measured by a variety of methods; for example, semiquantitative latex agglutination and quantitative high sensitivity immunoassay (eg, ELISA).
The newly developed highly sensitive automated D-dimer tests may be used to exclude PE and DVT: a negative test essentially rules out thrombosis, but a positive test does not confirm the diagnosis, and further testing (eg, ultrasound, CT angiography) is recommended. See Figure 9–23 and Table 8–20 for its use in pulmonary embolism evaluation.
Adam SS et al. D-dimer antigen: current concepts and future prospects. Blood 2009;113:2878. [PMID: 19008457]
Galioto NJ et al. Recurrent venous thromboembolism. Am Fam Physician 2011;83:293. [PMID: 21302870]
Green D. Interpreting coagulation assays. Blood Coagul Fibrinolysis 2010;21(Suppl 1):S3. [PMID: 20855988] |

		Dehydroepiandrosterone sulfate		

Test/Range/Collection	Physiologic Basis	Interpretation	Comments
Dehydroepiandrosterone sulfate (DHEA-S), serum or plasma Male: 40–500 mcg/dL Female: 20–320 mcg/dL SST, PPT, green, lavender/pink $$$$	DHEA is a 19-carbon endogenous steroid hormone secreted by the adrenal glands. It is converted to DHEA-S in the adrenals, liver, and small intestine. DHEA-S is albumin-bound in the circulation, and there is no diurnal variation in DHEA-S levels. Levels of DHEA-S are about 300 × higher than DHEA and more stable. It serves as the precursor of androgens and estrogens.	**Increased in:** Adrenal hyperplasia, adrenal cancer, congenital adrenal hyperplasia, polycystic ovarian syndrome. **Decreased in:** Adrenal insufficiency, hypopituitarism, rheumatoid arthritis (females), insulin, corticosteroids.	DHEAS measurement is typically used along with other steroid and peptide hormones to evaluate adrenal function, to help diagnose adrenal cortex tumors, and polycystic ovarian syndrome (in females). Orally ingested DHEA is converted to DHEA-S when passing through intestines and liver. People taking DHEA supplements have elevated blood levels of DHEA-S. Use by athletes is prohibited by the World Anti-doping Agency. Imrich R et al. Hypothalamic-pituitary-adrenal axis in rheumatoid arthritis. Rheum Dis Clin North Am 2010;36:721. [PMID: 21092849] Pugeat M et al. Recommendations for investigation of hyperandrogenism. Ann Endocrinol (Paris) 2010;71:2. [PMID: 20096825] Yildiz BO et al. The adrenal and polycystic ovary syndrome. Rev Endocr Metab Disord 2007;8:331. [PMID: 17932770]

Dexamethasone suppression test (low dose)		
Dexamethasone suppression test (low dose, overnight), serum or plasma 8:00 AM serum cortisol level: <5 mcg/dL [<140 nmol/L] SST, PPT, green $$ Give 1 mg dexamethasone at 11:00 PM. At 8:00 AM, draw serum/plasma cortisol level.	In normal patients, dexamethasone suppresses the 8:00 AM serum cortisol level below 5 mcg/dL. Patients with Cushing syndrome have 8:00 AM levels >10 mcg/dL (>276 nmol/L).	**Positive in:** Cushing syndrome (sensitivity is high in severe cases but less so in mild ones; specificity is 70–90% in patients with chronic illness or hospitalized patients)	Good screening test for Cushing syndrome. If this test is abnormal, use high-dose dexamethasone suppression test (see p. 122) to determine etiology. (See also Cushing syndrome algorithm, Figure 9–8.) Patients taking phenytoin may fail to suppress because of enhanced dexamethasone metabolism. Depressed patients may also fail to suppress morning cortisol level. Boscaro M et al. Approach to the patient with possible Cushing's syndrome. J Clin Endocrinol Metab 2009;94:3121. [PMID: 19734443] Elamin MB et al. Accuracy of diagnostic tests for Cushing's syndrome: a systematic review and metaanalyses. J Clin Endocrinol Metab 2008;93:1553. [PMID: 18334594] Nieman LK et al. The diagnosis of Cushing's syndrome: an Endocrine Society Clinical Practice Guideline. J Clin Endocrinol Metab 2008;93:1526. [PMID: 18334580]

Dexamethasone suppression test (high dose)			
Test/Range/Collection	Physiologic Basis	Interpretation	Comments
Dexamethasone suppression test (high-dose, overnight), serum or plasma 8:00 AM serum cortisol level: <5 mcg/dL [<140 nmol/L] SST, PPT, green $$	Suppression of plasma cortisol levels to <50% of baseline with dexamethasone indicates Cushing disease (pituitary-dependent ACTH hypersecretion) and differentiates this from adrenal and ectopic Cushing syndrome (see Cushing syndrome algorithm, Figure 9–8).	**Positive in:** Cushing disease (88–92% sensitivity; specificity 57–100%).	Test indicated only after a positive low-dose dexamethasone suppression test (see p. 121). Sensitivity and specificity depend on sampling time and diagnostic criteria. Measurement of urinary 17-hydroxycorticosteroids has been replaced in this test by measurement of serum cortisol. Bilateral sampling of the inferior petrosal sinuses for ACTH after administration of corticotrophin-releasing hormone has been used to identify the site of adenoma before surgery. Bertagna X et al. Cushing's disease. Best Pract Res Clin Endocrinol Metab 2009;23:607. [PMID: 19945026] Boscaro M et al. Approach to the patient with possible Cushing's syndrome. J Clin Endocrinol Metab 2009;94:3121. [PMID: 19734443] Pecori Giraldi F. Recent challenges in the diagnosis of Cushing's syndrome. Horm Res 2009;71(Suppl 1):123. [PMID: 19153521]

| Give 8 mg dexamethasone dose at 11:00 PM. At 8:00 AM, draw cortisol level. | | | |

Double-stranded DNA antibody		
Double-stranded-DNA antibody (ds-DNA Ab), serum <1:10 titer SST $$	IgG or IgM antibodies directed against host double-stranded DNA.	**Increased in:** Systemic lupus erythematosus (SLE; 60–70% sensitivity, 95% specificity) based on >1:10 titer. **Not increased in:** Drug-induced lupus.	Double-stranded DNA antibodies can be screened by an enzyme-linked immunosorbent assay (ELISA) assay, and, if positive, immunofluorescent antibody testing (IFA) is then performed. High titers are seen only in SLE. Titers of ds-DNA antibody correlate moderately well with occurrence of glomerulonephritis and renal disease activity. (See also Autoantibodies, Table 8–6.) Breda L et al. Laboratory tests in the diagnosis and follow-up of pediatric rheumatic diseases: an update. Semin Arthritis Rheum 2010;40:53. [PMID: 19246077] Munoz LE et al. Predictive value of anti-dsDNA autoantibodies: importance of the assay. Autoimmun Rev 2008;7:594. [PMID: 18603024]

	Drug abuse screen, urine		
Test/Range/Collection	Physiologic Basis	Interpretation	Comments
Drug abuse screen, urine (urine toxicology drug screen, urine drug screen) Negative $	Testing for drugs of abuse usually involves testing a single urine specimen for a number of drugs, eg, cocaine, opiates, barbiturates, amphetamines, benzodiazepines, cannabinoids, methadone, oxycodone, phencyclidine (PCP), tricyclic antidepressants. Screening tests are often immunoassays, which may not be specific for the tested drug. A positive test may warrant further confirmatory test by gas chromatography-mass spectrometry (GC/MS), the most widely accepted method of drug confirmation. Interpretation of results must take into account that urine concentrations can vary extensively with fluid intake and other biological variables. Adulteration of a urine specimen may also cause erroneous results.	**Positive in:** Chronic and casual drug users (sensitivity and specificity are assay-dependent).	It is important to know which drugs are included in the drug abuse screen and to understand that the test is qualitative and not quantitative. A single urine drug test detects only fairly recent drug use, and does not differentiate casual use from chronic drug use. The latter requires sequential drug testing and clinical evaluation. Urine drug testing does not determine the degree of impairment, the dose and frequency of drug taken, or the exact time of drug use. A negative result could be due to rapid metabolism/clearance of the drug, not taking drug as prescribed, or diversion of prescribed drugs to others. Cone EJ et al. Urine toxicology testing in chronic pain management. Postgrad Med 2009;121:91. [PMID: 19641275] Ropero-Miller JD et al. *Handbook of Workplace Drug Testing*, 2nd ed. Washington, DC: AACC Press, 2008. Tenore PL. Advanced urine toxicology testing. J Addict Dis. 2010;29:436. [PMID: 20924879]

Epstein-Barr virus antibodies		
Epstein-Barr virus antibodies, serum (EBV Ab) Negative SST $$	Antiviral capsid antibodies (anti-VCA) (IgM) often reach their peak at clinical presentation and last up to 3 months; anti-VCA IgG antibodies last for life. Early antigen antibodies (anti-EA) are next to develop, are most often positive at 1 month after presentation, typically last for 2–3 months, and may last up to 6 months in low titers. Anti-EA may also be found in some patients with Hodgkin disease, chronic lymphocytic leukemia, and some other malignancies. Anti-EB nuclear antigen (anti-EBNA) antibody begins to appear in a minority of patients in the third or fourth week but is uniformly present by 6 months.	**Increased in:** EB virus infection, infectious mononucleosis. Antibodies to the diffuse (D) form of antigen (detected in the cytoplasm and nucleus of infected cells) are greatly elevated in nasopharyngeal carcinoma. Antibodies to the restricted (R) form of antigen (detected only in the cytoplasm of infected cells) are greatly elevated in Burkitt lymphoma.	Most useful in diagnosing infectious mononucleosis in patients who have the clinical and hematologic criteria for the disease but who fail to develop the heterophile agglutinins (10%) (see Heterophile antibody). EBV antibodies cannot be used to diagnose "chronic" mononucleosis. Chronic fatigue syndrome is not caused by EBV. The best indicator of primary infection is a positive anti-VCA IgM (check for false positives caused by rheumatoid factor). Gulley ML et al. Laboratory assays for Epstein-Barr virus-related disease. J Mol Diagn 2008;10:279. [PMID: 18556771]

	Erythrocyte sedimentation rate		
Test/Range/Collection	**Physiologic Basis**	**Interpretation**	**Comments**
Erythrocyte sedimentation rate, whole blood (ESR) Males: <10 mm/h Females: <15 mm/h (laboratory-specific) Lavender $ Test must be run within 2 hours after sample collection.	In plasma, erythrocytes (red blood cells [RBCs]) usually settle slowly. However, if they aggregate for any reason (usually because of plasma proteins called acute-phase reactants, eg, fibrinogen), they settle rapidly. Sedimentation of RBCs occurs because their density is greater than plasma. ESR measures the distance in millimeters that erythrocytes fall during 1 hour.	**Increased in:** Infections (osteomyelitis, pelvic inflammatory disease (75%)), inflammatory disease (temporal arteritis, polymyalgia rheumatica, rheumatic fever), malignant neoplasms, paraproteinemias, anemia, pregnancy, chronic renal failure, GI disease (ulcerative colitis, regional ileitis). For endocarditis, sensitivity is approximately 93%. **Decreased in:** Polycythemia, sickle cell anemia, spherocytosis, anisocytosis, poikilocytosis, hypofibrinogenemia, hypogam-maglobulinemia, congestive heart failure, microcytosis, certain drugs (eg, high-dose corticosteroids).	There is often good correlation between ESR and C-reactive protein (CRP), but discordance between ESR and CRP has been noted in certain inflammatory disorders. Test is typically indicated for diagnosis and monitoring of temporal arteritis, systemic vasculitis and polymyalgia rheumatica. The test is not sensitive or specific for other conditions, although an extremely elevated ESR (eg, >100 mm/h) is useful in developing a rheumatic disease differential diagnosis. The ESR is higher in women, blacks, and older persons. A low value is of no diagnostic significance. The ESR should not be used to screen asymptomatic persons for disease because of its low sensitivity and specificity. Kale N et al. Diagnosis and management of giant cell arteritis: a review. Curr Opin Ophthalmol 2010;21:417. [PMID: 20811283] Keenan RT et al. Erythrocyte sedimentation rate and C-reactive protein levels are poorly coordinated with clinical measures of disease activity in rheumatoid arthritis, systemic lupus erythematosus and osteoarthritis patients. Clin Exp Rheumatol 2008;26:814. [PMID: 19032813] Rosa Neto NS et al. Screening tests for inflammatory activity: applications in rheumatology. Mod Rheumatol 2009;19:469. [PMID: 19697096] Wu AH et al. Antiquated tests within the clinical pathology laboratory. Am J Manag Care 2010;16:e220. [PMID: 21250398]

Erythropoietin		
Erythropoietin, serum or plasma (EPO) 5–30 mIU/mL [5–30 IU/L] SST, PPT $$$	Erythropoietin (EPO) is a glyco-protein hormone produced in the kidney (peritubular capillary endothelial cells) that induces RBC production by stimulating proliferation, differentiation, and maturation of erythroid precursors. Hypoxia is the usual stimulus for production of EPO. EPO has also been shown to have an important cytoprotective function in the neuronal and cardiovascular systems.	**Increased in:** Anemias associated with bone marrow hyporesponsiveness (aplastic anemia, iron deficiency anemia), hemolytic anemia, secondary polycythemia (high-altitude hypoxia, COPD, pulmonary fibrosis), EPO-producing tumors (cerebellar hemangioblastomas, pheochromocytomas, renal tumors), kidney transplant rejection, pregnancy, polycystic kidney disease, treatment with recombinant human EPO. **Decreased in:** Anemia of chronic disease, renal failure, inflammatory states, primary polycythemia (polycythemia vera) (39%), HIV infection with AZT treatment.	EPO levels are useful in differentiating primary from secondary polycythemia and in detecting recurrence of EPO-producing tumors. See diagnostic evaluation of polycythemia (Figure 9–21). Because virtually all patients with severe anemia due to chronic renal failure respond to EPO therapy, pre-therapy EPO levels are not necessary. Patients receiving recombinant human EPO as chronic therapy should have iron studies performed routinely. Landolfi R et al. Polycythemia vera. Intern Emerg Med 2010;5:375. [PMID: 20237866] Lippi G. Thrombotic complications of erythropoiesis-stimulating agents. Semin Thromb Hemost 2010;36:537. [PMID: 20632251] Marsden JT. Erythropoietin-measurement and clinical applications. Ann Clin Biochem 2006;43:97. [PMID: 16536911]

	Estradiol

Test/Range/Collection	Physiologic Basis	Interpretation	Comments
Estradiol (E2), serum Adult males: 10–40 pg/mL Adult females: Premenopausal: 30–400 pg/mL* Postmenopausal: 2–20 pg/mL Adult males: 37–147 pmol/L Adult females: Premenopausal: 110–1480 pmol/L* Postmenopausal: 7–73 pmol/L (*E2 levels vary widely through the menstrual cycle.) SST, red $$$$	In women, estradiol is produced primarily by the granulosa cells of the ovaries by aromatization of androstenedione to estrone, followed by conversion of estrone to estradiol by 17β-hydroxysteroid dehydrogenase. Smaller amounts of estradiol are also produced by the adrenal cortex and some peripheral tissues (eg, fat cells), and by the testes (in men). E2 is the predominant sex hormone in females. It is responsible for the development of secondary sex characteristics (eg, breast development). E2 levels in premenopausal women fluctuate during the menstrual cycle. They are low at menstruation (<50 pg/mL), rise with follicular development (peak 200–400 pg/mL), drop briefly at ovulation, rise again during the luteal phase, and then drop to menstrual levels. During pregnancy, estrogen levels, including estradiol, rise steadily toward term.	**Increased in:** Feminization, gynecomastia, precocious puberty, estrogen-producing tumors, hepatic cirrhosis, hyperthyroidism. **Decreased in:** Primary and secondary hypogonadism.	E2 measurement is of value, together with gonadotropins, in evaluating menstrual and fertility problems in adult females. It is also useful in the evaluation of feminization (including gynecomastia) and estrogen-producing tumors in males. E2 test is used in therapeutic monitoring of human menopausal gonadotropin therapy, estrogen replacement therapy, and antiestrogen therapy (eg, aromatase inhibitor therapy). It is also used for monitoring ovarian hyperstimulation during in vitro fertilization treatment. Johnson RE et al. Gynecomastia: pathophysiology, evaluation, and management. Mayo Clin Proc 2009;84:1010. [PMID: 19880691] Meczekalski B et al. Hypoestrogenism in young women and its influence on bone mass density. Gynecol Endocrinol 2010;26:652. [PMID: 20504098] Shulman DI et al. Use of aromatase inhibitors in children and adolescents with disorders of growth and adolescent development. Pediatrics 2008;121:e975. [PMID: 18381525]

Ethanol		
Ethanol, serum or plasma (EtOH) 0 mg/dL [mmol/L] SST, red, lavender, PPT $$ Do not use alcohol swab. Do not remove stopper.	Measures serum level of ethyl alcohol (ethanol).	**Present in:** Ethanol ingestion.	Whole blood alcohol concentrations are about 15% lower than serum concentrations. Each 100 mg/dL of ethanol contributes about 22 mosm/kg to serum osmolality (see Table 8–15). Legal intoxication in many states is defined as >80 mg/dL (>17 mmol/L). Lee H et al. Alcohol-induced blackout. Int J Environ Res Public Health 2009;6:2783. [PMID: 20049223] Leeman RF et al. Ethanol consumption: how should we measure it? Achieving consilience between human and animal phenotypes. Addict Biol 2010;15:109. [PMID: 20148775]

	Factor assays

Test/Range/Collection	Physiologic Basis	Interpretation	Comments
Factor assays (coagulation factors II, V, VII, VIII, IX, X, XI, and XII) Blood Blue 50–150% $$$ Deliver immediately to laboratory on ice. Stable for 2 hours. Freeze if assay is delayed >2 hours.	The partial thromboplastin time (PTT) and prothrombin time (PT) are the bases for factor assays. Factors VIII, IX, XI, and XII are PTT-based. Factors II, V, VII, and X are PT-based. The factor assay is based on the ability of patient plasma to correct the PTT or PT of specific factor-deficient plasma. Quantitative results are obtained from comparing with a standard curve made from dilutions of normal reference plasma.	**Decreased in:** Hereditary factor deficiency (eg, hemophilia A, B); acquired factor deficiency secondary to acquired factor-specific inhibitor (eg, factor VIII inhibitor), liver disease (except factor VIII) and DIC (consumptive coagulopathy); vitamin K deficiency and warfarin therapy (II, VII, IX, and X), etc. Severe factor II deficiency may occur in rare patients with lupus anticoagulant. Acquired factor X deficiency may occur in patients with amyloidosis. Patients with von Willebrand disease may have low factor VIII levels.	Although factor assays are typically PTT- or PT-based, chromogenic and immunogenic factor assays are also available for some factors including factors X and VIII. Heparin, hirudin, and argatroban can act as inhibitors and interfere with specific factor assays. Factor assay result needs to be interpreted with caution if non-parrellelism is present (eg, lupus anticoagulant, factor-specific inhibitor). Chromogenic assay is more reliable in this setting. Brenner B et al. Vitamin K-dependent coagulation factors deficiency. Semin Thromb Hemost 2009;35:439. [PMID: 19598072] Marbet GA. Quantification of coagulation factors and inhibitors. Still a special task. Hamostaseologie 2006;26:38. [PMID: 16444320] Verbruggen B et al. Improvements in factor VIII inhibitor detection: from Bethesda to Nijmegen. Semin Thromb Hemost 2009;35:752. [PMID: 20169511]

Factor II (prothrombin) mutation		
Factor II (prothrombin) G20210A mutation Blood Lavender $$$$	The factor II (prothrombin) 20210A mutation is a common genetic risk factor for thrombosis and is associated with elevated prothrombin levels. Higher concentrations of prothrombin lead to increased rates of thrombin generation, resulting in excessive growth of fibrin clots. It is an autosomal dominant disorder, with heterozygotes being at a 3- to 11-fold greater risk for thrombosis. Although homozygosity is rare, inheritance of two G20210A mutations would further increase the risk for developing thrombosis. The estimated frequency of factor II G20210A in white populations is between 1% and 6%. Prothrombin 20210 mutation is often ordered along with factor V Leiden analysis to help diagnose the cause of recurrent venous thrombosis and/or thromboembolism (VTE).	**Positive in:** Hypercoagulability secondary to factor II (prothrombin) G20210A mutation (sensitivity and specificity approach 100%).	If a patient is heterozygous for both the prothrombin G20210A and the factor V Leiden mutation, the combined heterozygosity leads to an earlier onset of thrombosis and tends to be more severe than single-gene heterozygosity. Polymerase chain reaction (PCR) is the most commonly used method for the detection of factor II G20210A mutation. Emadi A et al. Analytic validity of genetic tests to identify factor V Leiden and prothrombin G20210A. Am J Hematol 2010;85:264. [PMID: 20162544] Kyrle PA et al. Risk assessment for recurrent venous thrombosis. Lancet 2010;376:2032. [PMID: 21131039] Segal JB et al. Predictive value of factor V Leiden and prothrombin G20210A in adults with venous thromboembolism and in family members of those with a mutation: a systematic review. JAMA 2009;301:2472. [PMID: 19531787]

Test/Range/Collection	Physiologic Basis	Interpretation	Comments
Factor V (Leiden) mutation Blood Lavender $$$$	The Leiden mutation is a single nucleotide base mutation (G1691A) in the factor V gene, leading to an amino acid substitution (Arg506Glu) at one of the sites where coagulation factor V is cleaved by activated protein C (APC). This mutation results in a substantially reduced anticoagulant response to APC, because factor Va$_{Leiden}$ is inactivated about 10 times more slowly than normal factor Va. The frequency of factor V$_{Leiden}$ in white populations is between 2–15%. Factor V mutations may be present in up to half of the cases of unexplained venous thrombosis and are seen in more than 90% of patients with APC resistance.	**Positive in:** Hypercoagulability secondary to factor V$_{Leiden}$ mutation (sensitivity and specificity approach 100%).	The factor V Leiden mutation is the most common inherited risk factor for thrombosis and accounts for >90% of cases with APC resistance. The presence of the mutation is only a risk factor for thrombosis, not an absolute marker for disease. Homozygotes have a 50- to 100-fold increase in risk of thrombosis (relative to the general population), and heterozygotes have a 7-fold increase in risk. Polymerase chain reaction (PCR) is the most commonly used method for the detection of the Leiden mutation of factor V. Emadi A et al. Analytic validity of genetic tests to identify factor V Leiden and prothrombin G20210A. Am J Hematol 2010;85:264. [PMID: 20162544] Kyrle PA et al. Risk assessment for recurrent venous thrombosis. Lancet 2010;376:2032. [PMID: 21131039] Segal JB et al. Predictive value of factor V Leiden and prothrombin G20210A in adults with venous thromboembolism and in family members of those with a mutation: a systematic review. JAMA 2009;301:2472. [PMID: 19531787]

Factor VIII assay			
Factor VIII assay, plasma 50–150% of normal (varies with age) Blue $$$ Deliver immediately to laboratory on ice. Stable for 2 hours. Freeze if assay is delayed for >2 hours. $$$	Measures activity of factor VIII (antihemophilic factor), a key factor of the intrinsic clotting cascade. Clotting-based assay is commonly used. For patients with lupus anticoagulant, factor activity may be falsely low due to nonparallelism.	**Increased in:** Inflammatory states (acute-phase reactant), last trimester of pregnancy, oral contraceptives. **Decreased in:** Hemophilia A, von Willebrand disease (type 1, 3, 2N), DIC, acquired factor VIII inhibitor (acquired hemophilia).	Normal hemostasis requires at least 25% of factor VIII activity. Symptomatic hemophiliacs usually have levels ≤5%. Disease levels are defined as severe (<1%), moderate (1–5%), and mild (>5%). Factor VIII assays are used to guide replacement therapy in patients with hemophilia. Factor deficiency can be distinguished from factor inhibitor by an inhibitor screen and by nonparallelism on factor assays. Goodeve AC et al. Haemophilia A and von Willebrand's disease. Haemophilia 2010;16(Suppl 5):79. [PMID: 20590861] Kershaw G et al. Laboratory identification of factor inhibitors: the perspective of a large tertiary hemophilia center. Semin Thromb Hemost 2009;35:760. [PMID: 20169512] Spreafico M et al. Combined factor V and factor VIII deficiency. Semin Thromb Hemost 2009;35:390. [PMID: 19598067]

	Fecal fat

Test/Range/Collection	Physiologic Basis	Interpretation	Comments
Fecal fat, stool Random: <60 droplets of fat/high power field 72 hour: <7 g/d $$$ Qualitative: Random stool sample is adequate. Quantitative: Dietary fat should be at least 50–150 g/d for 2 days before collection. Then all stools should be collected for 72 hours and refrigerated.	In healthy people, most dietary fat is completely absorbed in the small intestine. Normal small intestinal lining, bile acids, and pancreatic enzymes are required for normal fat absorption.	**Increased in:** Malabsorption from small bowel disease (regional enteritis, celiac disease, tropical sprue), pancreatic insufficiency, diarrhea with or without fat malabsorption.	A random, qualitative fecal fat (so-called Sudan stain) is useful only if positive. Furthermore, it does not correlate well with quantitative measurements. Sudan stain appears to detect triglycerides and lipolytic by-products, whereas 72-hour fecal fat measures fatty acids from a variety of sources, including phospholipids, cholesteryl esters, and triglycerides. The quantitative method can be used to measure the degree of fat malabsorption initially and then after a therapeutic intervention. A normal quantitative stool fat reliably rules out pancreatic insufficiency and most forms of generalized small intestine disease. Besides fecal fat, fecal pancreatic elastase (see p. 225) can be used to evaluate pancreatic insufficiency with excellent sensitivity. Hammer HF. Pancreatic exocrine insufficiency: diagnostic evaluation and replacement therapy with pancreatic enzymes. Dig Dis 2010;28:339. [PMID: 20814209] Nandhakumar N et al. Interpretations: how to use faecal elastase testing. Arch Dis Child Educ Pract Ed 2010;95:119. [PMID: 20688857] Pezzilli R. Chronic pancreatitis: maldigestion, intestinal ecology and intestinal inflammation. World J Gastroenterol 2009;15:1673. [PMID: 19360910]

Fecal occult blood tests		
Fecal occult blood tests, stool Negative $ Dietary (meat, fish, turnips, horseradish) and medication (aspirin, nonsteroidal anti-inflammatory drugs) restrictions are often recommended to reduce false positive results, but available evidence does not suggest large effect on positivity rates in non-rehydrated testing. To avoid false-negatives, patients should avoid taking vitamin C. Patient collects two specimens from three consecutive bowel movements.	Measures blood in the stool using gum guaiac as an indicator reagent (gFOBT). In the Hemoccult test, gum guaiac is impregnated in a test paper that is smeared with stool using an applicator. Hydrogen peroxide is used as a developer solution. The resultant phenolic oxidation of guaiac in the presence of blood in the stool yields a blue color.	**Positive in:** Upper GI disease (peptic ulcer, gastritis, variceal bleeding, esophageal and gastric cancer), lower GI disease (diverticulosis, colonic polyps, colorectal cancer, inflammatory bowel disease, vascular ectasias, hemorrhoids).	Although fecal occult blood testing is an accepted screening test for colorectal cancer, the sensitivity and specificity of an individual test are low. The usefulness of fecal occult blood testing after digital rectal examination is low. Three randomized controlled trials have shown reductions in colon cancer mortality with yearly (33% reduction) or biennial (15–21% reduction) testing. About 1000 must be screened for 10 years to save one life. Quantitative fecal immunochemical test (FIT) is superior to gFOBT because there are no dietary and drug restrictions and it is more amenable to standardization and quality control. FIT screening is now preferred to gFOBT screening. Allison JE. FIT: A valuable but underutilized screening test for colorectal cancer—it's time for a change. Am J Gastroenterol 2010;105:2026. [PMID: 20816351]. U.S. Preventive Services Task Force. Screening for colorectal cancer: U.S. Preventive Services Task Force recommendation statement. Ann Intern Med 2008;149:627. [PMID: 18838716]. van Dam L et al. Performance improvements of stool-based screening tests. Best Pract Res Clin Gastroenterol 2010;24:479. [PMID: 20833351]

	Ferritin		
Test/Range/Collection	**Physiologic Basis**	**Interpretation**	**Comments**
Ferritin, serum or plasma Males: 16–300 ng/mL [mcg/L] Females: 4–161 ng/mL [mcg/L] SST, PPT, lavender/pink, green $$	Ferritin is the body's major iron storage protein. The serum ferritin level correlates with total body iron stores. The test is used to detect iron deficiency, to monitor response to iron therapy, and, in iron overload states, to monitor iron removal therapy. It is also used to predict homozygosity for hemochromatosis in relatives of affected patients. In the absence of liver disease and infection/inflammation, it is a more sensitive test for iron deficiency than serum iron and iron-binding capacity (transferrin saturation).	**Increased in:** Iron overload (hemochromatosis, hemosiderosis), acute or chronic liver disease, alcoholism, various malignancies (eg, leukemia, Hodgkin disease), chronic inflammatory disorders (eg, rheumatoid arthritis, adult Still disease), thalassemia minor, hyperthyroidism, HIV infection, non-insulin–dependent diabetes mellitus, and postpartum state. **Decreased in:** Iron deficiency (60–75%).	Serum ferritin is clinically useful in distinguishing between iron deficiency anemia (serum ferritin levels diminished) and anemia of chronic disease or thalassemia (levels usually normal or elevated). Test of choice for diagnosis of iron deficiency anemia. **Ferritin (ng/mL)** / **Likelihood Ratio (LR) for Iron Deficiency** >100 — 0.08 45–100 — 0.54 35–45 — 1.83 25–35 — 2.54 15–25 — 8.83 ≤15 — 52.00 Liver disease and conditions with acute phase response increase serum ferritin levels and may mask the diagnosis of iron deficiency. Serum soluble transferrin receptor (sTR) measurement is helpful in determining iron deficiency status. Serum ferritin < 1000 ng/mL may predict absence of cirrhosis in hemochromatosis. Bermejo F et al. A guide to diagnosis of iron deficiency and iron deficiency anemia in digestive diseases. World J Gastroenterol 2009;15:4638. [PMID: 19787826] Pasricha SR et al. Diagnosis and management of iron deficiency anaemia: a clinical update. Med J Aust 2010;193:525. [PMID: 21034387] Schmitt B et al. Screening primary care patients for hereditary hemochromatosis with transferrin saturation and serum ferritin level: systematic review for the American College of Physicians. Ann Intern Med 2005;143:522. [PMID: 16204165]

α-Fetoprotein

| α-Fetoprotein, serum (AFP)

0–15 ng/mL [mcg/L]

SST

$$

Avoid hemolysis. | α-fetoprotein (AFP) is a glycoprotein produced both early in fetal life and by some tumors. Serum AFP is a useful tumor marker. | **Increased in:** Hepatocellular carcinoma (72%), massive hepatic necrosis (74%), viral hepatitis (34%), chronic active hepatitis (29%), cirrhosis (11%), regional enteritis (5%), benign gynecologic diseases (22%), testicular carcinoma (embryonal) (70%), teratocarcinoma (64%), teratoma (37%), ovarian carcinoma (57%), endometrial carcinoma (50%), cervical cancer (53%), pancreatic cancer (23%), gastric cancer (18%), and colon cancer (5%).

Negative in: Seminoma. | The test is not sensitive or specific enough to be used as a general screening test for hepatocellular carcinoma (HCC). However, screening may be justified in populations at very high risk for hepatocellular cancer. Combined testing of AFP and des-gamma-carboxyprothrombin (DCP) increases the sensitivity of HCC diagnosis.

In hepatocellular cancer or germ cell tumors associated with elevated AFP, the test may be helpful in detecting recurrence after therapy.

AFP is also used to screen pregnant women at 15–20 weeks gestation for possible fetal neural tube defects. AFP level in maternal serum or amniotic fluid is compared with levels expected at a given gestational age.

Inagaki Y et al. Clinical and molecular insights into the hepatocellular carcinoma tumor marker des-gamma-carboxyprothrombin. Liver Int 2011;31:22. [PMID: 20874726]
Krantz DA et al. Screening for open neural tube defects. Clin Lab Med 2010;30:721. [PMID: 20638584]
Sturgeon CM et al. National Academy of Clinical Biochemistry Laboratory Medicine Practice Guidelines for use of tumor markers in liver, bladder, cervical, and gastric cancers. Clin Chem 2010;56:e1. [PMID: 20207771] |

Test/Range/Collection	Physiologic Basis	Interpretation	Comments
Fibrinogen	Fibrinogen is synthesized in the	**Increased in:** Inflammatory	Fibrinogen assay is typically performed in the
(functional), plasma	liver and has a half-life of about	states (acute-phase reactant), use	investigation of unexplained bleeding, prolonged PT
	4 days.	of oral contraceptives, pregnancy,	or PTT, or as part of a DIC panel.
150–400 mg/dL	Thrombin cleaves fibrinogen to	postmenopausal women, smok-	An elevated fibrinogen level has also been used as a
	form insoluble fibrin monomers,	ing, and exercise.	predictor of arterial thrombotic events.
[1.5–4.0 g/L]	which polymerize to form a clot.	**Decreased in:** Acquired defi-	Fibrinogen is generally measured by a clotting-based
		ciency: liver disease, consump-	functional (activity) assay. The Clauss assay, based
Panic: <75 mg/dL		tive coagulopathies such as DIC,	on a high concentration of thrombin added to diluted
		and thrombolytic therapy; heredi-	patient plasma, is the most commonly used method.
Blue		tary deficiency, resulting in an	Direct thrombin inhibitor therapy may interfere with
		abnormal (dysfibrinogenemia),	the assay.
$$		reduced (hypofibrinogenemia), or	Diagnosis of dysfibrinogenemia depends upon the
		absent fibrinogen	discrepancy between antigen (eg, enzyme-linked
		(afibrinogenemia).	immunosorbent assay, ELISA) and activity levels.
			Levi M et al. Guidelines for the diagnosis and management of
			disseminated intravascular coagulation. British Committee
			for Standards in Haematology. Br J Haematol 2009;145:24.
			[PMID: 19222477]
			Takagi H et al. Plasma fibrinogen and D-dimer concentra-
			tions are associated with the presence of abdominal aortic
			aneurysm: a systematic review and meta-analysis. Eur J Vasc
			Endovasc Surg 2009;38:273. [PMID: 19560946]

Fibrinogen (functional)

Fluorescent treponemal antibody-absorbed		
Fluorescent *Treponema pallidum* antibody-absorbed (FTA-ABS), serum Nonreactive SST $$	Detects specific antibodies against *Treponema pallidum*. Patient's serum is first diluted with nonpathogenic treponemal antigens (to bind nonspecific antibodies). The absorbed serum is placed on a slide that contains fixed *T. pallidum*. Fluorescein-labeled antihuman gamma globulin is then added to bind to and visualize (under a fluorescence microscope) the patient's antibody on treponemes.	**Reactive in:** Syphilis: primary (95%), secondary (100%), late latent (100%); also rarely positive in collagen vascular diseases in the presence of antinuclear antibody.	Historically, this test was used to confirm a reactive nontreponemal screening serologic test for syphilis such as RPR or VDRL. A new syphilis testing algorithm using treponemal tests for screening and nontreponemal serologic tests for confirmation has been proposed (see also Table 8–24). Once positive, the FTA-ABS may remain positive for life. However, one study found that at 36 months after treatment, 24% of patients had nonreactive FTA-ABS tests. Seña AC et al. Novel *Treponema pallidum* serologic tests: a paradigm shift in syphilis screening for the 21st century. Clin Infect Dis 2010;51:700. [PMID: 20687840] Tucker JD et al. Accelerating worldwide syphilis screening through rapid testing: a systematic review. Lancet Infect Dis 2010;10:381. [PMID: 20510278]

	Folic acid (RBC)		
Test/Range/Collection	Physiologic Basis	Interpretation	Comments
Folic acid (RBC), whole blood 165–760 ng/mL [370–1720 nmol/L] Lavender $$$	Folate is a vitamin necessary for methyl group transfer in thymidine formation, and hence DNA synthesis. Deficiency can result in megaloblastic anemia. The naturally occurring folate polyglutamates are hydrolyzed to monoglutamate forms before absorption by the small intestine. In the liver, folate monoglutamates are converted to N^5-methyltetrahydrofolate (MeTHF), which is excreted in bile. This methylated form of folate is reabsorbed from the gut but not taken up by the liver and therefore becomes the major circulating form of folate. Red cell folate has been considered ever more important because it reflects tissue folate level. Evidence from the literature indicates that serum/plasma folate measurements provide equivalent information when determining whether folate deficiency is present.	**Decreased in:** Tissue folate deficiency (from dietary folate deficiency), vitamin B_{12} deficiency (50–60%, since cellular uptake of folate depends on vitamin B_{12}).	A low red cell folate level may indicate either folate or vitamin B_{12} deficiency. A therapeutic trial of folate (and not red cell or serum folate testing) is indicated when the clinical and dietary history is strongly suggestive of folate deficiency and the peripheral smear shows hypersegmented polymorphonuclear leukocytes. However, the possibility of vitamin B_{12} deficiency must always be considered in the setting of megaloblastic anemia, since folate therapy treats the hematologic, but not the neurologic, sequelae of vitamin B_{12} deficiency. Folate deficiency has become a rare event in developed countries, and routine folate measurement is not recommended. Janus J et al. Evaluation of anemia in children. Am Fam Physician 2010;81:1462. [PMID: 20540485] Joelson DW et al. Diminished need for folate measurements among indigent populations in the post folic acid supplementation era. Arch Pathol Lab Med 2007;131:477. [PMID: 17516752] Kaferle J et al. Evaluation of macrocytosis. Am Fam Physician 2009;79:203. [PMID: 19202968]

Follicle-stimulating hormone

Follicle-stimulating hormone (FSH), serum or plasma
 	
Males: 1–10 mIU/mL
 	
Females: (mIU/mL)
  Follicular 4–13
  Luteal 2–13
  Midcycle 5–22
  Postmenopausal 20–138
  (laboratory-specific)
 	
SST, PPT, green
 	
$$
	FSH is stimulated by the hypothalamic hormone GnRH and is then secreted from the anterior pituitary in a pulsatile fashion. Levels rise during the preovulatory phase of the menstrual cycle and then decline. FSH is necessary for normal pubertal development and fertility in males and females.	**Increased in:** Primary (ovarian) gonadal failure, ovarian or testicular agenesis, castration, postmenopause, Klinefelter syndrome, drugs.
		
		Decreased in: Hypothalamic disorders, pituitary disorders, pregnancy, anorexia nervosa. Drugs: corticosteroids, oral contraceptives.
			Test indicated in the work-up of amenorrhea in women (see Amenorrhea algorithm, Figure 9–4); and delayed puberty, impotence, or infertility in men. Impotence work-up should begin with serum testosterone measurement. Basal FSH levels in premenopausal women depend on age, smoking history, and menstrual cycle length and regularity.
			Because of its variability, FSH is an unreliable guide to menopausal status during the transition into menopause.
			
			Deligeoroglou E et al. Evaluation and management of adolescent amenorrhea. Ann NY Acad Sci 2010;1205:23. [PMID: 20840249]
			Sills ES et al. Ovarian reserve screening in infertility: practical applications and theoretical directions for research. Eur J Obstet Gynecol Reprod Biol 2009;146:30. [PMID: 19487066]
			Su HI et al. Hormone changes associated with the menopausal transition. Minerva Ginecol 2009;61:483. [PMID: 19942836]

Test/Range/Collection	Physiologic Basis	Interpretation	Comments
Free Erythrocyte protoporphyrin, free, whole blood (FEP) <35 mcg/dL (method-dependent) Lavender $$$	Protoporphyrin is produced in the next to last step of heme biosynthesis. In the last step, iron is incorporated into protoporphyrin to produce heme. Enzyme deficiencies (ferrochelatase deficiency or inhibition), lack of iron, or presence of interfering substances (lead) can disrupt this process and cause elevated FEP as well as ZPP (zinc protoporphyrin).	**Increased in:** Decreased iron incorporation into heme (iron deficiency, anemia of chronic disease and chronic lead poisoning), erythropoietic protoporphyria.	FEP can be used to screen for lead poisoning in children provided that iron deficiency has been ruled out. However, FEP is not elevated until lead levels are >30 mcg/dL (1.45 mmol/L). Red cell ZPP is considered a better screening test for mild lead toxicity. Test does not discriminate between uroporphyrin, coproporphyrin, and protoporphyrin, but protoporphyrin is the predominant porphyrin measured. Iolascon A et al. Mutations in the gene encoding DMT1: clinical presentation and treatment. Semin Hematol 2009;46:358. [PMID: 19786204]
Fructosamine, serum or plasma 0.16–0.27 mmol/L SST, lavender, green $	Glycation of albumin produces fructosamine, a less expensive marker of glycemic control than HbA1c. The test is particularly useful if rapid monitoring of glycemic control is required (eg, during pregnancy) or if red cell life span is altered (eg, hemolysis, blood loss, kidney diseases).	**Increased in:** Diabetes mellitus, gestational diabetes.	Fructosamine correlates well with fasting plasma glucose (r = 0.74) but cannot be used to predict precisely the HbA1c. Fisher SJ. Commentary. Clin Chem 2011;57:157. [PMID: 21278360] Youssef D et al. Fructosamine—an underutilized tool in diabetes management: case report and literature review. Tenn Med 2008;101:31. [PMID: 19024248]

Gamma-glutamyl transpeptidase		
Gamma-glutamyl transpeptidase (GGT), serum or plasma 9–85 U/L [0.15–1.42 mckat/L] (laboratory-specific) SST, PPT, green $	GGT is an enzyme present in liver, kidney, and pancreas. It is induced by alcohol intake and is an extremely sensitive indicator of liver disease, particularly alcoholic liver disease.	**Increased in:** Liver disease: acute viral or toxic hepatitis, chronic or subacute hepatitis, alcoholic hepatitis, cirrhosis, biliary tract obstruction (intra-hepatic or extrahepatic), primary or metastatic liver neoplasm, and mononucleosis. Drugs (by enzyme induction): phenytoin, carbamazepine barbiturates, alcohol.	GGT is useful in follow-up of alcoholics undergoing treatment because the test is sensitive to modest alcohol intake. GGT is elevated in 90% of patients with liver disease. Elevated GGT activity has prognostic significance. GGT is used to confirm hepatic origin of elevated serum alkaline phosphatase. Aragon G et al. When and how to evaluate mildly elevated liver enzymes in apparently healthy patients. Cleve Clin J Med 2010;77:195. [PMID: 20200170] Targher G. Elevated serum gamma-glutamyltransferase activity is associated with increased risk of mortality, incident type 2 diabetes, cardiovascular events, chronic kidney disease and cancer—a narrative review. Clin Chem Lab Med 2010;48:147. [PMID: 19943812]

	Gastrin

Test/Range/Collection	Physiologic Basis	Interpretation	Comments
Gastrin, serum <100 pg/mL [ng/L] SST $$ Overnight fasting required.	Gastrin is secreted from G cells in the stomach antrum and stimulates acid secretion from the gastric parietal cells. Values fluctuate throughout the day but are lowest in the early morning.	**Increased in:** Gastrinoma (Zollinger-Ellison syndrome) (80–93% sensitivity), antral G cell hyperplasia, hypochlorhydria, achlorhydria, chronic atrophic gastritis, pernicious anemia. Drugs: antacids, cimetidine, and other H$_2$ blockers; omeprazole and other proton pump inhibitors. **Decreased in:** Antrectomy with vagotomy.	Gastrin is the first-line test for determining whether a patient with active ulcer disease has a gastrinoma. Gastric acid analysis is not indicated. Before interpreting an elevated level, be sure that the patient is not taking antacids, H$_2$ blockers, or proton pump inhibitors. Both fasting and post-secretin infusion levels may be required for diagnosis. Murugesan SV et al. Review article: Strategies to determine whether hypergastrinaemia is due to Zollinger-Ellison syndrome rather than a more common benign cause. Aliment Pharmacol Ther 2009;29:1055. [PMID: 19226290] Osefo N et al. Gastric acid hypersecretory states: recent insights and advances. Curr Gastroenterol Rep 2009;11:433. [PMID: 19903418]

Glomerular filtration rate, estimated		
Glomerular filtration rate, estimated (eGFR) (see Creatinine, serum or plasma) >60 mL/min/1.73 m²	The National Kidney Disease Education Program (NKDEP) recommends the use of the estimation of GFR from serum creatinine in adults (>18 years) with chronic kidney disease (CKD) and those at risk for CKD (diabetes mellitus, hypertension, and family history of kidney failure). Estimated GFR (eGFR) provides a clinically more useful measure of kidney function than creatinine alone. The recommended Modification of Diet in Renal Disease (MDRD) study equation (http://www.nkdep.nih.gov/lab-evaluation/gfr/estimating.shtml) involves the serum creatinine, urea nitrogen, and albumin concentrations, and the age, sex, and race of the patient. The new Chronic Kidney Disease Epidemiology Collaboration (CKD-EPI) equation (http://www.nephrologynow.com/publications/a-new-equation-to-estimate-glomerular-filtration-rate) can also be used to calculate the eGFR.	**Decreased in** CKD, kidney failure.	CKD is defined as either kidney damage or GFR <60 mL/min/1.73 m² for at least 3 months. Kidney damage is defined as pathologic abnormalities or markers of damage, including abnormalities in blood or urine tests (eg, albuminuria) or imaging studies. Kidney failure is defined as GFR <15 mL/min. Clinical laboratories are not routinely using the recommended equation, and its calculation may be too complex for direct clinical use. Levey AS et al. A new equation to estimate glomerular filtration rate. Ann Intern Med 2009;150:604. [PMID: 19414839]

Glucagon

Test/Range/Collection	Physiologic Basis	Interpretation	Comments
Glucagon, plasma 20–100 pg/mL [20–100 ng/L] (age- and laboratory-specific) Lavender $$$$ Fasting specimen collected in pre-chilled lavender tube is required. After drawing specimen, chill tube in wet ice for 10 minutes before centrifugation.	Glucagon is a peptide hormone secreted by the pancreatic alpha islet cells. Glucagon secretion is stimulated by low levels of blood glucose. It stimulates the production of glucose in the liver by glycogenolysis. Excessive glucagon secretion can lead to hyperglycemia. Glucagon-secreting tumors are associated with necrolytic migratory erythema, diabetes mellitus, thrombosis, and neuropsychiatric features.	**Increased in:** Glucagonoma and other glucagon-secreting tumors, familial hyperglucagonemia. **Decreased in:** Diabetes mellitus (type 1) with pronounced hypoglycemic features, chronic pancreatitis, post-pancreatectomy.	Useful as a tumor marker for diagnosis and follow-up of glucagon-secreting tumors. Results obtained with different glucagon assays can differ substantially. Different glucagon assays may exhibit variable cross-reactivity with different isoforms of glucagon, not all of which are biologically active. Serial measurements should, therefore, always be performed using the same assay. Kindmark H et al. Endocrine pancreatic tumors with glucagon hypersecretion: a retrospective study of 23 cases during 20 years. Med Oncol 2007;24:330. [PMID: 17873310] Öberg K. Pancreatic endocrine tumors. Semin Oncol 2010;37:594. [PMID: 21167379]

Glucose		
Glucose, serum or plasma 60–110 mg/dL [3.3–6.1 mmol/L] **Panic:** <40 or >500 mg/dL SST, PPT, gray $ Overnight fasting usually required.	Normally, the glucose concentration in extracellular fluid is closely regulated so that a source of energy is readily available to tissues and so that no glucose is excreted in the urine.	**Increased in:** Diabetes mellitus, Cushing syndrome (10–15%), chronic pancreatitis (30%). Drugs: corticosteroids, phenytoin, estrogen, thiazides. **Decreased in:** Pancreatic islet cell disease with increased insulin, insulinoma, adrenocortical insufficiency, hypopituitarism, diffuse liver disease, malignancy (adrenocortical, stomach, fibrosarcoma), infant of a diabetic mother, enzyme deficiency diseases (eg, galactosemia). Drugs: insulin, ethanol, propranolol; sulfonylureas, tolbutamide, and other oral hypoglycemic agents.	Diagnosis of diabetes mellitus requires a fasting plasma glucose of >126 mg/dL (7.0 mmol/L) on more than one occasion, a casual plasma glucose level ≥200 mg/dL (11.1 mmol/L) or HbA1c ≥ 6.5% along with symptoms of diabetes. Hypoglycemia is defined as a glucose of <50 mg/dL in men and <40 mg/dL in women. While random serum glucose levels correlate with home glucose monitoring results (weekly mean capillary glucose values), there is wide fluctuation within individuals. Thus, glycosylated hemoglobin levels are favored to monitor glycemic control. The American Diabetes Association recommends that adults age 45 years or older should be evaluated for diabetes by measuring fasting glucose levels. Long-term outcome studies are needed to provide evidence for this recommendation. Akhtar S et al. Scientific principles and clinical implications of perioperative glucose regulation and control. Anesth Analg 2010;110:478. [PMID: 20081134] American Diabetes Association. Diagnosis and classification of diabetes mellitus. Diabetes Care 2006;29(Suppl 1):S43. [PMID: 16373932] Moghissi ES. Reexamining the evidence for inpatient glucose control: new recommendations for glycemic targets. Am J Health Syst Pharm 2010;67(16 Suppl 8):S3. [PMID: 20689151]

	Glucose tolerance test		
Test/Range/Collection	**Physiologic Basis**	**Interpretation**	**Comments**
Glucose tolerance test (oral), serum Fasting: <100 mg/dL 1-hour: <200 mg/dL 2-hour: <140 mg/dL [Fasting: <5.6 mmol/L 1-hour: <11.0 mmol/L 2-hour: <7.7 mmol/L] SST, gray $$ Subjects should receive a 150- to 200-g/d carbohydrate diet for at least 3 days before the test. A 75-g glucose dose is dissolved in 300 mL of water for adults (1.75 g/kg for children) and given after an overnight fast. Serial determinations of plasma or serum venous blood glucoses are obtained at baseline, 1 hour, and 2 hours.	Oral glucose tolerance test (OGTT) determines the ability of a patient to respond appropriately to a glucose load.	**Increased glucose rise (decreased glucose tolerance) in:** Diabetes mellitus, impaired glucose tolerance, gestational diabetes, severe liver disease, hyperthyroidism, stress (infection), increased absorption of glucose from GI tract (hyperthyroidism, gastrectomy, gastroenterostomy, vagotomy, excess glucose intake), Cushing syndrome, pheochromocytoma. Drugs: diuretics, oral contraceptives, glucocorticoids, nicotinic acid, phenytoin. **Decreased glucose rise (flat glucose curve) in:** Intestinal disease (celiac sprue, Whipple disease), adrenal insufficiency (Addison disease, hypopituitarism), pancreatic islet cell tumors or hyperplasia.	Test is not generally required for diagnosis of diabetes mellitus. In screening for gestational diabetes, the glucose tolerance test is performed between 24 and 28 weeks of gestation. After a 50-g oral glucose load, a 2-hour postprandial blood glucose is measured as a screen. If the result is >140 mg/dL, then the full test with 100-g glucose load is done using the following reference ranges: Fasting: <105 mg/dL 1-hour: <190 mg/dL 2-hour: <165 mg/dL 3-hour: <145 mg/dL Hadar E et al. Establishing consensus criteria for the diagnosis of diabetes in pregnancy following the HAPO study. Ann N Y Acad Sci 2010;1205:88. [PMID: 20840258] Patel P et al. Diabetes mellitus: diagnosis and screening. Am Fam Physician 2010;81:863. [PMID: 20353144]

G6PD screen

| Glucose-6-phosphate dehydrogenase screen, whole blood (G6PD)

5–14 units/g Hb

[0.1–0.28 mckat/L]

Green or blue

$$ | G6PD is an enzyme in the hexose monophosphate shunt that is essential in generating reduced glutathione and NADPH, which protect hemoglobin from oxidative denaturation. Numerous G6PD isoenzymes have been identified. Inherited G6PD deficiency causes neonatal hyperbilirubinemia and chronic hemolytic anemia; exposure to oxidative stressors such as certain drugs or infection, can elicit significant acute hemolysis.

Most African Americans have G6PD-A(+) isoenzyme. 10–15% have G6PD-A(−), which has only 15% of normal enzyme activity. It is transmitted in an X-linked recessive manner.

Some Mediterranean people have the G6PD-B(−) variant, which has extremely low enzyme activity (1% of normal). | **Increased in:** Young erythrocytes (reticulocytosis).
Decreased in: G6PD deficiency. | In deficient patients, hemolytic anemia can be triggered by oxidant agents: antimalarial drugs (eg, chloroquine), nalidixic acid, nitrofurantoin, dapsone, phenacetin, vitamin C, and some sulfonamides. Patients from high risk groups (eg, African American and people from the Mediterranean region) should be screened for G6PD deficiency before taking an oxidant drug.

Hemolytic episodes can also occur in deficient patients who eat fava beans (favism), in patients with diabetic acidosis, and in infections.

G6PD deficiency may be the cause of hemolytic disease of newborns in Asians and Mediterraneans.

G6PD activity levels may be measured as normal during an acute episode, because only nonhemolyzed young red cells are assessed. If deficiency is still suspected, assay should be repeated in 2–3 months when cells of all ages are present.

Minucci A et al. Glucose-6-phosphate dehydrogenase laboratory assay: how, when, and why? IUBMB Life 2009;61:27. [PMID: 18942156]

Nkhoma ET et al. The global prevalence of G6PD deficiency: a systematic review and meta-analysis. Blood Cells Mol Dis 2009;42:267. [PMID: 19233695] |

	Glutamine		
Test/Range/Collection	Physiologic Basis	Interpretation	Comments
Glutamine, CSF, glass or plastic tube 6–15 mg/dL ***Panic:*** >40 mg/dL $$$	Glutamine is synthesized in the brain from ammonia and glutamic acid. Elevated CSF glutamine is associated with hepatic encephalopathy. It is considered as a mediator of ammonia neurotoxicity.	**Increased in:** Hepatic encephalopathy.	Test is not indicated if serum (or plasma) albumin, ALT, bilirubin, and alkaline phosphatase are normal or if there is no clinical evidence of liver disease. Hepatic encephalopathy is essentially ruled out if the CSF glutamine is normal. Albrecht J et al. Glutamine as a mediator of ammonia neurotoxicity: a critical appraisal. Biochem Pharmacol 2010;80:1303. [PMID: 20654582] Brusilow SW et al. Astrocyte glutamine synthetase: importance in hyperammonemic syndromes and potential target for therapy. Neurotherapeutics 2010;7:452. [PMID: 20880508] Lemberg A et al. Hepatic encephalopathy, ammonia, glutamate, glutamine and oxidative stress. Ann Hepatol 2009;8:95. [PMID: 19502650]

Glycohemoglobin (Hemoglobin A1c)

Glycohemoglobin, Hemoglobin A_{1c} (HbA$_{1c}$), blood 3.9–5.6% (method-dependent) Lavender, pink $$	During the life span of each RBC, glucose combines with hemoglobin to produce stable glycated hemoglobin. The level of glycated hemoglobin is related to the mean plasma glucose level during the previous 1–3 months. HbA$_{1c}$ level can be used to estimate the average blood glucose levels (eAG), ie, eAG = $28.7 \times A_{1c} - 46.7$. There are three glycated A hemoglobins: HbA$_{1a}$, HbA$_{1b}$, and HbA$_{1c}$. Some assays quantitate HbA$_{1c}$, some quantitate total HbA$_1$, and some quantitate all glycated hemoglobins, not just A. Hemoglobin variants may interfere with HbA$_{1c}$ determinations.	**Increased in:** Diabetes mellitus, splenectomy. Falsely high results can occur depending on the method used and may be due to presence of hemoglobin F or uremia. **Decreased in:** Any condition that shortens red cell life span (hemolytic anemias, congenital spherocytosis, acute or chronic blood loss, sickle cell disease, hemoglobinopathies).	HbA$_{1c}$ is useful for quantifying the risk of diabetic complications and for monitoring glycemic control. An increased HbA$_{1c}$ value (6.5% or higher) has been added as a diagnostic criterion for diabetes mellitus. There is a clear relationship between glycemic control as reflected by HbA$_{1c}$ and the progression of microvascular complications in both type I and type II diabetes. Intervention to lower blood glucose in clinical trials led to a reduction in the microvascular complications of diabetes. Executive summary: Standards of medical care in diabetes—2010. Diabetes Care 2010;33(Suppl 1):S4. [PMID: 20042774] Little RR et al. A review of variant hemoglobins interfering with hemoglobin A1c measurement. J Diabetes Sci Technol. 2009;3:446. [PMID: 20144281] Nathan DM et al. Translating the A1c assay into estimated average glucose values. Diabetes Care 2008;31:1473. [PMID: 18540046] Patel P et al. Diabetes mellitus: diagnosis and screening. Am Fam Physician 2010;81:863. [PMID: 20353144]

	Growth hormone		
Test/Range/Collection	**Physiologic Basis**	**Interpretation**	**Comments**
Growth hormone, serum or plasma (GH) 0–5 ng/mL [mcg/L] SST, PPT $$$	GH is a single-chain polypeptide of 191 amino acids that induces the generation of somatomedins, which directly stimulate collagen and protein synthesis. GH levels are subject to wide fluctuations during the day.	**Increased in:** Acromegaly (90% have GH levels >10 ng/mL). Laron dwarfism (defective GH receptor), starvation. Drugs: dopamine, levodopa. **Decreased in:** Pituitary dwarfism, hypopituitarism.	Nonsuppressibility of GH levels to <2 ng/mL after 100 g oral glucose and elevation of IGF-1 levels are the two most sensitive tests for acromegaly. Random determinations of GH are rarely useful in the diagnosis of acromegaly. For the diagnosis of hypopituitarism or GH deficiency in children, an insulin hypoglycemia test has been used. Failure to increase GH levels to >5 ng/mL after insulin (0.1 unit/kg) is consistent with GH deficiency. Pituitary dysfunction may occur after traumatic brain injury or post-partum hypotension (apoplexy). Bidlingmaier M et al. Measurement of human growth hormone by immunoassays: current status, unsolved problems and clinical consequences. Growth Horm IGF Res 2010;20:19. [PMID: 19818659] Chanson P et al. Pituitary tumours: acromegaly. Best Pract Res Clin Endocrinol Metab 2009;23:555. [PMID: 19945023]

Haptoglobin		
Haptoglobin, serum or plasma 46–316 mg/dL [0.5–3.2 g/L] SST, PPT, green, lavender $$	Haptoglobin is a glycoprotein synthesized in the liver that binds free hemoglobin. Its scavenging function counteracts the potentially harmful oxidative and nitric oxide-scavenging effects associated with "free" hemoglobin.	**Increased in:** Acute and chronic infection (acute-phase reactant), malignancy, biliary obstruction, ulcerative colitis, myocardial infarction, and diabetes mellitus. **Decreased in:** Newborns and children, posttransfusion, intravascular hemolysis, autoimmune hemolytic anemia, liver disease (10%). May be decreased following uneventful transfusion (10%) for unknown reasons.	Low haptoglobin is considered an indicator of hemolysis, but it is of uncertain clinical predictive value because of the greater prevalence of other conditions associated with low levels and because of occasional normal individuals who have very low levels. It thus has low specificity. High normal levels probably rule out significant intravascular hemolysis. Low haptoglobin levels aid in early recognition of the HELLP syndrome (**h**emolytic anemia, **e**levated **l**iver enzymes, and **l**ow **p**latelet count). Levy AP et al. Haptoglobin: basic and clinical aspects. Antioxid Redox Signal 2010;12:293. [PMID: 19659435] Quaye IK. Haptoglobin, inflammation and disease. Trans R Soc Trop Med Hyg 2008;102:735. [PMID: 18486167]

	Helicobacter pylori antibody		
Test/Range/Collection	**Physiologic Basis**	**Interpretation**	**Comments**
***Helicobacter pylori* antibody,** serum or plasma Negative SST, lavender/pink, green $$	*Helicobacter pylori* is a gram-negative spiral bacterium that is found on gastric mucosa. It induces acute and chronic inflammation in the gastric mucosa and a positive serologic antibody response. Serologic testing for *H. pylori* antibody (IgG and IgA) is by enzyme-linked immunosorbent assay (ELISA).	**Increased (positive) in:** Histologic (chronic or chronic active) gastritis due to *H. pylori* infection (with or without peptic ulcer disease). Sensitivity 98%, specificity 48%. Asymptomatic adults: 15–50%.	95% of patients with duodenal ulcers and >70% of those with gastric ulcers have chronic infection with *H. pylori* and associated histologic gastritis. All patients with peptic ulcers and positive *H. pylori* serology should be treated to eradicate *H. pylori* infection. Extragastric manifestations of *H. pylori* infection may include immune thrombocytopenic purpura (ITP) and idiopathic sideropenic anemia. The prevalence of *H. pylori*-positive serologic tests in asymptomatic adults is approximately 35% overall but is >50% in patients over age 60. Fewer than one in six adults with *H. pylori* antibody develop peptic ulcer disease. Treatment of asymptomatic adults with positive serology is not currently recommended. After successful eradication, serologic titers fall over a 3- to 6-month period but remain positive in up to 50% of patients at 1 year. The fecal antigen immunoassay and [¹³C] urea breath test have excellent sensitivity and specificity (>95%) for active infection. These tests are more cost-effective because they reduce unnecessary treatment of patients without active infection. Cover TL et al. *Helicobacter pylori* in health and disease. Gastroenterology 2009;136:1863. [PMID: 19457415] McColl KE. Clinical practice. *Helicobacter pylori* infection. N Engl J Med 2010;362:1597. [PMID: 20427808]

	Hematocrit	
Hematocrit, whole blood (Hct) Males: 39–49% Females: 35–45% (age-dependent) Lavender $	The Hct represents the percentage of whole blood volume composed of erythrocytes. Laboratory instruments calculate Hct from the erythrocyte count (RBC) and the mean corpuscular volume (MCV) by the formula: $$Hct = RBC \times MCV$$ Manual spun hematocrit (microhematocrit) is 1.5–3% higher than that from an automated hematology instrument and is less reliable.	**Increased in:** Hemoconcentration (as in dehydration, burns, vomiting), polycythemia (erythrocytosis), extreme physical exercise. **Decreased in:** Macrocytic anemia (liver disease, hypothyroidism, vitamin B_{12} deficiency, folate deficiency, myelodysplasia), normocytic anemia (early iron deficiency, anemia of chronic disease, hemolytic anemia, acute hemorrhage, bone marrow infiltrates), and microcytic anemia (iron deficiency, thalassemia). Hemodilution.	Conversion from hemoglobin (Hb) to hematocrit is roughly Hb × 3 = Hct. The Hct reported by clinical laboratories is not a spun Hct. The spun Hct may be spuriously high if the centrifuge is not calibrated, if the specimen is not spun to constant volume, or if there is "trapped plasma." In determining transfusion need, the clinical picture must be considered in addition to the Hct. Point-of-care instruments may not measure Hct accurately in all patients. In hemodialysis patients, erythropoiesis-stimulating agents have been used to maintain an Hct of 33–36% (hemoglobin of 11–12 g/dL) to reduce blood transfusions and improve quality of life, but recent data led to an FDA black box warning regarding a risk of myocardial infarction, stroke, and death associated with the use of these agents at higher than recommended doses. Christensen RD et al. The CBC: reference ranges for neonates. Semin Perinatol 2009;33:3. [PMID: 19167576] Harder L et al. The optimal hematocrit. Crit Care Clin 2010;26:335. [PMID: 20381724] McMullin MF. The classification and diagnosis of erythrocytosis. Int J Lab Hematol 2008;30:447. [PMID: 18823397]

	Hemoglobin A₂		
Test/Range/Collection	Physiologic Basis	Interpretation	Comments
Hemoglobin A₂, whole blood (HbA₂) 1.5–3.5% of total hemoglobin (Hb) Lavender $$	HbA₂ is a minor component of normal adult hemoglobin (<3.5% of total Hb).	**Increased in:** β-Thalassemia minor (HbA₂ levels 4–9% of total Hb, HbF 1–5%), β-thalassemia major (HbA₂ levels normal or increased, HbF 80–100%). **Decreased in:** Untreated iron deficiency, hemoglobin H disease, hemoglobin Lepore major (rare). Patients with the combination of iron deficiency and β-thalassemia may have a normal HbA₂ level.	Test is useful in the diagnosis of β-thalassemia minor (in absence of iron deficiency, which decreases HbA₂ and can mask the diagnosis). Quantitated by column chromatographic or automated HPLC techniques. Normal HbA₂ levels are seen in δ-thalassemia or very mild β-thalassemias. See thalassemia syndromes (Table 8–25). Mosca A et al. The role of haemoglobin A(2) testing in the diagnosis of thalassaemias and related haemoglobinopathies. J Clin Pathol 2009;62:13. [PMID: 19103851] Van Vranken M. Evaluation of macrocytosis. Am Fam Physician 2010;82:1117.

Hemoglobin electrophoresis		
Hemoglobin (Hb) electrophoresis, whole blood HbA: > 95% HbA$_2$: 1.5–3.5% HbF: <2% (age-dependent) Lavender, blue, or green $$	Hemoglobin electrophoresis is used as a screening test to detect and differentiate variant and abnormal hemoglobins. Alkaline and/or citrate agar electrophoresis is the commonly used method. Separation of hemoglobins is based on different rates of migration of charged hemoglobin molecules in an electric field. HPLC is a useful alternative method for hemoglobin analyses, and is routinely used for hemoglobinopathy screening.	Presence of HbS with HbA >HbS: sickle cell trait (HbAS) or sickle α-thalassemia; HbS and F, no HbA: sickle cell anemia (HbSS), sickle β^0-thalassemia, or sickle-HPFH (hereditary persistence of fetal hemoglobin); HbS >HbA and F: sickle β$^+$-thalassemia. Presence of HbC: HbA > HbC: HbC trait (HbAC); HbC and F, no HbA: HbC disease (HbCC), HbC-β^0-thalassemia, or HbC-HPFH; HbC >HbA: HbC β$^+$-thalassemia. Presence of HbS and HbC: HbSC disease. Presence of HbH: HbH disease. Increased HbA$_2$: β-thalassemia minor. Increased HbF: Hereditary persistence of fetal hemoglobin, sickle cell anemia, β-thalassemia, HbC disease, HbE disease.	Evaluation of a suspected hemoglobinopathy should include electrophoresis of a hemolysate to detect abnormal hemoglobins, quantitation of hemoglobins A$_2$ and F by column chromatography, and solubility test if HbS is detected. Interpretation of Hb electrophoresis results should be put in the clinical context, including the family history, serum iron studies, red cell morphology, hemoglobin, hematocrit, and red cell indices (eg, MCV). Molecular testing aids in genetic counseling of patients with thalassemia and combined hemoglobinopathies. Benson JM et al. History and current status of newborn screening for hemoglobinopathies. Semin Perinatol 2010;34:134. [PMID: 20207263] Langlois S et al. CCMG Prenatal Diagnosis Committee; SOGC Genetic Committee. Carrier screening for thalassemia and hemoglobinopathies in Canada. J Obstet Gynaecol Can 2008;30:950. [PMID: 19038079] Mosca A et al. The role of haemoglobin A(2) testing in the diagnosis of thalassaemias and related haemoglobinopathies. J Clin Pathol 2009;62:13. [PMID: 19103851]

	Hemoglobin, fetal		
Test/Range/Collection	Physiologic Basis	Interpretation	Comments
Hemoglobin, fetal, whole blood (HbF) Adult: < 2% (varies with age) Lavender, blue, or green $$	Fetal hemoglobin constitutes about 75% of total hemoglobin at birth and declines to 50% at 6 weeks, 5% at 6 months, and < 1.5% by 1 year. Within the first year, adult hemoglobin (HbA) becomes the predominant hemoglobin. Fetal to adult hemoglobin switching (HbF-to-HbA switch) is regulated by nuclear factors (eg, BCL11A).	**Increased in:** Hereditary disorders: eg, β-thalassemia major (20–100% of total Hb is HbF), β-thalassemia minor (2–5% HbF), HbE β-thalassemia (10–80% HbF), sickle cell anemia (5–20% HbF), hereditary persistence of fetal hemoglobin (10–40% HbF). Acquired disorders (< 10% HbF): aplastic anemia, megaloblastic anemia, paroxysmal nocturnal hemoglobinuria (PNH), leukemia (eg, juvenile myelomonocytic leukemia). **Decreased in:** Hemolytic anemia of the newborn.	Semiquantitative acid elution test (Kleihauer-Betke test) provides an estimate of fetal hemoglobin only and varies widely between laboratories. It is useful in distinguishing hereditary persistence of fetal hemoglobin (all RBCs show an increase in fetal hemoglobin) from β-thalassemia minor (only a portion of RBCs are affected). Enzyme-linked antiglobulin test and flow cytometry are also used to detect fetal red cells in the Rh(−) maternal circulation in suspected cases of Rh sensitization and to determine the amount of RhoGAM to administer (1 vial/15 mL fetal RBC). Prenatal diagnosis of hemoglobinopathies may be made from quantitative hemoglobin levels using HPLC or molecular diagnostic techniques. Mosca A et al. The relevance of hemoglobin F measurement in the diagnosis of thalassemias and related hemoglobinopathies. Clin Biochem 2009;42:1797. [PMID: 19580798] Sankaran VG et al. Advances in the understanding of haemoglobin switching. Br J Haematol 2010;149:181. [PMID: 20201948]

Hemoglobin, total		
Hemoglobin, total, whole blood (Hb) Males: 13.6–17.5 g/dL Females: 12.0–15.5 g/dL (age-dependent) [Males: 136–175 g/L] Females: 120–155 g/L] ***Panic:*** ≤ 7 g/dL Lavender $	Hemoglobin is the major protein of erythrocytes that transports oxygen from the lungs to peripheral tissues. It is measured by spectrophotometry on automated instruments after lysis of red cells and conversion of all hemoglobin to cyanmethemoglobin.	**Increased in:** Hemoconcentration (as in dehydration, burns, vomiting), polycythemia (erythrocytosis), extreme physical exercise. **Decreased in:** Macrocytic anemia (liver disease, hypothyroidism, vitamin B_{12} deficiency, folate deficiency, myelodysplasia), normocytic anemia (early iron deficiency, anemia of chronic disease, hemolytic anemia, acute hemorrhage, bone marrow infiltrates), and microcytic anemia (iron deficiency, thalassemia). Hemodilution.	The cyanmethemoglobin technique is the method of choice selected by the International Committee for Standardization in Hematology. The method measures all hemoglobin derivatives except sulfhemoglobin by hemolyzing the specimen and adding a reducing agent. As such, this method does not distinguish between intracellular versus extracellular hemoglobin (hemolysis). Cyanide-free hemoglobin method is also used on certain hematology analyzers. Hypertriglyceridemia and very high white blood cell counts can cause false elevations of Hb. Balducci L et al. Anemia, fatigue and aging. Transfus Clin Biol 2010;17:375. [PMID: 21067951] Janus J et al. Evaluation of anemia in children. Am Fam Physician 2010;81(12):1462. [PMID: 20540485] Moreno Chulilla JA et al. Classification of anemia for gastroenterologists. World J Gastroenterol 2009;15:4627. [PMID: 19787825]

Test/Range/Collection	Physiologic Basis	Interpretation	Comments
		Heparin anti-Xa assay	
Heparin anti-Xa assay, chromogenic, plasma Undetectable (<0.05 U/mL) Blue $$	The anti-Xa assay is a chromogenic assay that measures heparin level indirectly. Factor Xa is used as assay reagent. Heparin in patient's plasma binds with antithrombin and inhibits excess Xa. The quantity of residual Xa is then measured using a chromogenic substrate, and the released colored compound is measured spectrophotometrically. The quantity of residual Xa is inversely proportional to the amount of heparin present in plasma.	**Therapeutic ranges:** Unfractionated heparin: 0.35–0.70 U/mL. Low molecular weight heparin (LMWH): 0.40–1.10 U/mL. Note that the therapeutic ranges are laboratory- and method-specific.	The test can precisely determine the level of heparin in patient's plasma, and is used to monitor heparin therapy. PTT is the most commonly used test for monitoring unfractionated heparin therapy. For patients with documented lupus anticoagulant, PTT is unreliable and therefore heparin level by anti-Xa assay should be used. Low molecular weight heparin (LMWH) generally does not prolong the PTT, therefore the anti-Xa assay is used if monitoring is required (eg, in obesity with > 100 kg body weight, renal insufficiency, and pregnancy). Blood sample is typically collected 4 hours after subcutaneous injection. Dager WE et al. Systemic anticoagulation considerations in chronic kidney disease. Adv Chronic Kidney Dis 2010;17:420. [PMID: 20727512] Lehman CM et al. Comparative performance of three anti-factor Xa heparin assays in patients in a medical intensive care unit receiving intravenous, unfractionated heparin. Am J Clin Pathol 2006;126:416. [PMID: 16880140]

Heparin-associated antibody detection

Heparin-associated antibody detection (heparin-induced thrombocytopenia), serum or plasma Negative Red, lavender, blue $$	Heparin-induced thrombocytopenia (HIT) is a life-threatening disorder following exposure to unfractionated or (less commonly) low-molecular-weight heparin. The HIT antibodies are directed at heparin and platelet factor 4 (PF4) and may appear on exposure to heparin. The formed immune complexes propagate platelet activation, leading to release of more PF4 and thrombosis. However, only a minority of patients who form HIT antibodies actually develop thrombocytopenia and/or thrombosis (clinical HIT). An enzyme-linked immunosorbent assay (ELISA) method is typically used for the detection of heparin-associated antibodies.	**Positive in:** Heparin-induced thrombocytopenia, type II.	There are two types of HIT. Type I HIT is generally considered a benign condition and is not antibody-mediated. In type II HIT, thrombocytopenia is usually more severe and is antibody-mediated. Patients with type II HIT are at risk for developing arterial or venous thrombosis if heparin therapy is continued. The ELISA-based antigenic assay is very sensitive and is designed to detect antibody binding to PF4/heparin (usually IgG). However, the test is relatively nonspecific because it may also detect nonpathogenic IgA and IgM antibodies. Results should be used in conjunction with clinical findings, platelet counts, and other laboratory results. Functional assays (serotonin release assay, heparin-induced platelet aggregation study, and flow cytometry analysis) are more specific, but are technically demanding and usually done in reference laboratories. Arepally GM et al. Heparin-induced thrombocytopenia. Annu Rev Med 2010;61:77. [PMID: 20059332] Cuker A et al. ASH evidence-based guidelines: Is the IgG-specific anti-PF4/heparin ELISA superior to the polyspecific ELISA in the laboratory diagnosis of HIT? Hematology Am Soc Hematol Educ Program 2009;250. [PMID: 20008206] Otis SA et al. Heparin-induced thrombocytopenia: current status and diagnostic challenges. Am J Hematol 2010;85:700. [PMID: 20665476]

	Hepatitis A antibody

Test/Range/Collection	Physiologic Basis	Interpretation	Comments
Hepatitis A virus antibody, serum or plasma (Anti-HAV) Negative SST, PPT, green, blue $$	Hepatitis A is caused by a nonenveloped 27-nm RNA virus of the enterovirus-picornavirus group and is usually acquired by the fecal–oral route. IgM antibody is detectable within 1 week after symptoms develop and persists for 6 months. IgG antibody appears 4 weeks later than IgM and persists for years (see Figure 10–5 for time course of serologic changes). IgG antibody is positive after successful hepatitis A vaccination.	**Positive in:** Acute hepatitis A (IgM), convalescence from hepatitis A (IgG), after hepatitis A vaccination (IgG).	The most commonly used test for hepatitis A antibody is an immunoassay that detects total IgG and IgM antibodies. This test can be used to establish immune status. Specific IgM testing is necessary to diagnose acute hepatitis A. IgG antibody positivity is found in 40–50% of adults in the United States and Europe (higher rates in developing nations). Testing for anti-HAV (IgG) may reduce cost of HAV vaccination programs. Jacobsen KH et al. Hepatitis A virus seroprevalence by age and world region, 1990 and 2005. Vaccine 2010;28:6653. [PMID: 20723630] Jeong SH et al. Hepatitis A: clinical manifestations and management. Intervirology 2010;53:15. [PMID: 20068336]

Hepatitis B surface antigen		
Hepatitis B virus surface antigen, serum or plasma (HBsAg) Negative SST, PPT, green, blue $$	In hepatitis B virus infection, surface antigen is detectable 2–5 weeks before onset of symptoms, rises in titer, and peaks at about the time of onset of clinical illness. Generally it persists for 1–5 months, declining in titer and disappearing with resolution of clinical symptoms (see Figure 10–6 for time course of serologic changes).	**Increased in:** Acute hepatitis B, chronic hepatitis B (persistence of HBsAg for >6 months, positive HBcAb [total]) asymptomatic HBV carriers. May be undetectable in acute hepatitis B infection. If clinical suspicion is high, HBcAb (IgM) test is then indicated.	First-line test for the diagnosis of acute or chronic hepatitis B. If positive, HBV DNA testing is often performed to provide further information on the disease status. HBeAg is a marker of extensive viral replication found only in HBsAg-positive sera. Persistently HBeAg-positive patients are more infectious than HBeAg-negative patients and more likely to develop chronic liver disease. Fung J et al. Hepatitis B virus DNA and hepatitis B surface antigen levels in chronic hepatitis B. Expert Rev Anti Infect Ther 2010;8:717. [PMID: 20521898.] Wright TL. Introduction to chronic hepatitis B infection. Am J Gastroenterol 2006;101(Suppl):S1. [PMID: 16448446]

Test/Range/Collection	Physiologic Basis	Interpretation	Comments
		Hepatitis B surface antibody	**Hepatitis B core antibody**
Hepatitis B virus surface antibody (HBsAb, anti-HBs) Negative SST, lavender $$	Hepatitis B virus (HBV) is a DNA virus. This test detects antibodies to HBV surface antigen, which are thought to confer immunity to hepatitis B.	**Increased in:** Hepatitis B immunity due to HBV infection or prior hepatitis B vaccination. **Absent in:** Hepatitis B carrier state, nonexposure.	Test indicates immune status for HBV. It is not useful for the evaluation of acute or chronic hepatitis. (See Figure 10–6 for time course of serologic changes.) Kim HN et al. Hepatitis B vaccination in HIV-infected adults: current evidence, recommendations and practical considerations. Int J STD AIDS 2009;20(9):595. [PMID: 19710329] Mathew JL et al. Hepatitis B immunisation in persons not previously exposed to hepatitis B or with unknown exposure status. Cochrane Database Syst Rev 2008;16;(3):CD006481. [PMID: 18677780]
Hepatitis B virus core antibody, total, serum (HBcAb, anti-HBc) Negative SST $$	HbcAb (IgG and IgM) become positive (as IgM) about 2 months after exposure to hepatitis B virus. Its persistent positivity may reflect chronic hepatitis (IgM) or recovery (IgG). (See Figure 10–6 for time course of serologic changes.)	**Positive in:** Hepatitis B (acute and chronic), hepatitis B carriers, prior hepatitis B (immune) when IgG is present in low titer with or without HBsAb. **Negative:** After hepatitis B vaccination.	HBcAb (total) is useful in evaluation of acute or chronic hepatitis only if HBsAg is negative. An HBcAb (IgM) test is then indicated only if the HBcAb (total) is positive. HBcAb (IgM) may be the only serologic indication of acute HBV infection and occult HBV infection. HBcAb positive, HBsAg negative patients may reactivate their hepatitis B if given chemotherapy, and prophylaxis with HBV therapy should be considered in this setting. Urbani S. The role of anti-core antibody response in the detection of occult hepatitis B virus infection. Clin Chem Lab Med 2010;48:23. [PMID: 19919328]

Hepatitis B e antigen		
Hepatitis B e antigen/ antibody (HBeAg/Ab), serum or plsma Negative SST, PPT, green $$	HBeAg is a soluble protein secreted by HBV, related to HBcAg, indicating viral replication and infectivity. Two distinct serologic types of hepatitis B have been described, one with a positive HbeAg, and the other with a negative HBeAg and a positive anti-HBe antibody.	**Increased (positive) in:** HBV (acute, chronic) hepatitis.	The assumption has been that loss of HBeAg and accumulation of HBeAb are associated with decreased infectivity. Testing has proved unreliable, and tests are not routinely needed as indicators of infectivity. All patients positive for HBeAg must be considered infectious. Liaw YF et al. Hepatitis B e antigen seroconversion: a critical event in chronic hepatitis B virus infection. Dig Dis Sci 2010;55:2727. [PMID: 20238245] Ribeiro RM et al. Hepatitis B virus kinetics under antiviral therapy sheds light on differences in hepatitis B e antigen positive and negative infections. J Infect Dis 2010;202:1309. [PMID: 20874517]

Hepatitis B virus DNA, quantitative

Test/Range/Collection	Physiologic Basis	Interpretation	Comments
Hepatitis B virus DNA, quantitative (HBV-DNA), blood Quantification range 1.3–8.2 log IU/mL (20–170,000,000 IU/mL) (laboratory-specific) 1 IU/mL is approximately 5 copies/mL SST, PPT, lavender $$$$	The presence of HBV-DNA in serum or plasma confirms active hepatitis B infection and implies infectivity of serum. Current use of the assay is primarily for assessing responses of hepatitis B to therapy, such as peginterferon, tenofovir or entecavir. HBV-DNA is also used before and after liver transplantation to detect low-level viral replication, and for patients infected by mutant strains of HBV that do not make normal surface antigen. In patients with chronic hepatitis B, HBV DNA levels in blood correlate with the risk of cirrhosis and hepatocellular carcinoma, and thus have prognostic value. HBV-DNA can be detected using very sensitive techniques (eg, real-time PCR) even in patients thought to have recovered from HBV infection who are positive for anti-HBs and anti-HBc.	**Positive in:** Acute hepatitis B, chronic hepatitis B, silent HBV carriers, occult HBV infection.	Viral load fluctuates over time in most patients and may vary by as much as 10^2–10^4 in serial measurements. The World Health Organization has recognized an international standard, a genotype A subtype adw2 isolate, for HBV-DNA quantification. Assays are commonly reported in International Units (IU) based on comparison with the standard. However, correlation between copies/mL and IU is variable. Andersson KL et al. Monitoring during and after antiviral therapy for hepatitis B. Hepatology 2009;49(5 Suppl):S166. [PMID: 19399793] Fung J et al. Hepatitis B virus DNA and hepatitis B surface antigen levels in chronic hepatitis B. Expert Rev Anti Infect Ther 2010;8:717. [PMID: 20521898] Wong GL et al. Predictors of treatment response in chronic hepatitis B. Drugs 2009;69:2167. [PMID: 19852623]

Hepatitis C antibody			
Hepatitis C antibody, serum or plasma (HCAb, anti-HCV) Negative SST, PPT, green $$	Detects antibody to hepatitis C virus, which is a single-stranded RNA virus of the Flaviviridae family. The screening test (enzyme immunoassay [EIA]- or chemiluminescent immunoassay [CIA]-based) detects antibodies to proteins expressed by putative structural (HC34) and nonstructural (HC31, C100-3) regions of the HCV genome. The presence of these antibodies indicates that the patient has been infected with HCV, may harbor infectious HCV, and may be capable of transmitting HCV. A recombinant immunoblot assay (RIBA), equivalent to Western blot, is available as a confirmatory test. HCV RNA tests are preferred for confirming active infection if the screening test is positive. See Figure 10–7 for hepatitis C serologic changes.	**Increased in:** Acute hepatitis C (only 20–50%; seroconversion may take 3 months or more), posttransfusion chronic hepatitis (70–90%), blood donors (0.5–1%), non–blood-donating general public (2–3%), hemophiliacs (75%), intravenous drug users (40–80%), hemodialysis patients (1–30%), male homosexuals (4%).	Sensitivity of screening assays for HCV infection is 86%, specificity 99.5%. Seropositivity for hepatitis C documents previous exposure, not necessarily acute infection. Samples that are weakly positive (signal-to-cutoff ratio <3.8 for EIA assay or <8 for CIA assay) require reflex HCV-RNA or RIBA testing. Samples that are negative on screening test usually require no further testing. However, HCV-RNA is generally obtained if there is high clinical suspicion of HCV despite a negative anti-HCV, especially in immunocompromised persons or in the setting of acute hepatitis. Anti-HCV and the RIBA often do not become positive during an acute infection; HCV RNA test is required if clinically indicated. Chevaliez S et al. How to use virological tools for optimal management of chronic hepatitis C. Liver Int 2009;29(Suppl 1):9. [PMID: 19207960] Ghany MG et al. Diagnosis, management, and treatment of hepatitis C: an update. Hepatology 2009;49:1335. [PMID: 19330875] Pham TN et al. Occult hepatitis C virus infection: what does it mean? Liver Int 2010;30:502. [PMID: 20070513]

Test/Range/Collection	Physiologic Basis	Interpretation	Comments
Hepatitis C RNA (HCV RNA), quantitative (HCV viral load)	Detection of HCV RNA is used to confirm active infection and to monitor treatment with interferon-based therapy. Widely used methods include reverse-transcriptase PCR (RT-PCR) and branched DNA (b-DNA) transcription-mediated amplification (TMA).	**Positive in:** Hepatitis C.	RNA is very susceptible to degradation; thus, improper specimen handling can cause false-negative results. Assays are generally reported in IU/mL, with standardization using WHO reference material. A less than 2 log (or 100-fold) decrease in viral load after 12 weeks of treatment indicates lack of response to therapy.
Negative (detection limit: 12 IU/mL, assay-specific)			Chevaliez S et al. How to use virological tools for optimal management of chronic hepatitis C. Liver Int 2009;29(Suppl 1):9. [PMID: 19207960]
$$$$			Le Guillou-Guillemette H et al. Detection and quantification of serum or plasma HCV RNA: mini review of commercially available assays. Methods Mol Biol 2009;510:3. [PMID: 19009249]
PPT, SST, or lavender.			Teoh NC et al. Individualisation of antiviral therapy for chronic hepatitis C. J Gastroenterol Hepatol 2010;25:1206. [PMID: 20594246]
Separate serum or plasma and freeze at −20°C within 2 hours. Analysis should be done within 2 hours.			

Hepatitis C virus genotyping

Hepatitis C virus genotyping		
Hepatitis C virus genotyping PPT, SST, or lavender $$$$ Separate serum or plasma from cells within 2 hours of collection.	HCV genotyping is a tool used to optimize antiviral treatment regimens. HCV RNA is assayed using reverse transcription polymerase chain reaction (RT-PCR) to amplify a specific portion of the 5' untranslated region (5' UTR) of the hepatitis C virus. The amplified nucleic acid is sequenced bidirectionally. Another technique is the line probe assay (LiPA) that uses genotype-specific probes to detect sequence variations in the 5' UTR and the core region of the viral genome. The test may be unsuccessful if the HCV RNA viral load is less than 1,000 HCV RNA copies per mL.	**Positive in:** Hepatitis C. Isolates of hepatitis C virus are grouped into six major genotypes. These genotypes are subtyped according to sequence characteristics and are designated as 1a, 1b, 2a, 2b, 3a, 3b, 4, 5a, and 6a.	Genotyping to identify the HCV subtype is performed to determine potential responses to therapy with interferon and ribavirin. Patient prognosis and disease course may be genotype dependent. Compared with hepatitis C genotypes 2 and 3, genotypes 1 and 4 are more resistant to eradication in response to pegylated interferon and ribavirin therapy. Chevaliez S et al. How to use virological tools for optimal management of chronic hepatitis C. Liver Int 2009;29(Suppl 1):9. [PMID: 19207960] Teoh NC et al. Individualisation of antiviral therapy for chronic hepatitis C. J Gastr oenterol Hepatol 2010;25:1206. [PMID: 20594246] Zeuzem S et al. Management of hepatitis C virus genotype 2 or 3 infection: treatment optimization on the basis of virological response. Antivir Ther 2009;14:143. [PMID: 19430089]

	Hepatitis D antibody

Test/Range/Collection	Physiologic Basis	Interpretation	Comments
Hepatitis D virus antibody, serum (anti-HDV) Negative SST, red $$	This antibody is a marker for acute or persisting infection with the delta agent, a defective RNA virus that can infect only HBsAg-positive patients. HBV plus hepatitis D virus (HDV) infection may be more severe than HBV infection alone. Antibody to HDV ordinarily persists for about 6 months after acute infection. Further persistence indicates carrier status.	**Positive in:** Hepatitis D.	Test only indicated in HBsAg-positive patients. Chronic HDV hepatitis occurs in 80–90% of HBsAg carriers who are superinfected with delta virus. Rizzetto M. Hepatitis D: thirty years after. J Hepatol 2009;50:1043. [PMID: 19285743] Wedemeyer H et al. Peginterferon plus adefovir versus either drug alone for hepatitis delta. N Engl J Med 2011;364:322. [PMID: 21268724]

Hepatitis E antibody		
Hepatitis E antibody, serum (anti-HEV) Negative Red, SST $$$	Hepatitis E virus (HEV) is a small single-stranded RNA virus that causes hepatitis. The virus has a single serotype but 4 genotypes; genotypes 1 and 2 infect only humans, whereas genotypes 3 and 4 primarily infect other mammals, particularly pigs, but occasionally cause human disease as well. The virus is acquired through the fecal-oral route, usually through contaminated water supplies. HEV can also be transmitted by blood transfusion. Perinatal transmission from infected mother to infant has also been reported. HEV generally causes a self-limited acute infection. Chronic hepatitis does not develop after acute infection, except in transplant or immunocompromised patients (eg, HIV).	**Positive in:** Acute hepatitis E (IgM), convalescence from hepatitis E (IgG).	Both anti-HEV IgM and anti-HEV IgG ELISA assays are available. False positive or negative result may occur. Detection of HEV RNA in serum or stool is the gold standard test for acute hepatitis E and has been used for both epidemiologic and diagnostic purposes. Blood donation screening with microarrays has been proposed. Aggarwal R. Hepatitis E: Historical, contemporary and future perspectives. J Gastroenterol Hepatol 2011;26 (Suppl 1):72. [PMID: 21199517] Mushahwar IK. Hepatitis E virus: molecular virology, clinical features, diagnosis, transmission, epidemiology, and prevention. J Med Virol 2008;80:646. [PMID: 18297720]

Test/Range/Collection	Physiologic Basis	Interpretation	Comments
Heterophile antibody, serum (Monospot, Paul-Bunnell test) Negative SST, red $	Infectious mononucleosis (IM) is an acute saliva-transmitted infectious disease due to the Epstein-Barr virus (EBV). The virus preferentially infects B cells and causes immune responses including the activation of T cells. Heterophile (Paul-Bunnell) anti-bodies (IgM) appear in 60% of mononucleosis patients within 1–2 weeks and in 80–90% within the first month. They are not specific for EBV but are found only rarely in other disorders. The monospot test, a form of the heterophile antibody test, is a rapid test for infectious mononu-cleosis due to EBV. The test relies on the agglutination of horse RBCs by heterophile antibodies in patient's serum. Titers are substantially diminished by 3 months after primary infec-tion and are not detectable by 6 months.	**Positive in:** Infectious mono-nucleosis (IM) (90–95%). **Negative in:** Heterophile-negative mononucleosis: CMV, heterophile-negative EBV, toxoplasmosis, hepatitis viruses, HIV-1 seroconversion, listeriosis, tularemia, brucellosis, cat-scratch disease, Lyme disease, syphilis, rickettsial infections, medications (phenytoin, sul-fasalazine, dapsone), collagen vascular diseases (especially systemic lupus erythematosus), subacute infective endocarditis.	The test is used as an aid in the diagnosis of IM. The three classic laboratory features of IM are lympho-cytosis, a significant number (>10–20%) of atypical lymphocytes (reactive T cells) on Wright-stained peripheral blood smear, and positive heterophile test. If heterophile test is negative in the setting of hemato-logic and clinical evidence of a mononucleosis-like illness, a repeat test in 1–2 weeks may be positive. EBV serology (anti-VCA, anti-EBNA, anti-EA) may also be indicated, especially in children and teenage patients who may have negative heterophile tests. Bravender T. Epstein-Barr virus, cytomegalovirus, and infectious mononucleosis. Adolesc Med State Art Rev 2010;21:251. [PMID: 21047028] Gulley ML et al. Laboratory assays for Epstein-Barr virus-related disease. J Mol Diagn 2008;10:279. [PMID: 18556771]

Histoplasma capsulatum antigen		
***Histoplasma capsulatum* antigen,** urine, serum, CSF (HPA) Negative SST (serum) $$ Deliver urine, CSF in a clean plastic or glass container tube. Urine is the best specimen for the test.	Histoplasmosis is the most common systemic fungal infection and typically starts as a pulmonary infection with influenza-like symptoms. This may heal, progress, or lie dormant with reinfection occurring at a later time. Heat-stable *H. capsulatum* polysaccharide is detected by enzyme immunoassay antigen (EIA) using alkaline phosphatase or horseradish peroxidase-conjugated antibodies. EIA has replaced the previously used radioimmunoassay (RIA) as the mainstream method.	**Increased in:** Disseminated histoplasmosis (90–97% in urine, 50–78% in blood, and approximately 42% in CSF), localized disease (16% in urine), blastomycosis (urine and serum), coccidioidomycosis (CSF).	Histoplasmosis is usually seen in the Mississippi and Ohio River valleys but may appear elsewhere. Detection of *Histoplasma* antigenemia or antigenuria is recommended for the diagnosis of disseminated histoplasmosis and may be useful in the early acute stage of pulmonary histoplasmosis before the appearance of antibodies. The test can also be used to monitor therapy or to follow relapse in immuno-compromised patients. EIA for *H. capsulatum var capsulatum* polysaccharide antigen in urine is a useful test in diagnosis of disseminated histoplasmosis and in assessing efficacy of treatment or in detecting relapse, especially in AIDS patients and when serologic tests for antibodies may be negative. It is not useful for ruling out localized pulmonary histoplasmosis. In bronchoalveolar lavage fluid, HPA has 70% sensitivity for the diagnosis of pulmonary histoplasmosis. The antigenuria test's high sensitivity and specificity have dispelled the confusion in interpreting antibody test results. Kauffman CA. Diagnosis of histoplasmosis in immunosuppressed patients. Curr Opin Infect Dis 2008;21:421. [PMID: 18594296] Kauffman CA. Histoplasmosis. Clin Chest Med 2009;30:217. [PMID: 19375629] Pasqualotto AC et al. *Histoplasma capsulatum* recovery from the urine and a short review of genitourinary histoplasmosis. Mycopathologia 2009;167:315. [PMID: 19184526]

Test/Range/Collection	Physiologic Basis	Interpretation	Comments
***Histoplasma capsulatum* precipitins,** serum Negative SST (acute and convalescent samples, collected 2–3 weeks apart) $$	This test screens for *Histoplasma* antibodies by detecting precipitins to specific antigens ("H" and "M" bands) by immunodiffusion (ID). "M" precipitin is present in approximately 70% of acute and chronic histoplasmosis cases. Only 10% of patients have both "M" and "H" precipitins. Positive H band indicates active infection, but is rarely found alone; M band indicates acute or chronic infection or prior skin testing. Presence of both is highly suggestive of active histoplasmosis.	**Positive in:** Previous, chronic, or acute histoplasma infection, recent histoplasmin skin testing. Cross-reactions at low levels in patients with blastomycosis and coccidioidomycosis.	Test is useful as a screening test or as an adjunct to complement fixation test (see below) in diagnosis of systemic histoplasmosis. Kauffman CA. Diagnosis of histoplasmosis in immunosuppressed patients. Curr Opin Infect Dis 2008;21:421. [PMID: 18594296] Kauffman CA. Histoplasmosis. Clin Chest Med 2009;30:217. [PMID: 19375629] Versalovic J et al (editors): *Manual of Clinical Microbiology*, 10th ed. ASM Press, 2011.

***Histoplasma capsulatum* precipitins**

Histoplasma capsulatum CF antibody

Histoplasma capsulatum complement fixation (CF) antibody, serum, CSF <1:4 titer SST $$ Submit paired sera—one specimen collected within 1 week after onset of illness and another 2 weeks later.	The standard method for the diagnosis of histoplasmosis remains culture isolation and identification of the organism. However, culture often requires 2–4 weeks. Antibody detection offers a more rapid alternative and is valuable in the diagnosis of acute, chronic, disseminated, and meningeal histoplasmosis. Antibodies in primary pulmonary infections are generally found within 4 weeks after exposure and frequently are present at the time symptoms appear. Two types of CF test are available based on mycelial antigen and yeast phase antigen. The yeast phase test is considerably more sensitive. Latex agglutination (LA) and enzyme-linked immunosorbent assay (ELISA) tests are also available but are less reliable.	**Increased in:** Previous, chronic, or acute histoplasma infection (75–80%), recent histoplasmin skin testing (20%), other fungal disease, leishmaniasis. Cross-reactions in patients with blastomycosis and coccidioidomycosis.	Elevated CF titers >1:16 are suggestive of infection. Titers >1:32 or rising titers are usually indicative of active infection. Histoplasmin skin test is not recommended for diagnosis because it interferes with subsequent serologic tests. The CF test is usually positive in CSF from patients with chronic meningitis. About 3.5–12% of clinically normal persons have positive titers, usually less than 1:16. Kauffman CA. Diagnosis of histoplasmosis in immunosuppressed patients. Curr Opin Infect Dis 2008;21:421. [PMID: 18594296] Kauffman CA. Histoplasmosis. Clin Chest Med 2009;30:217. [PMID: 19375629] Pizzini CV et al. Evaluation of a Western blot test in an outbreak of acute pulmonary histoplasmosis. Clin Diagn Lab Immunol 1999;6:20. [PMID: 9874658] Versalovic J et al (editors): Manual of Clinical Microbiology, 10th ed. ASM Press, 2011.

	HIV antibody

Test/Range/Collection	Physiologic Basis	Interpretation	Comments
HIV antibody, serum or plasma Negative SST, PPT, lavender, green $$	This test detects antibody against the human immunodeficiency virus-1 (HIV-1), the etiologic agent of most HIV infections in the US. Antibodies become detectable approximately 22–27 days after acute infection. Early detection is crucial for the institution of highly active antiretroviral therapy (HAART). HIV antibody test is considered positive only when a repeatedly reactive enzyme immunoassay (EIA) is confirmed by a Western blot (WB) analysis. Immunofluorescent antibody (IFA) test is also performed in some laboratories for screening and/or as a substitute for the Western blot test. Rapid HIV antibody tests are available and provide timely detection of antibody to HIV in cases of needlestick injury or exposure to potentially HIV-contaminated materials.	**Positive in:** HIV infection: EIA sensitivity > 99% after first 2–4 months of infection, specificity 99%. When combined with confirmatory test, specificity is 99.995%.	Although Western blot test is currently the most sensitive and specific assay for HIV serodiagnosis, it is highly dependent on the proficiency of the laboratory performing the test and on the standardization of the procedure. The CDC recommends that all pregnant women be offered HIV testing. Several rapid HIV antibody screening tests are available in the US; specimen types include whole blood, serum, plasma and oral fluids. An HIV Ag/Ab combination assay is also available, which is designed to detect HIV infection early during the seroconversion window. Butto S et al. Laboratory diagnostics for HIV infection. Ann Ist Super Sanita 2010;46:24. [PMID: 20348616] Chappel RJ et al. Immunoassays for the diagnosis of HIV: meeting future needs by enhancing the quality of testing. Future Microbiol 2009;4:963. [PMID: 19824789] Chu C et al. Diagnosis and initial management of acute HIV infection. Am Fam Physician 2010;81:1239. [PMID: 20507048] Pandori MW et al. Assessment of the ability of a fourth-generation immunoassay for human HIV antibody and p24 antigen to detect both acute and recent HIV infections in a high-risk setting. J Clin Microbiol 2009;47:2639. [PMID: 19535523]

HIV RNA, quantitative		
HIV RNA, quantitative (viral load), plasma <40 [copies per mL] (assay-specific) Lavender, PPT $$$$	Monitoring HIV-1 RNA level (viral load) in plasma of infected patients is used to assess disease progression and patient response to antiviral therapy. Currently, there are three FDA-approved commercially developed assays to monitor HIV viral load. Assays are based on RT-PCR target amplification (Roche Amplicor HIV Monitor and Abbott m2000) or branched-chain DNA (bDNA) signal amplification (Versant HIV-1 RNA 3.0 Assay bDNA). The HIV viral load assays are intended for use in conjunction with clinical presentation and other laboratory markers of disease progression.	The real-time PCR based assays (eg, Abbott m2000, Roche Amplicor) have a broad dynamic range from 40–75 copies/mL to 1×10^7 copies/mL. The bDNA-based assay (Versant HIV-1 RNA) has a measurement range of 75–500,000 copies per mL.	The clinical significance of changes in HIV-1 viral load has not been fully established; however, a threefold change (0.5 log) in copies/mL may be significant. Caution should be taken in the interpretation of any single viral load determination. d'Ettorre G et al. The role of HIV-DNA testing in clinical practice. New Microbiol 2010;33:1. [PMID: 20402409] Hamers RL et al. Dried fluid spots for HIV type-1 viral load and resistance genotyping: a systematic review. Antivir Ther 2009;14:619. [PMID: 19704164] Korenromp EL et al. Clinical prognostic value of RNA viral load and CD4 cell counts during untreated HIV-1 infection—a quantitative review. PLoS One 2009;4:e5950. [PMID: 19536329] Rouet F et al. In-house HIV-1 RNA real-time RT-PCR assays: principle, available tests and usefulness in developing countries. Expert Rev Mol Diagn 2008;8:635. [PMID: 18785811]

	HIV resistance testing	
Test/Range/Collection	**Physiologic Basis**	**Interpretation**

Comments
Phenotypic resistance tests (eg, PhenoSense GT from Monogram Biosciences) rely on PCR amplification of viral protease and reverse transcriptase (RT) gene sequence in lieu of viral isolation. The test involves cloning and expression of the amplified viral RNA in an HIV-1 vector that lacks these regions and contains luciferase reporter gene in place of the viral envelope gene. The replication of the recombinant virus in the presence of various antiviral agents is monitored by the amount of expressed luciferase. Genotypic resistance assays (eg, line probe assay) detect specific mutations in the viral genome that are associated with resistance to various antiretroviral agents. The initial step of the assay is PCR amplification of viral protease and a 250–400 codon segment of HIV RT gene. This is followed by either direct sequencing or by hybridization-based detection of the amplified products to assess the presence of mutations associated with resistance to antiretroviral agents. Bogoch I et al. First-line regimen failure of antiretroviral therapy: a clinical and evidence-based approach. Curr Opin HIV AIDS 2009;4:493. [PMID: 20048716] Grant PM et al. The use of resistance testing in the management of HIV-1-infected patients. Curr Opin HIV AIDS 2009;4:474. [PMID: 20048713] MacArthur RD. Understanding HIV phenotypic resistance testing: usefulness in managing treatment-experienced patients. AIDS Rev 2009;11:223. [PMID: 19940949] Taylor S et al. Using HIV resistance tests in clinical practice. J Antimicrob Chemother 2009;64:218. [PMID: 19535382]

HIV resistance testing

Lavender, PPT

$$$$

Testing for resistance to antiretroviral agents is considered to be standard of care and is widely used in the management of HIV-infected persons. It is an important tool in optimizing the efficacy of combination therapy to treat HIV infection. The identification of resistance mutations allows selection of antiviral agents with maximum therapeutic benefit and minimum toxic side effects.

Both phenotypic and genotypic resistance tests are available.

Positive in: HIV-1 infection with drug resistance.

HLA typing		
HLA (human leukocyte antigen) typing, serum and blood (HLA) SST (2 mL) and yellow (40 mL) $$$$ Specimens must be <24 hours old. Refrigerate serum, but not blood in yellow tubes.	The human leukocyte antigen (HLA) system consists of four closely linked loci (HLA–A, –B, –C, and –DR) located on the short arm of chromosome 6. The previous gold standard technique for HLA phenotyping was the complement-dependent cytotoxicity test. This is a complement-mediated serologic assay in which antiserum containing specific anti-HLA antibodies is added to peripheral blood lymphocytes. Cell death indicates that the lymphocytes carried the specific targeted antigen. The three HLA-A, –B, and –C are determined in this manner. The HLA-D locus (DR or D-related) is determined by mixed lymphocyte culture. DNA-based methods for HLA genotyping have largely replaced traditional HLA testing based on serologic assays.	**Useful in:** Evaluation of transplant candidates and potential donors and for paternity and forensic testing.	HLA typing is usually performed for matching transplantation candidates and potential donors, in blood product matching (eg, platelets), and in paternity testing. It is also helpful in diagnosis of certain diseases (eg, B27 for ankylosing spondylitis) and prevention of adverse drug reactions associated with particular HLA antigens (eg, B*5701 for abacavir sensitivity). Howell WM et al. The HLA system: immunobiology, HLA typing, antibody screening and crossmatching techniques. J Clin Pathol 2010;63:387. [PMID: 20418230] Leffell MS et al. The role of the histocompatibility laboratory in desensitization for transplantation. Curr Opin Organ Transplant 2009;14:398. [PMID: 19417655] Lu Y et al. Multiplex HLA-typing by pyrosequencing. Methods Mol Biol 2009;496:89. [PMID: 18839107] Tinckam K. Histocompatibility methods. Transplant Rev (Orlando) 2009;23:80. [PMID: 19298939]

	HLA-B27 typing		
Test/Range/Collection	**Physiologic Basis**	**Interpretation**	**Comments**
HLA-B27 typing, whole blood Negative Yellow $$$ Specimens must be <24 hours old.	The HLA-B27 allele is found in approximately 8% of the US white population. It occurs less frequently in the African American population. PCR-based HLA-B27 testing is available.	There is an increased incidence of spondyloarthritis among patients who are HLA-B27–positive. HLA-B27 is present in 88% of Caucasian patients with ankylosing spondylitis. It is also associated with the development of reactive arthritis (formerly known as Reiter syndrome) (80%) following infection with enteric organisms, such as *Yersinia, Shigella,* or *Salmonella.*	The best diagnostic test for ankylosing spondylitis is a lumbar spine film and not HLA-B27 typing. HLA-B27 testing is not usually clinically indicated. Sheehan NJ. HLA-B27: What's new? Rheumatology (Oxford) 2010;49:621. [PMID: 20083539] Zamecki KJ et al. HLA typing in uveitis: use and misuse. Am J Ophthalmol 2010;149:189.e2. [PMID: 20103052]

Homocysteine

Homocysteine, plasma or serum Males: 4–12 mcmol/L Females: 4–10 mcmol/L (method- and age-dependent) SST, green (Fasting specimen is required; plasma or serum must be separated from cells within 1 hour of collection.) $$	Homocysteine is a naturally occurring, sulfur-containing amino acid produced during catabolism of methionine, an essential amino acid. It is metabolized by two major pathways: remethylation and transsulfuration. Several vitamins function as cofactors and substrates in these pathways: folic acid and vitamin B_{12} regulate the remethylation pathway catalyzed by methylenetetrahydrofolate reductase (MTHFR) and methionine synthase, respectively, whereas vitamin B_6 is a cofactor for cystathione β-synthase, a key enzyme in the transsulfuration pathway. Deficiencies in one or more of these vitamins can lead to acquired hyperhomocysteinemia. Homocystinuria is a rare autosomal recessive disorder that usually results from defective activity of cystathione β-synthase.	**Increased in:** Homocystinuria due to defects in cystathionine β-synthase, methionine synthase or intracellular cobalamin metabolism. MTHFR C677T mutation, deficiency of folic acid or B vitamins (eg B_{12}, B_6), cigarette smoking, chronic alcohol ingestion, renal failure, systemic lupus erythematosus, hypothyroidism, diabetes mellitus, certain medications (eg, methotrexate, nicotinic acid, theophylline, L-dopa), and advanced age. **Decreased in:** Down syndrome, hyperthyroidism.	Hyperhomocysteinemia is typically defined as a total homocysteine level above the 95th percentile of a control population, which in most studies is approximately 15 mcmol/L. Hyperhomocysteinemia may be classified as moderate (16–30), intermediate (31–100), and severe (>100 mcmol/L). Clinical and epidemiologic studies have demonstrated that hyperhomocysteinemia is an independent risk factor for atherosclerosis and coronary heart disease and for arterial and venous thromboembolism. Nevertheless, due to the lack of definitive evidence for clinical treatment outcome benefits from reducing homocysteine levels, routine screening for hyperhomocysteinemia is not recommended. It is reasonable to determine levels of fasting homocysteine in high-risk patients, especially those with strong family history of premature atherosclerosis or with arterial occlusive diseases, as well as their family members. For patients with elevated homocysteine concentration, it is important to check their vitamin status. Clarke R et al. B-Vitamin Treatment Trialists' Collaboration. Effects of lowering homocysteine levels with B vitamins on cardiovascular disease, cancer, and cause-specific mortality: meta-analysis of 8 randomized trials involving 37,485 individuals. Arch Intern Med 2010;170:1622. [PMID: 20937919] Di Minno MN et al. Homocysteine and arterial thrombosis: challenge and opportunity. Thromb Haemost 2010;103:942. [PMID: 20352150] Khandanpour N et al. Homocysteine and peripheral arterial disease: systematic review and meta-analysis. Eur J Vasc Endovasc Surg 2009;38:316. [PMID: 19560951]

Test/Range/Collection	Physiologic Basis	Interpretation	Comments
5-Hydroxyindoleacetic acid			**5-Hydroxyindoleacetic acid**
5-Hydroxyindoleacetic acid, urine (5-HIAA) 2–8 mg/24 hr [10–40 mcmol/d] Urine bottle containing hydrochloric acid $$	Serotonin (5-hydroxytryptamine) is a neurotransmitter that is metabolized by monoamine oxidase (MAO) to 5-HIAA and then excreted into the urine. Serotonin is secreted by most carcinoid tumors, which arise from neuroendocrine cells in locations derived from the embryonic gut. Biochemical diagnosis of gastrointestinal carcinoids is established by demonstrating elevation of urinary 5-HIAA or plasma chromogranin A or serotonin.	**Increased in:** Metastatic carcinoid tumor (foregut, midgut, and bronchial). Nontropical sprue (slight increase). Diet: Bananas, walnuts, avocado, eggplant, pineapple, plums. Drugs: reserpine. **Negative in:** Rectal carcinoids (usually), renal insufficiency. Drugs: MAO inhibitors, phenothiazines. Test is often falsely positive because pretest probability is low. Using 5-HIAA/Cr ratio may improve performance.	Urinary 5-HIAA excretion is used as a biochemical tumor marker for clinical diagnosis, to monitor treatment effects, and as a prognostic predictor. A very high concentration of urinary 5-HIAA is an indicator that a gastrointestinal carcinoid tumor is malignant. Because most carcinoid tumors drain into the portal vein and serotonin is rapidly cleared by the liver, the carcinoid syndrome (flushing, bronchial constriction, diarrhea, hypotension, and cardiac valvular lesions) is a late manifestation of carcinoid tumors, appearing only after hepatic metastasis has occurred. Gheorariya V et al. Carcinoid tumors of the gastrointestinal tract. South Med J 2009;102:1032. [PMID: 19738517] Pasieka JL. Carcinoid tumors. Surg Clin North Am 2009;89:1123. [PMID: 19836488]

IgG index

IgG index, serum and CSF 0.29–0.59 ratio SST or red (serum), glass or plastic tube (CSF) $$$ Collect serum and CSF simultaneously.	This test compares CSF IgG and albumin levels with serum levels. The formula used for CSF IgG index calculation is: (CSF IgG/ CSF albumin)/(serum IgG/serum albumin). An increased ratio allegedly reflects synthesis of IgG within the central nervous system.	**Increased in:** Multiple sclerosis (80–90%), neurosyphilis, subacute sclerosing panencephalitis, other inflammatory and infectious CNS diseases.	Test is reasonably sensitive but not specific for multiple sclerosis. There is no predictable correlation between the IgG index values and the oligoclonal IgG band number in patients with multiple sclerosis (see Oligoclonal bands, p. 220). Luque FA et al. Cerebrosinal fluid analysis in multiple sclerosis. Int Rev Neurobiol 2007;79:341. [PMID: 17531849]

Test/Range/Collection	Physiologic Basis	Interpretation	Comments
Immunofixation electrophoresis (IFE), serum or urine Negative SST (serum) $$$	IFE is used to identify specific immunoglobulin (Ig) classes. Proteins are separated electrophoretically on several tracks on a gel. Antisera specific to individual classes of molecules are added to each track. If specific classes of heavy or light chain are present, insoluble complexes form with the antisera, which can then be stained and detected.	**Positive in:** Presence of identifiable monoclonal protein: plasma cell neoplasms (myeloma, Waldenström macroglobulinemia, heavy chain disease, primary amyloidosis, monoclonal gammopathy of undetermined significance, plasmacytoma), lymphoma, leukemia. The most common M-protein seen in myeloma is the IgG type, followed by IgA and light chain only.	IFE is indicated to define an overt or suspicious Ig spike seen on serum protein electrophoresis (SPEP) or urine protein electrophoresis (UPEP), to differentiate a polyclonal from a monoclonal increase (eg, M-protein in serum, Bence Jones protein in urine), and to identify the nature of a monoclonal increase. The IFE detection limit for M-protein is approximately 25 mg/dL. Immuno-subtraction capillary zone electrophoresis (CZE) is an alternative test to IFE, and is increasingly used in clinical laboratories. Kyle RA et al. Monoclonal gammopathy of undetermined significance and smoldering multiple myeloma. Curr Hematol Malig Rep 2010;5:62. [PMID: 20425398] Nau KC et al. Multiple myeloma: diagnosis and treatment. Am Fam Physician 2008;78:853. [PMID: 18841734]

Immunofixation electrophoresis

Immunoglobulins

Immunoglobulins, serum (Ig)		

Immunoglobulins, serum (Ig)

IgA: 0.78–3.67 g/L

IgG: 5.83–17.6 g/L

IgM: 0.52–3.35 g/L

SST

$$$

IgG makes up about 85% of total serum immunoglobulins and predominates late in immune responses. It is the only immunoglobulin to cross the placenta. IgM antibody predominates early in immune responses.

Secretory IgA plays an important role in host defense mechanisms by blocking transport of microbes across mucosal surfaces.

↑ **IgG:** *Polyclonal:* Autoimmune diseases (eg, SLE, rheumatoid arthritis), sarcoidosis, chronic liver diseases, some parasitic diseases, chronic or recurrent infections.

Monoclonal: Multiple myeloma (IgG type), lymphomas, or other malignancies.

↑ **IgM:** *Polyclonal:* Isolated infections such as viral hepatitis, infectious mononucleosis, early response to bacterial or parasitic infection.

Monoclonal: Waldenström macroglobulinemia, lymphoma.

↑ **IgA:** *Polyclonal:* Chronic liver disease, chronic infections (especially of the GI and respiratory tracts).

Monoclonal: Multiple myeloma (IgA).

↓ **IgG:** Immunosuppressive therapy, genetic (severe combined immunodeficiency disease [SCID]), Wiskott-Aldrich syndrome, common variable immunodeficiency).

↓ **IgM:** Immunosuppressive therapy.

↓ **IgA:** Inherited IgA deficiency (ataxia telangiectasia, combined immunodeficiency disorders).

Protein electrophoresis (PEP, serum and/or urine) followed by IFE detects monoclonal immunoglobulin (paraprotein in serum, Bence Jones protein in urine).

Quantitative immunoglobulin levels are indicated in the evaluation of immunodeficiency. In X-linked agammaglobulinemia (also known as Bruton agammaglobulinemia), immunoglobulins of all classes are nearly undetectable, and there is a complete lack of circulating B cells.

IgG deficiency is associated with recurrent and occasionally severe pyogenic infections.

The most common form of multiple myeloma is the IgG type, followed by IgA type. Myeloma of IgM, IgD, or IgE type is rare. Quantitation of the serum paraprotein is used for treatment monitoring and patient follow-up.

Berenson JR et al. Monoclonal gammopathy of undetermined significance: a consensus statement. Br J Haematol 2010;150:28. [PMID: 20507313]

Nau KC et al. Multiple myeloma: diagnosis and treatment. Am Fam Physician 2008;78:853. [PMID: 18841734]

Wood PM. Primary antibody deficiency syndromes. Curr Opin Hematol 2010;17:356. [PMID: 20442656]

	Inhibitor screen (1:1 mix)		
Test/Range/Collection	**Physiologic Basis**	**Interpretation**	**Comments**
Inhibitor screen (1:1 mix), plasma Negative Blue $$ Fill tube completely.	Test is useful for evaluating a prolonged PTT and/or PT. (Presence of heparin should first be excluded.) Patient's plasma is mixed with pooled normal plasma (1:1 mix) and PTT and/or PT are performed. If the patient has a factor deficiency, the post-mixing PTT/PT will be normal (correction). If an inhibitor is present, the post-mixing PTT/PT will still be prolonged (no correction) immediately and/or after incubation.	**Positive in:** Presence of inhibitor: Antiphospholipid antibodies (lupus anticoagulant, LAC), factor-specific antibodies, or both. **Negative in:** Factor deficiencies. See evaluation of isolated prolongation of PTT (Figure 9–22).	Lupus anticoagulant is a nonspecific inhibitor, which prolongs PTT on inhibitor screen (1:1 mix study) both immediately and after 1–2 hours' incubation. 1- to 2-hour incubation period is often needed to detect factor-specific antibodies with low *in vitro* affinities (eg, post-mixing PTT is normal immediately, but is prolonged after incubation). Ledford-Kraemer MR. Laboratory testing for lupus anticoagulants: pre-examination variables, mixing studies, and diagnostic criteria. Semin Thromb Hemost 2008;34:380. [PMID: 18814072] Tripodi A. Testing for lupus anticoagulants: all that a clinician should know. Lupus 2009;18:291. [PMID: 19276296] Verbruggen B et al. Improvements in factor VIII inhibitor detection: from Bethesda to Nijmegen. Semin Thromb Hemost 2009;35:752. [PMID: 20169511]

Insulin antibody		
Insulin antibody, serum Negative SST, red $$$	This assay quantitatively measures human serum autoantibodies to endogenous insulin or antibodies to exogenous insulin. Insulin antibodies develop in nearly all diabetics treated with insulin. Most antibodies are IgG and do not cause clinical problems. Occasionally, high-affinity antibodies can bind to exogenous insulin and cause insulin resistance.	**Increased in:** Insulin therapy, type 1 diabetes mellitus before treatment (secondary to autoimmune pancreatic B-cell destruction).	Insulin antibodies interfere with most assays for total insulin and C-peptide. Free insulin and free C-peptide can be measured instead in patients with insulin antibodies. Insulin antibody test is not sensitive or specific for the detection of surreptitious insulin use; use C-peptide level instead. If anti-insulin antibody is present in a child with diabetes who is not insulin-treated, the diagnosis of type 1 diabetes is confirmed. The detection of anti-insulin antibody in insulin-treated patients is of no diagnostic utility. Anti-insulin antibody only roughly correlates with insulin requirements in patients with diabetes. Bingley PJ. Clinical applications of diabetes antibody testing. J Clin Endocrinol Metab 2010;95:25. [PMID: 19875480]

Test/Range/Collection	Physiologic Basis	Interpretation	Comments
Insulin, immunoreactive, serum or plasma 6–35 mcU/mL [42–243 pmol/L] SST, PPT, lavender $$ Fasting sample required. Measure glucose concurrently.	Measures levels of insulin, either endogenous or exogenous.	**Increased in:** Insulin-resistant states (eg, obesity, type 2 diabetes mellitus, uremia, glucocorticoids, acromegaly), liver disease, surreptitious use of insulin or oral hypoglycemic agents, insulinoma (pancreatic islet cell tumor). **Decreased in:** Type 1 diabetes mellitus, hypopituitarism.	Measurement of serum insulin level has little clinical value except in the diagnosis of fasting hypoglycemia. An insulin-to-glucose ratio >0.3 is presumptive evidence of insulinoma. C-peptide should be used as well as serum insulin to distinguish insulinoma from surreptitious insulin use, since C-peptide will be absent with exogenous insulin use. Neal JM et al. Insulin immunoassays in the detection of insulin analogues in factitious hypoglycemia. Endocr Pract 2008;14:1006. [PMID: 19095600]
Insulin-like growth factor-1, plasma (IGF-1, previously known as somatomedin C) 123–463 ng/mL (age- and sex-dependent) Lavender $$$$	Insulin-like growth factor-1 is a growth hormone (GH)-dependent plasma peptide produced by the liver. It mediates the growth-promoting effect of GH. It has an anabolic, insulin-like action on fat and muscle and stimulates collagen and protein synthesis. Its level is relatively constant throughout the day. Its concentration is regulated by genetic factors, nutrient intake, GH, and other hormones such as T4, cortisol, and sex steroids.	**Increased in:** Acromegaly (level correlates with disease activity better than GH level). **Decreased in:** Pituitary dwarfism, hypopituitarism, Laron dwarfism (end-organ resistance to GH), fasting for 5–6 days, poor nutrition, hypothyroidism, cirrhosis. Values may be normal in GH-deficient patients with hyperprolactinemia or craniopharyngioma.	IGF-1 is a sensitive test for acromegaly. Normal IGF-1 levels rule out active acromegaly. In acromegaly, IGF-1 levels are useful for assessing the relative degree of GH excess, because changes in IGF-1 correlate with changes in symptoms and soft tissue growth. IGF-1 is also very useful in monitoring the symptomatic response to therapy. IGF-1 can be decreased in adult GH deficiency, but it is not a sensitive test. Bidlingmaier M. Pitfalls of insulin-like growth factor I assays. Horm Res 2009;71(Suppl 1):30. [PMID: 19153502] Frystyk J et al. The current status of IGF-1 assays—a 2009 update. Growth Horm IGF Res 2010;20:8. [PMID: 19818658]

Intrinsic factor blocking antibody		
Intrinsic factor blocking antibody (IFBA), serum Negative SST, red $$$$	Vitamin B_{12} (cobalamin) deficiency can lead to megaloblastic anemia and neurologic deficits. The most common cause of B_{12} deficiency in developed countries is pernicious anemia (PA). Pernicious anemia is an autoimmune disorder that results in diminished or absent gastric acid, pepsin, and intrinsic factor (IF) production. Most PA patients have autoantibodies against gastric parietal cells or IF, with the latter being very specific but present in only 50–60% of cases. Parietal cell antibodies are more sensitive but less specific. Measurement of serum B_{12}, either preceded or followed by serum methylmalonic acid (MMA) test, is the first step in diagnosing pernicious anemia (PA). If these tests support B_{12} deficiency, then intrinsic factor blocking antibody (IFBA) testing may be indicated to confirm PA as the etiology.	**Positive in:** Pernicious anemia (sensitivity 50–50%, specificity >95%).	A positive IFBA test supports very strongly a diagnosis of PA. Since the diagnostic sensitivity of IFBA testing for PA is 50–60%, an indeterminate or negative IFBA test does not exclude the diagnosis of PA. In these patients, either PA or another etiology, such as malnutrition, may be present. Measurement of serum gastrin levels will help in these cases. In patients with PA, fasting serum gastrin is elevated (>200 pg/mL) as a compensatory response to the achlorhydria that is present in this condition. Do not order IFBA testing in patients who received a vitamin B12 injection within the previous 2 weeks because high levels of vitamin B_{12} can interfere with the assay. Lahner E et al. Pernicious anemia: new insights from a gastroenterological point of view. World J Gastroenterol 2009;15:5121. [PMID: 19891010] Ward PC. Modern approaches to the investigation of vitamin B_{12} deficiency. Clin Lab Med 2002;22:435. [PMID: 12134470]

Iodine

Test/Range/Collection	Physiologic Basis	Interpretation	Comments
Iodine, 24-hr urine 90–1000 mcg/24 hr [0.7–7.9 mcmol/24 hr] Requires refrigerated aliquot of >10 mL of well-mixed 24-hour urine collection. Do not freeze. $$$$	Iodine is a trace mineral essential for the production of thyroid hormones. Symptoms and signs of iodine deficiency include thyroid goiter, mental retardation, and stunted growth in children. 90% of ingested iodine is excreted in urine. The measurement of urinary iodine excretion serves as an index and estimate of dietary iodine intake.	**Increased in:** Excess iodine intake, iodine-containing drug therapy or contrast media exposure. **Decreased in:** Deficiency in dietary iodine.	Test is used to detect iodine deficiency. Plant foods are poor source of iodine so vegetarians are at risk for iodine deficiency, especially if they avoid iodine enriched salt. Useful for monitoring iodine excretion rate as an index of daily iodine replacement therapy, and for correlating total body iodine load with ^{131}I-uptake studies in assessing thyroid function. Values >1000 mcg/24 hr may indicate dietary excess, but more frequently suggest recent drug or contrast media exposure. Als C et al. Quantification of urinary iodine: a need for revised thresholds. Eur J Clin Nutr 2003;57:1181. [PMID: 12947440] Veiberg P et al. Estimation of iodine intake from various urinary iodine measurements in population studies. Thyroid 2009;19:1281. [PMID: 19888863]

Iron		
Iron (Fe), serum or plasma 50–175 mcg/dL [9–31 mcmol/L] SST, PPT $ Hemolyzed sample unacceptable	Plasma iron concentration is determined by absorption from the intestine; storage in the intestine, liver, spleen, bone marrow; rate of breakdown or loss of hemoglobin; and rate of synthesis of new hemoglobin. The key regulator of iron homeostasis is hepcidin. Hepcidin excess or deficiency contributes to the dysregulation of iron homeostasis in hereditary and acquired iron disorders.	**Increased in:** Hemosiderosis (eg, multiple transfusions, excess iron administration), acute Fe poisoning (children), hemolytic anemia, pernicious anemia, aplastic or hypoplastic anemia, viral hepatitis, lead poisoning, thalassemia, hemochromatosis. Drugs: estrogens, ethanol, oral contraceptives. **Decreased in:** Iron deficiency, nephrotic syndrome, chronic renal failure, many infections, active hematopoiesis, remission of pernicious anemia, hypothyroidism, malignancy (carcinoma), postoperative state, kwashiorkor.	Absence of stainable iron on bone marrow aspirate differentiates iron deficiency from other causes of microcytic anemia (eg, thalassemia, sideroblastic anemia, some chronic disease anemias) but the procedure is invasive and expensive. Serum iron, iron-binding capacity, transferrin saturation, serum ferritin or soluble transferrin receptor may obviate the need for bone marrow examination. Serum iron, transferrin saturation and ferritin are useful in screening family members for hereditary hemochromatosis. Recent transfusion confounds the test results. Pasricha SR et al. Diagnosis and management of iron deficiency anaemia: a clinical update. Med J Aust 2010;193:525. [PMID: 21034387] Pietrangelo A. Hepcidin in human iron disorders: therapeutic implications. J Hepatol 2011;54:173. [PMID: 20932599] Van Vranken M. Evaluation of macrocytosis. Am Fam Physician 2010;82:1117. [PMID: 21121557]

	Iron-binding capacity		
Test/Range/Collection	Physiologic Basis	Interpretation	Comments
Iron-binding capacity, total, serum (TIBC) 250–460 mcg/dL [45–82 mcmol/L] SST, PPT, green $$	Iron is transported in plasma complexed to transferrin, which is synthesized in the liver. Total iron-binding capacity is calculated from transferrin levels measured immunologically. Each molecule of transferrin has two iron-binding sites; so its iron-binding capacity is 1.47 mg/g. Normally, transferrin carries an amount of iron representing about 16–60% of its capacity to bind iron (eg, % saturation of iron-binding capacity is 16–60%).	**Increased in:** Iron deficiency anemia, late pregnancy, infancy, acute hepatitis. Drugs: oral contraceptives. **Decreased in:** Hypoproteinemic states (eg, nephrotic syndrome, starvation, malnutrition, cancer), hemochromatosis, thalassemia, hyperthyroidism, chronic infections, chronic inflammatory disorders, chronic liver disease, other chronic disease.	TIBC correlates with serum transferrin, but the relationship is not linear over a wide range of transferrin values and is disrupted in diseases affecting transferrin-binding capacity or other iron-binding proteins. Increased % transferrin saturation with iron is seen in iron overload (iron poisoning, hemolytic anemia, sideroblastic anemia, thalassemia, hemochromatosis, pyridoxine deficiency, aplastic anemia, RBC transfusions). Decreased % transferrin saturation with iron is seen in iron deficiency (usually saturation <16%). Transferrin levels can also be used to assess nutritional status. Recent transfusion confounds the test results. Pasricha SR et al. Diagnosis and management of iron deficiency anaemia: a clinical update. Med J Aust 2010;193:525. [PMID: 21034387] Van Vranken M. Evaluation of microcytosis. Am Fam Physician 2010;82:1117. [PMID: 21121557]

Islet cell antibodies		
Islet cell antibodies (ICAs), IgG, serum Negative aST U$$$	Islet cell antibodies (ICAs) are associated with type 1 diabetes or insulin-dependent diabetes mellitus (IDDM). ICAs attack pancreatic islet cells, leading to insulin deficiency. ICAs are present in the serum of patients during the prediabetic phase and predict development of type 1 disease. ICAs are detected on thin frozen sections of human pancreas by indirect immunofluorescence assay (IFA), which measures a variety of autoantibodies and is semi-quantitative. ICAs include antibodies directed against several islet cell autoantigens, including insulin, glutamic acid decarboxylase (GAD), insulinoma-associated protein 2 (IA2), and efflux zinc transporter (ZnT8). Radioimmunoassays are available for evaluating specific insulin, GAD and IA2 autoantibodies, which are more reliable markers for the prediabetic state.	**Increased in:** Type 1 diabetes mellitus; individuals at risk for developing type 1 diabetes mellitus.	Useful in assessing risk and predicting onset of type 1 diabetes. Measurements of insulin Ab, GAD Ab, and IA2 Ab are useful adjuncts to measuring ICAs. Predictive value for the development of type I diabetes in first-degree relatives of patients with type 1 diabetes increases to 90–100% when the ICAs are strongly and persistently positive. ICAs are present in combination with insulin Ab or GAD antibodies, or when 2 or more of GAD, IA2, and insulin autoantibodies are present. Although not required for diagnosis, an assay for ICAs can be useful in aiding the differential diagnosis of type 1 (eg, latent autoimmune diabetes) versus type 2 diabetes. ICAs are present in 85% of newly diagnosed type 1 diabetic patients, but are rarely detected in type 2 diabetic patients. Bingley PJ. Clinical applications of diabetes antibody testing. Clin Endocrinol Metab 2010;95:25. [PMID: 19875480] Bonifacio E et al. Advances in prediction and natural history of type1 diabetes. Endocrinol Metab Clin North Am 2010;39:513. [PMID: 20723817] Winter WE et al. Type 1 diabetes islet autoantibody markers. Diabetes Technol Ther 2002;4:817. [PMID: 12614488]

	JAK2 (V617F) mutation		
Test/Range/Collection	**Physiologic Basis**	**Interpretation**	**Comments**
***JAK2* (V617F) mutation**, blood or bone marrow Lavender $$$$	*JAK2* stands for the Janus Kinase 2. Detection of the *JAK2* V617F mutation provides a qualitative diagnostic marker for the non-chronic myelogenous leukemia subgroup of myeloproliferative disorders, including polycythemia vera (PV), essential thrombocythemia (ET), and chronic idiopathic myelofibrosis (CIMF). The V617F mutation, a valine-to-phenylalanine substitution at codon 617, leads to constitutive tyrosine phosphorylation activity, which is believed to confer independence and/or hypersensitivity of myeloid progenitors to cytokines (eg, erythropoietin).	**Positive in:** PV (~80%), ET (50%), CIMF (40%).	A positive result identifies a *JAK2* V617F mutation and is strongly supportive of a diagnosis of PV, ET, or CIMF. It is particularly useful for establishing a diagnosis of PV in patients with marked erythrocytosis (eg, hemoglobin > 18.5 g/dL in males or > 16.5 g/dL in females). A negative result does not rule out the possibility of diagnosis of PV, ET, or CIMF. Reflex testing for *JAK2* exon 12/13 mutations and *MPL* W515 mutation is often indicated. See diagnostic evaluation for polycythemia and thrombocytosis (Figures 9–21 and 9–26). Kilpivaara O et al. *JAK2* and *MPL* mutations in myeloproliferative neoplasms: discovery and science. Leukemia 2008;22:1813. [PMID: 18754026] Koppikar P et al. *JAK2* and *MPL* mutations in myeloproliferative neoplasms. Acta Haematol 2008;119:218. [PMID: 18565540] Spivak JL. Narrative review: Thrombocytosis, polycythemia vera, and *JAK2* mutations: the phenotypic mimicry of chronic myeloproliferation. Ann Intern Med 2010;152:300. [PMID: 20194236] Tefferi A. Novel mutations and their functional and clinical relevance in myeloproliferative neoplasms: *JAK2*, *MPL*, *TET2*, *ASXL1*, *CBL*, *IDH* and *IKZF1*. Leukemia 2010;24:1128. [PMID: 20428194]

Kappa and lambda free light chains

Kappa and lambda free light chains, quantitative, serum

Free kappa (κ): 0.57–2.63 mg/dL

Free lambda (λ): 0.33–1.94 mg/dL

Free kappa/lambda ratio: 0.26–1.65

[Free kappa: 5.7–26.3 × 10^3 g/L]

[Free lambda: 3.3–19.4 × 10^3 g/L]

SST, red

$

Plasma cells produce 1 of the 5 heavy chains (A, M, G, D, E) together with kappa (κ) or lambda (λ) molecules. There is an excess free light chain (FLC) production over heavy chain synthesis. Serum kappa FLCs are normally monomeric, while lambda FLCs tend to be dimeric, joined by disulphide bonds. The half-lives of serum FLCs are short (kappa 2–4 hours; lambda 3–6 hours).

Increased, with abnormal κ/λ ratio: Multiple myeloma including intact Ig producing myeloma, light-chain-only myeloma and "nonsecretory" myeloma, primary amyloidosis (light-chain amyloidosis, AL), plasmacytoma, and high-risk monoclonal gammopathy of undetermined significance (MGUS).

Increased, with normal κ/λ ratio: Infection, renal impairment that is unrelated to plasma cell disorder.

The serum FLC assay, in combination with serum protein electrophoresis (SPEP) and immunofixation, yields high sensitivity in disease screening and may eliminate the need for 24-hr urine studies for diagnosis of plasma cell dyscrasias.

The baseline FLC levels are of prognostic value in all plasma cell dyscrasias.

Because of short half-lives, FLC concentrations allow more rapid assessment of the effects of treatment than do those of intact monoclonal Ig (eg, the half-life of IgG is 21 days, and of IgA, 5 days).

FLC molecules at high levels are frequently nephrotoxic. The FLC measurements thus can guide patient management.

Dispenzieri A et al. International Myeloma Working Group guidelines for serum-free light chain analysis in multiple myeloma and related disorders. Leukemia 2009;23:215. [PMID: 19020545]

Ozsan GH et al. Serum free light chain analysis in multiple myeloma and plasma cell dyscrasias. Expert Rev Clin Immunol 2011;7:65. [PMID: 21162651]

Kappa and lambda free light chains (*continued*)		
Test/Range/Collection	Physiologic Basis	Interpretation	Comments
	The serum Ig FLC nephelometric immunoassay measures levels of free kappa and lambda light chains. Serum levels of FLC are dependent on the balance between production by plasma cells and renal clearance. When there is increased polyclonal Ig production and/or renal impairment, both kappa and lambda FLC concentrations can increase up to 30–40 fold. However, the κ/λ ratio remains unchanged. In contrast, plasma cell dyscrasias produce an excess of only one of the light-chain types (monoclonal), often with suppression of the alternate light chain, so κ/λ ratios become highly abnormal, either increased or decreased.		

Lactate dehydrogenase		
Lactate dehydrogenase (LDH), serum or plasma 88–230 U/L [1.46–3.82 mckat/L] (laboratory-specific) SST, PPT $ Hemolyzed specimens are unacceptable.	LDH is an enzyme that catalyzes the interconversion of lactate and pyruvate in the presence of NAD/NADH. It is widely distributed in body cells and fluids. Because LDH is highly concentrated in RBCs, spuriously elevated serum levels occur if RBCs are hemolyzed during specimen collection.	**Increased in:** Tissue necrosis, especially in acute injury of cardiac muscle, RBCs, kidney, skeletal muscle, liver, lung, and skin. Commonly elevated in various carcinomas, in *Pneumocystis jiroveci* pneumonia (78–94%) and non-Hodgkin lymphomas. Marked elevations occur in hemolytic anemias, megaloblastic anemia (vitamin B_{12} and/or folate deficiency), PV, thrombotic thrombocytopenic purpura (TTP), hepatitis, cirrhosis, obstructive jaundice, renal disease, musculoskeletal disease, and CHF. Drugs causing hepatotoxicity (eg, acetaminophen) or hemolysis. **Decreased in:** Drugs: clofibrate, fluoride (low dose).	LDH is an important prognostic marker for various non-Hodgkin lymphomas. It also correlates with disease transformation in patients with low-grade lymphomas. Serum LDH is a useful prognostic biomarker in metastatic melanoma although serum S100B protein may be superior in predicting prognosis and response to treatment. LDH is not a useful liver function test, and it is not specific enough for the diagnosis of hemolytic or megaloblastic anemias. In diagnosis of myocardial infarction, serum LDH has been replaced by cardiac-specific troponin I levels. LDH isoenzymes are not clinically useful. De Jone D et al. Predicting transformation in follicular lymphoma. Leuk Lymphoma 2009;50:1406. [PMID: 19606378] Gilligan TD et al. American Society of Clinical Oncology Clinical Practice Guideline on uses of serum tumor markers in adult males with germ cell tumors. J Clin Oncol 2010;28:3388. [PMID: 20530278] Gogas H et al. Biomarkers in melanoma. Ann Oncol 2009;20(Suppl 6):vi8. [PMID: 19617299] Kyrtsonis MC et al. Staging systems and prognostic factors as a guide to therapeutic decisions in multiple myeloma. Semin Hematol 2009;46:110. [PMID: 19389494]

Test/Range/Collection	Physiologic Basis	Interpretation	Comments
Lactate, venous blood 0.5–2.0 meq/L [mmol/L] Gray $$$ Collect on ice in gray-top tube containing fluoride to inhibit *in vitro* glycolysis and lactic acid production.	Severe tissue anoxia leads to anaerobic glucose metabolism with production of lactic acid (type A lactic acidosis). In other disorders, lactic acidosis (type B) occurs with no clinical evidence of inadequate tissue oxygen delivery. Lactate is a useful laboratory marker for monitoring tissue perfusion status in critically ill patients, particularly those with sepsis and septic shock.	**Increased in:** Lactic acidosis, ethanol ingestion, sepsis, shock, liver disease, diabetic ketoacidosis, muscular exercise, hypoxia, regional hypoperfusion (bowel ischemia), prolonged use of a tourniquet (spurious elevation), MELAS (mitochondrial myopathy, encephalopathy, lactic acidosis, and stroke-like episodes), type I glycogen storage disease, fructose 1,6-diphosphatase deficiency (rare), pyruvate dehydrogenase deficiency, non-Hodgkin and Burkitt lymphoma (rare). Drugs: phenformin, metformin (debated), isoniazid toxicity, nucleoside reverse-transcriptase inhibitors.	Lactic acidosis should be suspected when there is a markedly increased anion gap (>18 meq/L) in the absence of other causes (eg, renal failure, ketosis, ethanol, methanol, or salicylate). Lactic acidosis is characterized by lactate levels >5 mmol/L and serum pH <7.35. However, hypoalbuminemia may mask the anion gap and concomitant alkalosis may raise the pH. Blood lactate levels may indicate whether perfusion is being restored by therapy. Dell'Aglio DM et al. Acute metformin overdose: examining serum pH, lactate level, and metformin concentrations in survivors versus nonsurvivors: a systematic review of the literature. Ann Emerg Med 2009;54:818. [PMID: 19556031] Jansen TC et al. Blood lactate monitoring in critically ill patients: a systematic health technology assessment. Crit Care Med 2009;37:2827. [PMID: 19707124]

Lactate

	Lead	
Lead, whole blood (Pb) Child (<6 yr): <10 mcg/dL Child (>6 yr): <25 mcg/dL [Child (<6 yr): <0.48 mcmol/L] Child (>6 yr): <1.21 mcmol/L] Adult: <40 mcg/dL [Adult: <1.93 mcmol/L] Industrial workers' limit: <50 mcg/dL [Industrial workers' limit: <2.42 mcmol/L] Navy $$ Use trace metal-free navy blue top tube with heparin.	Lead salts are absorbed through: ingestion, inhalation, or the skin. About 5–10% of ingested lead is found in blood, and 95% of this is in erythrocytes; 80–90% is taken up by bone, where it is relatively inactive. Lead poisons enzymes by binding to protein disulfide groups, leading to cell death. Lead levels fluctuate. Several specimens may be needed to rule out lead poisoning. There is substantial individual variability in vulnerability to lead.	**Increased in:** Lead poisoning, including abnormal ingestion (especially lead-containing paint, water from lead plumbing, moonshine whiskey), occupational exposures (metal smelters, miners, welders, storage battery workers, auto manufacturers, ship builders, paint manufacturers, printing workers, pottery workers, gasoline refinery workers, demolition and tank cleaning workers), retained bullets.	Cognition may be impaired by modest elevations of blood lead concentrations. Neurologic impairment may be detectable in children with lead levels of 15 mcg/dL and in adults at 30 mcg/dL; full-blown symptoms appear at >60 mcg/dL. Most chronic lead poisoning leads to a moderate anemia with basophilic stippling of erythrocytes on peripheral blood smear. Acute poisoning is rare and associated with abdominal pain and constipation. Recent studies have demonstrated that harmful effects can occur in children with blood lead levels less than the current limit of 10 mcg/dL, and a new cutoff value of 5 mcg/dL has been recommended. Janus J et al. Evaluation of anemia in children. Am Fam Physician 2010;81:1462. [PMID: 20540485] Warniment C et al. Lead poisoning in children. Am Fam Physician 2010;81:751. [PMID: 20229974]

Test/Range/Collection	Physiologic Basis	Interpretation	Comments
Legionella antibody, serum <1:32 titer SST $$$ Submit paired sera, one collected within 2 weeks of illness and another 2–3 weeks later.	*Legionella pneumophila* is a weakly staining gram-negative bacillus that causes Pontiac fever (acute influenza-like illness) and legionnaires disease (a pneumonia that may progress to a severe multisystem illness). It does not grow on routine bacteriologic culture media. There are at least 6 serogroups of *L. pneumophila* and at least 22 species of *Legionella*. Indirect immunofluorescent assays for *L. pneumophila* serogroup 1 (IgM and/or IgG) and serogroups 1–6 (IgM and/or IgG) are both available.	**Increased in:** *Legionella* infection (80% of patients with pneumonia have a fourfold rise in titer); cross-reactions with other infectious agents (*Yersinia pestis* [plague], *Francisella tularensis* [tularemia], *Bacteroides fragilis*, *Mycoplasma pneumoniae*, *Leptospira interrogans*, campylobacter serotypes).	The test provides only a retrospective laboratory diagnosis because it generally takes more than 3 weeks to mount a detectable antibody response. More than a fourfold rise in titer to >1:128 in specimens gathered more than 3 weeks apart indicates recent infection. A single titer of >1:256 is considered diagnostic. About 50–60% of cases of legionellosis may have a positive direct fluorescent antibody test. Culture can have a sensitivity of 50%. All three methods may increase sensitivity to 90%. This test is species-specific. Polyvalent antiserum is needed to test for all serogroups and species. Urine *Legionella* antigen testing, in adjunct to cultures, may provide a rapid turnaround for results. The urine antigen test is very specific, but the sensitivity ranges from 70% to 90% because it detects primarily serogroup 1 infections. Diederen BM. Legionella spp. and Legionnaires' disease. J Infect 2008;56:1. [PMID: 17980914]

Leukemia/lymphoma phenotyping by flow cytometry		
Leukemia/lymphoma phenotyping by flow cytometry Blood, bone marrow aspirates, fine-needle aspirates, fresh tissue biopsies, body fluids. Lavender or yellow (blood, bone marrow), green (bone marrow) Specimen should be delivered within 24 hours. $$$	Immunophenotyping by multi-parameter flow cytometry is an integral part of the diagnosis and classification systems for leukemias and malignant lymphomas. The majority of immunophenotyping markers are the cluster of differentiation antigens, or CD antigens. Other commonly used markers include glycophorin A, HLA-DR, immunoglobulin (Ig) light chains, MPO (myeloperoxidase), TdT (terminal deoxynucleotidyl transferase), and ZAP-70 (zeta-chain associated protein kinase 70). Detection of certain cellular antigens also has prognostic (eg, ZAP-70) and therapeutic (eg, CD20, CD33, CD52) significance.	**Abnormal phenotype profile present in:** Acute myeloid leukemias, acute lymphoblastic leukemias, B- and T-cell non-Hodgkin lymphomas, plasma cell myeloma. **Markers expressed mainly in hematopoietic precursors:** HLA-DR TdT, CD34; **B cells:** CD19, CD20, CD22, CD24, CD10, CD79, Ig heavy chains (γ, α, μ, δ), and light chains (κ, λ); **T cells:** CD3, CD7. CD5, CD2, CD4, CD8; **myeloid cells:** MPO, CD13, CD33, CD11, CD117. **Markers that suggest megakaryocytic differentiation:** CD41, CD42, CD61; **erythroid differentiation:** glycophorin, hemoglobin A; **monocytic differentiation:** CD14, CD15, CD64, CD68; **NK cells:** CD16, CD56; **hairy cell leukemia:** CD103 on clonal B cells.	Each leukemia/lymphoma has a unique diagnostic immunophenotype (Table 8–13). An interpretative report should be generated for each specimen analyzed. Multicolor analysis may be performed, allowing for an accurate definition of the surface and cytoplasmic antigen profile of specific cells. Two simultaneous hematologic malignancies may be detected within the same tissue site. Morphologic features remain the cornerstone of the evaluation of leukemia/lymphoma, but ancillary studies including immunophenotyping, cytogenetics, and/or molecular genetic testing are needed in most, if not all, cases. Craig FE et al. Flow cytometric immunophenotyping for hematologic neoplasms. Blood 2008;111:3941. [PMID: 18198345] Kumar S et al. Immunophenotyping in multiple myeloma and related plasma cell disorders. Best Pract Res Clin Haematol 2010;23:433. [PMID: 21112041] Peters JM et al. Multiparameter flow cytometry in the diagnosis and management of acute leukemia. Arch Pathol Lab Med 2011;135:44. [PMID: 21204710]

Lipase			
Test/Range/Collection	Physiologic Basis	Interpretation	Comments
Lipase, serum or plasma 0–160 U/L [0–2.66 mckat/L] (laboratory-specific) SST, PPT $$	Lipases are responsible for hydrolysis of glycerol esters of long-chain fatty acids to produce fatty acids and glycerol. Lipases are produced in the liver, intestine, tongue, stomach, and many other cells. Assays are highly dependent on the substrate used.	**Increased in:** Acute, recurrent, or chronic pancreatitis, pancreatic pseudocyst, pancreatic malignancy, peritonitis, biliary disease, hepatic disease, diabetes mellitus (especially diabetic ketoacidosis), intestinal disease, gastric malignancy or perforation, cystic fibrosis, inflammatory bowel disease (Crohn disease and ulcerative colitis).	Serum lipase may be a more reliable test than serum amylase for the initial diagnosis of acute pancreatitis, because of its increased sensitivity in acute alcoholic pancreatitis and because lipase remains elevated longer than amylase. The specificity of lipase and amylase in acute pancreatitis is similar, although both are poor. Simultaneous measurement of serum amylase and lipase does not improve diagnostic accuracy. Measurement of serum lipase does not help in determining the severity or cause of acute pancreatitis, and daily measurements are of no value in assessing the patient's clinical progress or ultimate prognosis. Test sensitivity is not very good for chronic pancreatitis or pancreatic cancer. For chronic pancreatic insufficiency, fecal pancreatic elastase (p. 225) has excellent sensitivity. Hasibeder WR et al. Critical care of the patient with acute pancreatitis. Anaesth Intensive Care 2009;37:190. [PMID: 19400483] Shah AM et al. Acute pancreatitis with normal serum lipase: a case series. JOP 2010;11:369. [PMID: 20601812]

Luteinizing hormone		
Luteinizing hormone, serum or plasma (LH) Males: 1–10 mIU/mL Females: (mIU/mL) Follicular 1–18 Luteal 0.4–20 Midcycle peak 24–105 Postmenopausal 15–62 (laboratory-specific) SST, PPT, green $$	LH is stimulated by the hypothalamic hormone gonadotropin-releasing hormone (GnRH). It is secreted from the anterior pituitary and acts on the gonads. LH is the principal regulator of steroid biosynthesis in the ovary and testis.	**Increased in:** Primary hypogonadism, polycystic ovary syndrome, postmenopause, endometriosis, after depot leuprolide injection, immunoassay result may be falsely elevated in pregnancy. **Decreased in:** Pituitary or hypothalamic failure, anorexia nervosa, bulimia, advanced prostate cancer, severe stress, malnutrition, Kallman syndrome (gonadotropin deficiency associated with anosmia). Drugs: digoxin, oral contraceptives, phenothiazines.	In male hypogonadism, serum LH and FSH levels can distinguish between primary (hypergonadotropic) and secondary (hypogonadotropic) hypogonadism. Hypogonadism associated with aging (andropause) may present a mixed picture, with low testosterone levels and low to low-normal gonadotropin levels. Repeated measurement may be required to diagnose gonadotropin deficiencies. Elevated serum LH levels are a common feature in polycystic ovary syndrome, but measurement of total testosterone is the test of choice to diagnose polycystic ovary syndrome. Arnold IJ et al. Inactivating mutations of luteinizing hormone beta-subunit or luteinizing hormone receptor cause oligo-amenorrhea and infertility in women. Horm Res 2009;71:75. [PMID: 19129711]

	Lyme disease antibody		
Test/Range/Collection	Physiologic Basis	Interpretation	Comments
Lyme disease antibodies, total, serum ELISA: negative (<1:8 titer) Western blot: nonreactive SST $	Test detects the presence of antibody to *Borrelia burgdorferi*, the etiologic agent in Lyme disease, an inflammatory disorder transmitted by the ticks *Ixodes dammini*, *I pacificus*, and *I scapularis* in the northeastern and midwestern, western, and southeastern United States, respectively. Detects IgM antibody, which develops within 3–6 weeks after the onset of rash or IgG, which develops within 6–8 weeks after the onset of disease. IgG antibody may persist for months.	**Positive in:** Lyme disease, asymptomatic individuals living in endemic areas, immunization with recombinant outer-surface protein A (OspA) Lyme disease vaccine, syphilis (*Treponema pallidum*), tick-borne relapsing fever (*Borrelia hermsii*). **Negative in:** First 5 weeks of *Borrelia* infection or after antibiotic therapy.	Test is less sensitive in patients with only a rash. Because culture or direct visualization of the organism is difficult, serologic diagnosis (by enzyme-linked immunosorbent assay, ELISA) is indicated, although sensitivity and specificity and standardization of procedure between laboratories need improvement. Positive serologic testing (IgM and/or IgG) on specimens < 4 weeks after appearance of skin rash need to be confirmed by Western blots. However, IgM Western blot in the chronic stage (> 4 weeks after disease onset) is generally not recommended. Cross-reactions may occur with syphilis (should be excluded by RPR and treponemal antibody assays). Aguero-Rosenfeld ME. Lyme disease: laboratory issues. Infect Dis Clin North Am 2008;22:301. [PMID: 18452803] Stanek G et al. Lyme borreliosis: a European perspective on diagnosis and clinical management. Curr Opin Infect Dis 2009;22:450. [PMID: 19571749]

Magnesium		
Magnesium, serum or plasma (Mg²⁺) 1.8–3.0 mg/dL [0.75–1.25 mmol/L] ***Panic:*** <0.5 or >4.5 mg/dL [<0.2 or >1.85 mmol/L] Red, green $	Magnesium is primarily an intracellular cation (second most abundant, 60% found in bone); it is a necessary cofactor in numerous enzyme systems, particularly ATPases. By regulating enzymes controlling intracellular calcium, Mg^{2+} affects smooth muscle vasoconstriction, important to the underlying pathophysiology of several critical illnesses. In extracellular fluid, it influences neuromuscular response and irritability. Magnesium concentration is determined by intestinal absorption, renal excretion, and exchange with bone and intracellular fluid.	**Increased in:** Dehydration, tissue trauma, renal failure, hypoadrenocorticism, hypothyroidism. Drugs: aspirin (prolonged use), lithium, magnesium salts, progesterone, triamterene. **Decreased in:** Chronic diarrhea, enteric fistula, starvation, chronic alcoholism, total parenteral nutrition with inadequate replacement, hypoparathyroidism (especially post-parathyroid surgery), acute pancreatitis, chronic glomerulonephritis, hyperaldosteronism, diabetic ketoacidosis, CHF, critical illness, Gitelman syndrome (hereditary hypomagnesemia–hypocalciuria), hereditary isolated magnesium wasting, induced hypothermia. Drugs: albuterol, amphotericin B, calcium salts, cisplatin, citrates (blood transfusion), cyclosporine, diuretics, ethacrynic acid.	Magnesium deficiency correlates with higher mortality and poorer clinical outcome in the ICU and is directly implicated in hypokalemia, hypocalcemia, tetany, and dysrhythmia. Hypomagnesemia is associated with tetany, weakness, disorientation, and somnolence. A magnesium deficit may exist with little or no apparent change in serum level. Prolonged hypomagnesemia can cause refractory hypokalemia as well as functional hypoparathyroidism. There is a progressive reduction in serum magnesium level during normal pregnancy (related to hemodilution). James MF. Magnesium in obstetrics. Best Pract Res Clin Obstet Gynaecol 2010;24:327. [PMID: 20005782] Kramer JH et al. Neurogenic inflammation and cardiac dysfunction due to hypomagnesemia. Am J Med Sci 2009;338:22. [PMID: 19593099] Moe SM. Disorders involving calcium, phosphorus, and magnesium. Prim Care 2008;35:215. [PMID: 18486714] Rude RK et al. Skeletal and hormonal effects of magnesium deficiency. J Am Coll Nutr 2009;28:131. [PMID: 19828898]

Test/Range/Collection	Physiologic Basis	Interpretation	Comments
			Mean corpuscular hemoglobin
Mean corpuscular hemoglobin, blood (MCH) 26–34 pg Lavender $	MCH indicates the amount of hemoglobin per RBC in absolute units. MCH is calculated from measured values of hemoglobin (Hb) (g/dL) and RBC ($\times 10^{12}$/L) by the formula: $MCH = (Hb/RBC) \times 10$	**Increased in:** Macrocytosis, hemochromatosis. **Decreased in:** Microcytosis (iron deficiency, thalassemia), hypochromia (lead poisoning), sideroblastic anemia, anemia of chronic disease).	Low MCH can mean hypochromia or microcytosis or both. High MCH is evidence of macrocytosis. Janus J et al. Evaluation of anemia in children. Am Fam Physician 2010;81:1462. [PMID: 20540485] Langlois S et al. Carrier screening for thalassemia and hemoglobinopathies in Canada. J Obstet Gynaecol Can 2008;30:950. [PMID: 19038079]
			Mean corpuscular hemoglobin concentration
Mean corpuscular hemoglobin concentration, blood (MCHC) 31–36 g/dL [310–360 g/L] Lavender $	MCHC is the average hemoglobin concentration in RBCs. It is calculated from hemoglobin concentration of whole blood (Hb, g/dL) and hematocrit (MCV $\times$ RBC): $MCHC = \dfrac{Hb}{MCV \times RBC}$	**Increased in:** Marked spherocytosis (hereditary spherocytosis or immune hemolysis). Spuriously increased in autoagglutination, hemolysis (with spuriously high Hb or low MCV or RBC), lipemia, cellular dehydration syndromes, hereditary xerocytosis. **Decreased in:** Hypochromic anemia (iron deficiency, thalassemia, lead poisoning), sideroblastic anemia, anemia of chronic disease. Spuriously decreased with markedly high white blood cell count.	The MCHC value may be misleading in the presence of a dimorphic population of RBCs. An X et al. Disorders of red cell membrane. Br J Haematol 2008;141:367. [PMID: 18341630] Urrechaga E. The new mature red cell parameter, low haemoglobin density of the Beckman-Coulter LH750: clinical utility in the diagnosis of iron deficiency. Int J Lab Hematol 2010;32:e144. [PMID: 19220525]

Mean corpuscular volume		
Mean corpuscular volume, blood (MCV) 80–100 fL Lavender $	MCV is the average volume of the red cells, and it is measured by automated hematology instrument based on electrical impedance or forward light scatter.	**Increased in:** Liver disease (alcoholic and nonalcoholic), alcohol abuse, HIV/AIDS, hemochromatosis, megaloblastic anemia (folate, vitamin B_{12} deficiencies), myelodysplasia, reticulocytosis, chemotherapy, post splenectomy, hypothyroidism, newborns. Spurious increase in autoagglutination, high white blood cell count. Drugs: methotrexate, phenytoin, zidovudine. **Decreased in:** Iron deficiency, thalassemia, sideroblastic anemia, lead poisoning, hereditary spherocytosis, and some anemias of chronic disease.	MCV can be normal in combined iron and folate deficiency. In patients with two red cell populations (macrocytic and microcytic), MCV may be normal. MCV is an insensitive test in the evaluation of anemia. It is not uncommon for patients with iron deficiency anemia or pernicious anemia to have a normal MCV. A low MCV can be used as an indication of iron depletion in frequent blood donors and a guide to phlebotomy therapy for hemochromatosis. See anemias (Figure 9–5; Tables 8–2, 8–3). Janus J et al. Evaluation of anemia in children. Am Fam Physician 2010;81:1462. [PMID: 20540485] Kaferle J et al. Evaluation of macrocytosis. Am Fam Physician 2009;79:203. [PMID: 19202968] Moreno Chulilla JA et al. Classification of anemia for gastroenterologists. World J Gastroenterol 2009;15:4627. [PMID: 19787825] Van Vranken M. Evaluation of macrocytosis. Am Fam Physician 2010;82:1117. [PMID: 21121557]

Test/Range/Collection	Physiologic Basis	Interpretation	Comments
Metanephrines, free (unconjugated), plasma <1.40 nmol/L Lavender, PPT $$$	Catecholamines (norepinephrine and epinephrine), secreted in excess by pheochromocytomas, are metabolized within tumor cells by the enzyme catechol-O-methyltransferase to meta-nephrines (normetanephrine and metanephrine), and these can be detected in plasma. Measurement of plasma concentrations of free (unconjugated) metanephrines offers several advantages for the detection of pheochromocytoma: independence of short-term changes noted in catecholamine secretion in response to change of posture, exercise, or intraoperative stress; good correlation with tumor mass; and only minor interference from drugs. In diagnosis of pheochromocytoma, determination of plasma free metanephrines is often more reliable and efficient than other biochemical tests.	**Increased in:** Pheochromocytoma (sensitivity 99%; specificity 89–94%).	The plasma free metanephrines test has been recommended as one of the first-line biochemical tests for the diagnosis of pheochromocytoma. (See Pheochromocytoma algorithm, Figure 9–20.) Sensitivity of plasma free metanephrines (99%) is higher than that of urinary fractionated metanephrines (97%), plasma catecholamines (84%), and urinary vanillylmandelic acid (64%). Specificity of plasma free metanephrines is 89–94% compared with urinary vanillylmandelic acid (95%), urinary total metanephrines (93%), urinary catecholamines (88%), plasma catecholamines (81%), and urinary fractionated metanephrines (69%). Plasma catecholamines are often spuriously increased when drawn in the hospital setting. Eisenhofer G et al. Current progress and future challenges in the biochemical diagnosis and treatment of pheochromocytomas and paragangliomas. Horm Metab Res 2008;40:329. [PMID: 18491252] Ilias I et al. Diagnosis, localization and treatment of pheochromocytoma in MEN 2 syndrome. Endocr Regul 2009;43:89. [PMID: 19856714] Nieman LK. Approach to the patient with an adrenal incidentaloma. J Clin Endocrinol Metab 2010;95:4106. [PMID: 20823463]

Metanephrines		
Metanephrines, urine 0.3–0.9 mg/24 hr [1.6–4.9 mcmol/24 hr] Urine bottle containing hydrochloric acid $$$ Collect 24-hour urine.	Catecholamines (norepinephrine and epinephrine), secreted in excess by pheochromocytomas, are metabolized by the enzyme catechol-*O*-methyltransferase to metanephrines (normetaphrine and metanephrine), and these are excreted in the urine.	**Increased in:** Pheochromocytoma (98% sensitivity, 93% specificity), neuroblastoma, ganglioneuroma. Drugs: Monoamine oxidase inhibitors.	Urinary metanephrines are often the first-line biochemical tests for the diagnostic evaluation of pheochromocytoma. (see Pheochromocytoma algorithm, Figure 9–20). Because <0.1% of persons with hypertension have a pheochromocytoma, routine screening of all such people would yield a positive predictive value of <10%. Avoid overutilization of tests. Do not order urine vanillylmandelic acid, urine catecholamines, and plasma metanephrines and catecholamines at the same time. Donckier JF et al. Phaeochromocytoma: state-of-the-art. Acta Chir Belg 2010;110:140. [PMID: 20514823]

	Methanol

Test/Range/Collection	Physiologic Basis	Interpretation	Comments
Methanol, whole blood Negative Green or lavender $$	Methanol is extensively metabolized by alcohol dehydrogenase to formaldehyde and by aldehyde dehydrogenase to formic acid, the major toxic metabolite. Serum methanol levels > 20 mg/dL are toxic and levels > 40 mg/dL are life-threatening.	**Increased in:** Methanol intoxication.	Methanol intoxication is associated with metabolic acidosis and an osmol gap (see Table 8–15). Methanol is commonly ingested in its pure form or in cleaning or copier solutions. Acute ingestion causes an optic neuritis that may result in blindness. Methanol poisoning can be fatal. Fomepizole, a competitive alcohol dehydrogenase inhibitor, can be used to treat methanol poisoning and can obviate the need for hemodialysis. Quantitative measurement of the serum methanol level using gas chromatography is expensive, time-consuming, and not always available. Because methanol is osmotically active and measurement of serum osmolality is easily performed, the osmol gap is often used as a screening test. See Table 8–15. Jammalamadaka D et al. Ethylene glycol, methanol and isopropyl alcohol intoxication. Am J Med Sci 2010;339:2761. [PMID: 20090509] Reddy NJ et al. Delayed neurological sequelae from ethylene glycol, diethylene glycol and methanol poisonings. Clin Toxicol (Phila) 2010;48:967. [PMID: 21192754]

Methemoglobin		
Methemoglobin, whole blood (MetHb) <0.15 g/dL [<23.25 mmol/L] or <1.5% of total Hb Blood gas syringe (heparinized) (Lavender or green for total hemoglobin only) $$ Don't remove the stopper or cap, analyze promptly.	Methemoglobin has its heme iron in the oxidized ferric state and thus cannot combine with and transport oxygen. Methemoglobin can be assayed spectrophotometrically by measuring the decrease in absorbance at 630–635 nm due to the conversion of methemoglobin to cyanmethemoglobin with cyanide. CO-oximetry is the gold standard and is useful for rapid quantitation of methemoglobin.	**Increased in:** Hereditary methemoglobinemia: structural hemoglobin variants (hemoglobin M) (rare), NADH-MetHb reductase (cytochrome b_5 reductase) deficiency. Acquired methemoglobinemia: Oxidant drugs such as sulfonamides, dapsone, sulfasalazine, silver sulfadiazine, primaquine, isoniazid, nitrites, nitroglycerin, nitrates, aniline dyes, phenacetin, hydralazine, topical anesthetics (eg, benzocaine, prilocaine), ifosfamide chemotherapy, chloramine toxicity during hemodialysis, infants with diarrhea or urinary tract infections (due to oxidant stress).	Levels of 1.5 g/dL (about 10% of total Hb) result in visible cyanosis. The diagnosis can be suspected by the characteristic chocolate brown color of a freshly obtained blood sample. Patients with levels of about 35% have headache, weakness, and breathlessness (tachycardia, tachypnea). Levels >70% are usually fatal. Administration of methylene blue facilitates the reduction of MetHb to Hb in the enzyme deficiency state and ameliorates the cyanosis but it has no effect in reducing Hb M variants or in relieving the cyanosis that they cause. do Nascimento TS et al. Methemoglobinemia: from diagnosis to treatment. Rev Bras Anestesiol 2008;58:651. [PMID: 19082413] Percy MJ et al. Recessive congenital methaemoglobinaemia: cytochrome b(5) reductase deficiency. Br J Haematol 2008;141:298. [PMID: 18318771]

	MTHFR mutation		
Test/Range/Collection	Physiologic Basis	Interpretation	Comments
Methylenetetrahydrofolate reductase (*MTHFR*) mutation Blood Lavender $$$$	5,10-Methylenetetrahydrofolate reductase (MTHFR) plays a key role in folate metabolism. MTHFR enzyme deficiency leads to hyperhomocysteinemia. Increased plasma homocysteine is a risk factor for arteriosclerotic vascular disease and thrombosis. Two mutations in the human *MTHFR* gene, C667T and A1298C, result in moderate impairment of MTHFR activity. *MTHFR* mutation test is ordered along with other inherited clotting risk testing, such as factor V Leiden and prothrombin 20210 mutation tests.	**Positive in:** Individuals with *MTHFR* C677T and/or A1298C mutations (sensitivity and specificity approach 100%).	The *MTHFR* mutation assay is indicated for patients with early-onset arteriosclerotic vascular disease or thrombosis, particularly those with hyperhomocysteinemia or significant family histories. See recommended testing for venous thrombosis (Figure 9–27). Both C677T and A1298C mutations should be examined when assessing genetic risk factors for hyperhomocysteinemia. Only those who are homozygous for C677T mutation or compound heterozygous for the C677T/A1298C mutations have significantly elevated plasma homocysteine levels. Double homozygotes have not been reported. The assay is typically polymerase chain reaction (PCR) based. Cattaneo M. Hyperhomocysteinemia and venous thromboembolism. Semin Thromb Hemost 2006;32:716. [PMID: 17024599] Khandanpour N et al. Peripheral arterial disease and methylenetetrahydrofolate reductase (*MTHFR*) C677T mutations: a case-control study and meta-analysis. J Vasc Surg 2009;49:711. [PMID: 19157768]

Methylmalonic acid

| Methylmalonic acid (MMA), serum or plasma

0–0.4 mcmol/L
(0–4.7 mcg/dL)

SST, red, lavender, green

$$ | Elevation of serum methylmalonic acid (MMA) in cobalamin (B_{12}) deficiency results from impaired conversion of methylmalonyl-CoA to succinyl-CoA, a pathway involving methylmalonyl-CoA mutase as its enzyme and adenosylcobalamin as its coenzyme. Serum MMA is used to indirectly evaluate vitamin B_{12} status, mainly for confirming B_{12} deficiency in patients with low serum B_{12} levels. | **Increased in:** Vitamin B_{12} (cobalamin) deficiency (95%), pernicious anemia, renal insufficiency, pregnancy, elderly (5–15%). | Explanation of high frequency (5–15%) of increased serum MMA in the elderly with low or normal serum vitamin B_{12} levels is unclear. Benefits of B_{12} supplementation in this situation are unclear.
Normal MMA levels can exclude vitamin B_{12} deficiency in the presence of unexplained low B_{12} levels found in lymphoid disorders.
Test is usually normal in HIV patients who may have low serum vitamin B_{12} levels without actual vitamin B_{12} deficiency; these patients usually have low vitamin B_{12}-binding protein.
For individuals with mildly elevated MMA levels (0.40–2.00 mcmol/L), vitamin B_{12} treatment normalizes MMA level but has no significant effect on hemoglobin, MCV, or anemic, neurologic, or gastroenterologic symptoms, at least in the short term.
Urine MMA (reference interval: 0–3.6 mmol/mol creatinine) test is also available for evaluating B_{12} status as well as monitoring patients with methylmalonic aciduria.
Kaferle J et al. Evaluation of macrocytosis. Am Fam Physician 2009;79:203. [PMID: 19202968]
Selhub J et al. The use of blood concentrations of vitamins and their respective functional indicators to define folate and vitamin B12 status. Food Nutr Bull 2008;29(2 Suppl):S67. [PMID: 18709882] |

Test/Range/Collection	Physiologic Basis	Interpretation	Comments
Metyrapone test (overnight)			
Metyrapone test (overnight), plasma or serum 8 AM cortisol: <10 mcg/dL [<280 nmol/L] 8 AM 11-deoxycortisol: >7 mcg/dL [>202 nmol/L] SST, lavender, or green $$$ Give 2.0–3.0 g metyrapone orally (dependent on body weight) at 12:00 midnight. Draw serum cortisol and 11-deoxycortisol levels at 8:00 AM.	The metyrapone stimulation test assesses both pituitary and adrenal reserve and is mainly used to diagnose secondary adrenal insufficiency (see Adrenocortical Insufficiency algorithm, Figure 9–3). Metyrapone is a drug that inhibits adrenal 11 β-hydroxylase and blocks cortisol synthesis. The consequent fall in cortisol increases release of ACTH and hence production of corticosteroids formed proximal to the block (eg, 11-deoxycortisol).	**Decreased in:** An 8 AM 11-deoxycortisol level ≤7 mcg/dL indicates primary or secondary adrenal insufficiency.	The overnight metyrapone test assesses the integrity of the entire hypothalamic–pituitary–adrenal axis. It can be useful in assessing the HPA axis post-hypophysectomy, in diagnosing secondary adrenal insufficiency in AIDS patients, or in corticosteroid-treated patients to assess the extent of suppression of the pituitary–adrenal axis. The use of an extended metyrapone test in the differential diagnosis of ACTH-dependent Cushing syndrome (pituitary versus ectopic) has been questioned. Test is not useful in panic disorder, posttraumatic stress disorder, or fibromyalgia syndrome. Kazlauskaite R et al. Pitfalls in the diagnosis of central adrenal insufficiency in children. Endocr Dev 2010;17:96. [PMID: 19955760] Santhanam P et al. Diagnostic predicament of secondary adrenal insufficiency. Endocr Pract 2010;16:686. [PMID: 20439244]

β₂-Microglobulin

β₂-Microglobulin,
serum or plasma (β₂-M)

<0.2 mg/dL

[<2.0 mg/L]

SST, green, lavender

$$$

β₂-Microglobulin is a low-molecular-weight protein that is the light chain of the class I MHC antigens. It is present on the surface of all nucleated cells and in all body fluids. It is almost totally reabsorbed and catabolized by the proximal renal tubules.

It is increased in many conditions that are accompanied by high cell turnover and/or immune activation.

Increased in: Inflammatory conditions (eg, inflammatory bowel disease), infections (eg, HIV, CMV), graft rejection, autoimmune disorders, lymphoid malignancies, multiple myeloma, chronic renal failure, lymphoproliferative, myeloproliferative, and myelodysplastic disorders.

Because of its accumulation with renal dysfunction and its ability to become glycosylated, form fibrils, and deposit in tissues, β₂M is a cause of dialysis-associated amyloidosis.

Of tests used to predict progression to AIDS in HIV-infected patients, CD4 cell number has the most predictive power, followed closely by β₂M.

Serum β₂M levels are elevated in many hematological and lymphoid malignancies. An association has been found between serum β₂M levels and tumor burden in some disorders, particularly multiple myeloma, making it a valuable prognostic marker in these conditions.

Drüeke TB et al. Beta2-microglobulin. Semin Dial 2009;22:378. [PMID: 19708985]

Gupta SM et al. Evaluation of beta2 microglobulin level as a marker to determine HIV/AIDS progression. J Commun Dis 2004;36:166. [PMID: 16509252]

Heegaard NH. Beta(2)-microglobulin: from physiology to amyloidosis. Amyloid 2009;16:151. [PMID: 19657763]

	Mitochondrial antibodies		
Test/Range/Collection	Physiologic Basis	Interpretation	Comments
Mitochondrial antibodies (AMA), serum Negative (<1.0 U) SST $$	Originally demonstrated using immunofluorescence approaches, antimitochondrial antibodies can now be detected using commercially available enzyme-linked immunosorbent assays (ELISAs). Although ELISAs are more practical, they are slightly less sensitive than immunofluorescence techniques. In AMA-negative patients with a high suspicion of primary biliary cirrhosis (PBC), antimitochondrial autoantibodies can be sought using recombinant autoantigens.	**Increased in:** Primary biliary cirrhosis (85–95%), chronic active hepatitis (25–28%), occasionally in CREST syndrome and other autoimmune diseases; lower titers in viral hepatitis, infectious mononucleosis, neoplasms, cryptogenic cirrhosis (25–30%).	Primarily used to distinguish PBC (antibodies present) from extrahepatic biliary obstruction (antibodies absent). The antigens recognized by AMA have been designated M1–M9. AMA from patients with PBC recognize the M2 antigen complex, which includes enzymes of the 2-pyruvate dehydrogenase (PDH-E2) and 2-oxoglutarate dehydrogenase. The titer or levels of AMA do not indicate disease activity or prognosis in patients with PBC. AMA subtype profiles do not predict prognosis in patients with PBC. Hohenester S et al. Primary biliary cirrhosis. Semin Immunopathol 2009;31:283. [PMID: 19603170] Mendes F et al. Antimitochondrial antibody-negative primary biliary cirrhosis. Gastroenterol Clin North Am 2008;37:479. [PMID: 18499032] Muratori L et al. Antimitochondrial antibodies and other antibodies in primary biliary cirrhosis: diagnostic and prognostic value. Clin Liver Dis 2008;12:261. [PMID: 18456179]

Neutrophil cytoplasmic antibodies		
Neutrophil cytoplasmic antibodies, serum (ANCA) Negative SST, red $$$	Measurement of autoantibodies in serum against cytoplasmic constituents of neutrophils. (See also Autoantibodies, Table 8–6.) Dual testing by standard indirect immunofluorescence for serum cytoplasmic ANCA (cANCA) and perinuclear ANCA (pANCA) with reflex testing of myeloperoxidase (MPO) and proteinase 3 (PR3) antibodies is often recommended. In some laboratories, ANCA testing is performed with MPO and PR3 antibodies as a single panel.	**Positive in:** Granulomatosis with polyangiitis (formerly Wegener granulomatosis), systemic vasculitis, pauci-immune crescentic glomerulonephritis, paraneoplastic vasculitis, Churg-Strauss angitis, microscopic polyangiitis, drug-induced vasculitis, ulcerative colitis.	In the patient with systemic vasculitis, elevated ANCA levels imply active disease and high likelihood of recurrence. However, ANCA levels can be persistently elevated and should be used in conjunction with other clinical indices in treatment decisions. For ANCA-associated vasculitis, ANCA sensitivity, specificity, positive predictive value, and negative predictive value vary with method and population studied. Beauvillain C et al. Antineutrophil cytoplasmic autoantibodies: how should the biologist manage them? Clin Rev Allergy Immunol 2008;35:47. [PMID: 18176846] Tervaert JW et al. Fifty years of antineutrophil cytoplasmic antibodies (ANCA) testing: do we need to revise the international consensus statement on testing and reporting on ANCA? APMIS Suppl 2009;127:55. [PMID: 19515141] Wiik AS. Autoantibodies in ANCA-associated vasculitis. Rheum Dis Clin North Am 2010;36:479. [PMID: 20688245] Wiik A. Clinical and pathophysiological significance of anti-neutrophil cytoplasmic autoantibodies in vasculitis syndromes. Mod Rheumatol 2009;19:590. [PMID: 19730973]

	N-telopeptide, cross-linked		
Test/Range/Collection	**Physiologic Basis**	**Interpretation**	**Comments**
N-telopeptide, cross-linked (NTx), urine Adults: 20–100 units 7–17 years old: 20–700 units (NTx Units = nmol Bone Collagen Equivalents/ mmol creatinine or nM BCE/mM creatinine) (age-specific and laboratory-specific) 24-hour urine. Collect without preservative. $$$$	Approximately 90% of the organic matrix of bone is type I collagen that is cross-linked at the N- and C-terminal ends of the molecule. Cross-linked N-terminal fragment of type I collagen (NTx) is a specific marker of increased bone resorption. Urine NTx test is preferred over serum test. The intra-individual coefficient of variation of urine NTx measurements is approximately 30%. Part of this variation is due to diurnal fluctuations, and a 24-hour collection is thus preferred.	**Increased in:** Osteoporosis, osteomalacia, rickets, Paget disease, hyperparathyroidism, hyperthyroidism, fractures, childhood growth, multiple myeloma, and cancer with bone metastasis.	Test may be useful for monitoring of antiresorptive treatment in patients with osteopenia, osteoporosis, Paget disease, or other disorders. Not useful during childhood growth and during fracture healing. Biologic variability of urine levels of NTx may limit its clinical usefulness. Also see C-telopeptide, beta-cross-linked (p. 116). Civitelli R et al. Bone turnover markers: understanding their value in clinical trials and clinical practice. Osteoporos Int 2009;20:843. [PMID: 19190842] Delmas PD et al. The use of biochemical markers of bone turnover in osteoporosis. Committee of Scientific Advisors of the International Osteoporosis Foundation. Osteoporos Int 2000;11:S2. [PMID: 11193237]

Nuclear antibody		
Nuclear antibody, serum (anti-nuclear antibody, ANA) <1:20 SST $$	Heterogeneous antibodies to nuclear antigens (DNA and RNA, histone, and nonhistone proteins). Nuclear antibody is measured in serum by layering the patient's serum over human epithelial cells and detecting the antibody with fluorescein conjugated polyvalent antihuman immunoglobulin. Enzyme-linked immunosorbent assay (ELISA) is also available for ANA detection, but has lower sensitivity for systemic lupus erythematosus (SLE) compared with immunofluorescence assay.	**Elevated in:** Patients over age 65 (35–75%, usually in low titers), SLE (98%), drug-induced lupus (100%), Sjögren syndrome (80%), rheumatoid arthritis (30–50%), scleroderma (60%), mixed connective tissue disease (100%), Felty syndrome, mononucleosis, hepatic or biliary cirrhosis, hepatitis, leukemia, myasthenia gravis, dermato-myositis, polymyositis, chronic renal failure.	A negative ANA test does not completely rule out SLE, but alternative diagnoses should be considered. The pattern of ANA staining may give some clues to diagnoses, but because the pattern also changes with serum dilution, it is not routinely reported. Only the rim (peripheral) pattern is highly specific (for SLE). Not useful as a screening test. Should be used only when there is clinical evidence of a connective tissue disease. Breda L et al. Laboratory tests in the diagnosis and follow-up of pediatric rheumatic diseases: an update. Semin Arthritis Rheum 2010;40:53. [PMID: 19246077] Satoh M et al. Clinical interpretation of antinuclear antibody tests in systemic rheumatic diseases. Mod Rheumatol 2009;19:219. [PMID: 19277826] Watts JB. Rational use of laboratory testing in the initial evaluation of soft tissue and joint complaints. Prim Care 2010;37:673. [PMID: 21050950]

	Oligoclonal bands

Test/Range/Collection	Physiologic Basis	Interpretation	Comments
Oligoclonal bands, serum and CSF Negative SST or red (serum), glass or plastic tube (CSF) $$ Collect serum and CSF simultaneously.	Electrophoretic examination of IgG found in CSF may show oligoclonal bands not found in serum. It is considered positive for CSF oligoclonal bands if there are two or more bands in the CSF that are not present in the serum. This suggests local production in CSF of limited species of IgG. The pathogenesis of oligoclonal bands in multiple sclerosis is still obscure.	**Positive in:** Multiple sclerosis, CNS syphilis, subacute sclerosing panencephalitis, progressive multifocal leukoencephalopathy, Guillain-Barré syndrome, other CNS inflammatory diseases.	Test is indicated when multiple sclerosis is suspected clinically. Identical serum and CSF oligoclonal bands ("mirror pattern"), or no oligoclonal bands, suggest systemic immune activation. IgG index (see p. 183) is a more reliable test analytically, but neither test is specific for multiple sclerosis. There is no predictable correlation between the IgG index and the oligoclonal band number in the CSF of multiple sclerosis patients. Quantification of oligoclonal bands in CSF is an insensitive prognostic indicator and should not be used to influence treatment decisions. Awad A et al. Analyses of cerebrospinal fluid in the diagnosis and monitoring of multiple sclerosis. J Neuroimmunol 2010;219:1. [PMID: 19782408]

Osmolality, serum

| Osmolality, serum or plasma (Osm)

285–293 mosm/kg H$_2$O [mmol/kg H$_2$O]

Panic: <240 or >320 mosm/kg H$_2$O

SST, PPT

$$$ | Test measures the osmotic pressure of serum by the freezing point depression method. Plasma and urine osmolality are more useful indicators of degree of hydration than BUN, hematocrit, or serum proteins. Serum osmolality can be estimated by the following formula:

$$Osm = 2(Na^+) + \frac{BUN}{2.8} + \frac{Glucose}{18}$$

where Na$^+$ is in meq/L and BUN and glucose are in mg/dL. | **Increased in:** Diabetic ketoacidosis, nonketotic hyperosmolar hyperglycemic coma, hypernatremia secondary to dehydration (diarrhea, severe burns, vomiting, fever, hyperventilation, inadequate water intake, central or nephrogenic diabetes insipidus, or osmotic diuresis), hypernatremia with normal hydration (hypothalamic disorders, defective osmostat), hypernatremia with overhydration (iatrogenic or accidental excessive NaCl or NaHCO$_3$ intake), alcohol or other toxic ingestion (see Comments), hypercalcemia; tube feedings. Drugs: corticosteroids, mannitol, glycerin.

Decreased in: Pregnancy (third trimester), hyponatremia with hypovolemia (adrenal insufficiency, renal losses, diarrhea, vomiting, severe burns, peritonitis, pancreatitis), hyponatremia with normovolemia (SIADH), hyponatremia with hypervolemia (CHF, cirrhosis, nephrotic syndrome, postoperative state). Drugs: chlorthalidone, cyclophosphamide, thiazides. | If the difference between calculated and measured serum osmolality is greater than 10 mosm/kg H$_2$O, suspect the presence of a low-molecular-weight toxin (ethanol, methanol, isopropyl alcohol, ethylene glycol, acetone, ethyl ether, paraldehyde, or mannitol), ethanol being the most common. (See Table 8–15 for further explanation.)

Every 100 mg/dL of ethanol increases serum osmolality by 22 mosm/kg H$_2$O (ethanol/4.6).

Whereas the osmolal gap may overestimate the blood alcohol level, a normal serum osmolality excludes ethanol intoxication.

Measurement of serum osmolality is an important first step in the laboratory evaluation of the hyponatremic patient. The simultaneous measurement of plasma ADH (vasopressin) and plasma osmolality in a dehydration test is the most powerful diagnostic tool in the differential diagnosis of polyuria/polydipsia.

Decaux G et al. Clinical laboratory evaluation of the syndrome of inappropriate secretion of antidiuretic hormone. Clin J Am Soc Nephrol 2008;3:1175. [PMID: 18434618]

Jammalamadaka D et al. Ethylene glycol, methanol and isopropyl alcohol intoxication. Am J Med Sci 2010;339:276. [PMID: 20090509]

Schrier RW et al. Diagnosis and management of hyponatremia in acute illness. Curr Opin Crit Care 2008;14:627. [PMID: 19005303] |

Osmolality, urine

Test/Range/Collection	Physiologic Basis	Interpretation	Comments
Osmolality, urine (Urine Osm) Random: 100–900 mosm/ kg H_2O [mmol/kg H_2O] Urine container $$	Test measures renal tubular concentrating ability. Urine osmolality and specific gravity usually change in parallel with each other. When large molecules such as glucose and protein are present, however, the results diverge. Specific gravity is increased more, due to the weight of the molecules, whereas urine osmolality is increased less, reflecting the number of molecules.	**Increased in:** Hypovolemia. Drugs: anesthetic agents (during surgery), carbamazepine, chlorpropamide, cyclophosphamide, metolazone, vincristine. **Decreased in:** Diabetes insipidus, primary polydipsia, exercise, starvation. Drugs: acetohexamide, demeclocycline, glyburide, lithium, tolazamide.	In the hypoosmolar state (serum osmolality < 280 mosm/kg), urine osmolality is used to determine whether water excretion is normal or impaired. A urine osmolality value of < 100 mosm/kg indicates complete and appropriate suppression of antidiuretic hormone secretion. With average fluid intake, normal random urine osmolality is 100–900 mosm/kg H_2O. After 12-hour fluid restriction, normal random urine osmolality is >850 mosm/kg H_2O. Decaux G et al. Clinical laboratory evaluation of the syndrome of inappropriate secretion of antidiuretic hormone. Clin J Am Soc Nephrol 2008;3:1175. [PMID: 18434618] Jefferson JW. A clinician's guide to monitoring kidney function in lithium-treated patients. J Clin Psychiatry 2010;71:1153. [PMID: 20923621] Reddy P et al. Diagnosis and management of hyponatraemia in hospitalised patients. Int J Clin Pract 2009;63:1494. [PMID: 19769706]

Osteocalcin

Osteocalcin, serum or plasma Adults: 10–50 ng/mL 7–17-years-old: 25–300 ng/mL (age-specific) SST, red, lavender, pink or green $$$$	Osteocalcin is a noncollagen protein of 49 amino acids in bone matrix, produced by osteoblasts. Its production is dependent on vitamin K and is stimulated by 1,25-dihydroxy vitamin D. Osteocalcin is released into the circulation from the matrix during bone resorption and is considered a marker of bone turnover. Both intact osteocalcin (amino acids 1–49) and the large N-terminal/midregion (N-MID) fragment (amino acids 1–43) are present in blood. Intact osteocalcin is unstable due to protease cleavage between amino acids 43 and 44. The N-MID-fragment, resulting from cleavage, is more stable. The test detects both the stable N-MID-fragment and intact osteocalcin.	**Increased in:** Osteoporosis, osteomalacia, rickets, Paget disease, hyperparathyroidism, renal osteodystrophy, thyrotoxicosis, fractures, acromegaly, and cancer with bone metastasis. **Decreased in:** Hypoparathyroidism, hypothyroidism, and growth hormone deficiency.	Test may be useful for monitoring and assessing effectiveness of antiresorptive therapy in patients treated for osteopenia, osteoporosis, Paget disease, or other disorders in which osteocalcin levels are elevated. Test can also be used as an adjunct in the diagnosis of conditions associated with increased bone turnover, including Paget disease, cancer accompanied by bone metastases, primary hyperparathyroidism, and renal osteodystrophy. Osteocalcin is cleared by the kidneys. In patients with renal failure, the osteocalcin levels can be elevated as a result of impaired clearance and renal osteodystrophy. Civitelli R et al. Bone turnover markers: understanding their value in clinical trials and clinical practice. Osteoporos Int 2009;20:843. [PMID: 19190842] Delmas PD et al. The use of biochemical markers of bone turnover in osteoporosis. Committee of Scientific Advisors of the International Osteoporosis Foundation. Osteoporos Int 2000;11:S2. [PMID: 11193237] Garnero P. Biomarkers for osteoporosis management: utility in diagnosis, fracture risk prediction and therapy monitoring. Mol Diagn Ther 2008;12:157. [PMID: 18510379]

Test/Range/Collection	Physiologic Basis	Interpretation	Comments
Oxygen, partial pressure			
Oxygen, partial pressure (PO₂), whole blood 83–108 mm Hg [11.04–14.36 kPa] Heparinized syringe $$$ Collect arterial blood in a heparinized syringe. Send to laboratory immediately on ice.	Test measures the partial pressure of oxygen (oxygen tension) in arterial blood. Partial pressure of oxygen is critical because it determines (along with hemoglobin and blood supply) tissue oxygen supply.	**Increased in:** Oxygen therapy. **Decreased in:** Ventilation/perfusion mismatching (asthma, COPD, atelectasis, pulmonary embolism, pneumonia, interstitial lung disease, airway obstruction by foreign body, shock); alveolar hypoventilation (kyphoscoliosis, neuromuscular disease, head injury, stroke); right-to-left shunt (congenital heart disease). Drugs: barbiturates, opioids.	% Saturation of hemoglobin (Hb) (SO₂) is the percent of total Hb that is combined with O₂; SO₂ is dependent on the oxygen partial pressure. % Saturation on blood gas reports is calculated, not measured. It is calculated from PO₂ and pH using reference oxyhemoglobin dissociation curves for normal adult hemoglobin (lacking methemoglobin, carboxyhemoglobin, etc). At PO₂ < 60 mm Hg, the oxygen saturation (and content) cannot be reliably estimated from the PO₂. Therefore, oximetry should be used to determine % saturation directly. Ayers P et al. Diagnosis and treatment of simple acid-base disorders. Nutr Clin Pract 2008;23:122. [PMID: 18390779] Toffaletti J et al. Misconceptions in reporting oxygen saturation. Anesth Analg 2007;105(6 Suppl):S5. [PMID: 18048899]

Pancreatic elastase		

| Pancreatic elastase, fecal

>200 mcg/g

$$$

Collect >1 g of random formed stool in clean, leak proof plastic container. Freeze immediately. | Fecal pancreatic elastase-1 is a protease synthesized by pancreatic acinar cells. The ELISA-based quantitative assay is a sensitive, specific, and noninvasive test for exocrine pancreatic insufficiency, superior to chymotrypsin. Sensitivity is 100% for severe, 77–100% for moderate, and 0–60% for mild pancreatic insufficiency, respectively. Specificity is 93% except for patients with small intestinal disease, eg, Crohn's disease and gluten-sensitive enteropathy. | **Decreased in:** Exocrine pancreatic insufficiency (mild-moderate 100–200 mcg/g; severe <100 mcg/g). | Fecal elastase-1 is a marker of pancreatic exocrine secretion. There is a direct correlation between pancreatic elastase-1 levels in pancreatic fluid and stool. It is a superior marker to fecal chymotrypsin and fecal fat (see p. 134).

Beharry S et al. How useful is fecal pancreatic elastase-1 as a marker of exocrine pancreatic disease? J Pediatr 2002;141:84. [PMID: 12091856]

Herzig KH et al. Fecal pancreatic elastase-1 levels in older individuals without gastrointestinal diseases or diabetes mellitus. BMC Geriatr 2011;11:4. [PMID: 21266058]

Nandhakumar N et al. Interpretations: how to use faecal elastase testing. Arch Dis Child Educ Pract Ed 2010;95:119. [PMID: 20688857] |

	Parathyroid hormone		
Test/Range/Collection	Physiologic Basis	Interpretation	Comments
Parathyroid hormone, serum or plasma (PTH) Intact PTH: 11–54 pg/mL [1.2–5.7 pmol/L] (laboratory-specific) SST, lavender, green $$$$ Fasting sample preferred; simultaneous measurement of serum calcium and phosphorus is also required.	PTH is secreted from the parathyroid glands. It mobilizes calcium from bone, increases distal renal tubular reabsorption of calcium, decreases proximal renal tubular reabsorption of phosphorus, and stimulates 1,25-hydroxy vitamin D synthesis from 25-dihydroxy vitamin D by renal 1α-hydroxylase. The "intact" PTH molecule (84 amino acids) has a circulating half-life of about 5 minutes. Carboxyl terminal and mid-molecule fragments make up 90% of circulating PTH. They are biologically inactive, cleared by the kidney, and have half-lives of about 1–2 hours. The amino terminal fragment is biologically active and has a half-life of 1–2 minutes. Measurement of PTH by immunoassay depends on the specificity of the antibodies used. Intact PTH assays using two antibodies ("sandwich" immunoassay) are the standard assays. The second- and third-generation intact PTH assays are less prone to interference from large PTH fragments (eg, amino acids 7–84), and the enhanced assays measure only the biologically intact PTH molecule (amino acids 1–84).	**Increased in:** Primary hyperparathyroidism, secondary hyperparathyroidism due to renal disease, vitamin D deficiency. Drugs: lithium, furosemide, propofol, phosphates. **Decreased in:** Hypoparathyroidism, sarcoidosis, hyperthyroidism, hypomagnesemia, malignancy with hypercalcemia, nonparathyroid hypercalcemia.	PTH results must always be evaluated in light of concurrent serum calcium levels. PTH tests differ in sensitivity and specificity from assay to assay and from laboratory to laboratory. Carboxyl terminal antibody measures intact, carboxyl terminal and midmolecule fragments. It is 85% sensitive and 95% specific for primary hyperparathyroidism. Amino terminal antibody measures intact and amino terminal fragments. It is about 75% sensitive for hyperparathyroidism. Intact PTH assays are preferred because they detect PTH suppression in nonparathyroid hypercalcemia. Intact PTH is a better indicator of hyperparathyroidism in renal failure. Sensitivity of immunometric assays is 85–90% for primary hyperparathyroidism. Intraoperative quick PTH monitoring in patients undergoing parathyroidectomy can be used to confirm cure and predict long-term operative success in most cases. A low intraoperative PTH level during thyroid surgery is a predictor of postoperative hypocalcemia resulting from parathyroid gland ischemia. See diagnostic algorithms for hypercalcemia and hypocalcemia (Figures 9–13 and 9–15). Eastell R et al. Diagnosis of asymptomatic primary hyperparathyroidism: Proceedings of the Third International Workshop. J Clin Endocrinol Metab 2009;94:340. [PMID: 19193909] Souberbielle JC et al. Interpretation of serum parathyroid hormone concentrations in dialysis patients: what do the KDIGO guidelines change for the clinical laboratory? Clin Chem Lab Med 2010;48:769. [PMID: 20298134] Souberbielle JC et al. Parathyroid hormone measurement in CKD. Kidney Int 2010;77:93. [PMID: 19812537]

Parathyroid hormone-related protein		
Parathyroid hormone-related protein (PTHrP), plasma Assay-specific (pmol/L or undetectable) Lavender Tube containing anticoagulant and protease inhibitors; specimen drawn without a tourniquet. $$	Parathyroid hormone-related protein (PTHrP) is a 139- to 173-amino acid protein with amino terminal homology to PTH. The homology explains the ability of PTHrP to bind to the PTH receptor and have PTH-like effects on bone and kidney. PTHrP induces increased plasma calcium, decreased plasma phosphorus, and increased urinary cAMP. PTHrP is found in keratinocytes, fibroblasts, placenta, brain, pituitary gland, adrenal gland, stomach, liver, testicular Leydig cells, and mammary glands. Its physiologic role in these diverse sites is unknown. PTHrP is secreted by solid malignant tumors (lung, breast, kidney; other squamous tumors) and produces humoral hypercalcemia of malignancy. PTHrP can act as an oncoprotein to regulate the growth and proliferation of many common malignancies and is a marker of cancers that metastasize to bone. PTHrP analysis is by immunoradiometric assay (IRMA). Assay of choice is amino terminal–specific IRMA. Two-site IRMA assays require sample collection in protease inhibitors because serum proteases destroy immunoreactivity.	**Increased in:** Humoral hypercalcemia of malignancy (80% of solid tumors).	Assays directed at the amino terminal portion of PTHrP are not influenced by renal failure. Increases in PTHrP concentrations are readily detectable with most current assays in the majority of patients with humoral hypercalcemia of malignancy. About 20% of patients with malignancy and hypercalcemia have low PTHrP levels because their hypercalcemia is caused by local osteolytic processes. Lumachi F et al. Cancer-induced hypercalcemia. Anticancer Res 2009;29:1551. [PMID: 19443365] Santarpia L et al. Hypercalcemia in cancer patients: pathobiology and management. Horm Metab Res 2010;42:153. [PMID: 19960404]

	Partial thromboplastin time

Test/Range/Collection	Physiologic Basis	Interpretation	Comments
Partial thromboplastin time, activated, plasma (aPTT) 25–35 seconds (laboratory-specific) ***Panic:*** ≥60 seconds (off heparin) Blue $$ Do not contaminate specimen with heparin.	The aPTT is a clot-based test in which phospholipid reagent, an activator substance, and calcium are added to the patient's plasma, and the time for a fibrin clot to form is measured. PTT evaluates the intrinsic and common coagulation pathways and adequacy of all coagulation factors except XIII and VII. PTT is usually abnormal if any factor level drops below 25–40% of normal, depending on the PTT reagent used. PTT is commonly used to monitor unfractionated heparin therapy.	**Increased in:** Deficiency of any individual coagulation factor except Factors XIII and VII, presence of nonspecific inhibitor (eg, lupus anticoagulant), specific factor inhibitor, von Willebrand disease (PTT may also be normal), hemophilia A and B, DIC. Drugs: heparin, direct thrombin inhibitor (eg, hirudin, argatroban), warfarin. See evaluation of isolated prolongation of PTT (Figure 9–22) and bleeding disorders (Figure 9–7, Table 8–7). **Decreased in:** Hypercoagulable states (eg, increased factor VIII levels).	PTT cannot be used to monitor very high doses of heparin (eg, cardiac bypass surgery) because the clotting time is beyond the analytical measurement range of PTT. For patients with documented lupus anticoagulant, PTT can not be used to monitor heparin therapy. Chromogenic anti-Xa assay is used instead. Patients receiving low molecular weight heparin usually have normal PTT values. PTT may be normal in patients with von Willebrand disease and chronic DIC. Heparin contamination is a very common cause of an unexplained prolonged PTT. Heparin neutralization with heparinase may be needed to rule out this possibility. PTT may be falsely prolonged if anticoagulant volume is not adjusted for increased hematocrit (eg, polycythemia vera) or if the specimen tube is not fully filled. Baudo F et al. Diagnosis and treatment of acquired haemophilia. Haemophilia 2010;16:102. [PMID: 20536992] Devreese K et al. Challenges in the diagnosis of the antiphospholipid syndrome. Clin Chem 2010; 56:930. [PMID: 20360130] Devreese K et al. Laboratory diagnosis of the antiphospholipid syndrome: a plethora of obstacles to overcome. Eur J Haematol 2009;83:1. [PMID: 19226362] Tripodi A. Testing for lupus anticoagulants: all that a clinician should know. Lupus 2009;18:291. [PMID: 19276296]

pH

pH, whole blood Arterial: 7.35–7.45 Venous: 7.31–7.41 Heparinized syringe $$$ Specimen must be collected in heparinized syringe and immediately transported on ice to lab without exposure to air.	pH assesses the acid–base status of blood, an extremely useful measure of integrated cardiorespiratory function. The essential relationship between pH, P_{CO_2}, and bicarbonate (HCO_3^-) is expressed by the Henderson–Hasselbalch equation (at 37°C): $$pH = 6.1 + \log\left[\frac{HCO_3^-}{P_{CO_2} \times 0.03}\right]$$ Arteriovenous pH difference is 0.01–0.03 but is greater in patients with CHF and shock.	**Increased in:** *Respiratory alkalosis:* Hyperventilation (eg, anxiety), sepsis, liver disease, fever, early salicylate poisoning, and excessive artificial ventilation. *Metabolic alkalosis:* Loss of gastric HCl (eg, vomiting, potassium depletion, excessive alkali administration (eg, bicarbonate, antacids) diuretics, volume depletion. **Decreased in:** *Respiratory acidosis:* Decreased alveolar ventilation (eg, COPD, respiratory depressants), neuromuscular diseases (eg, myasthenia gravis). *Metabolic acidosis* (bicarbonate deficit): Increased formation of acids (eg, ketosis [diabetes mellitus, alcohol, starvation], lactic acidosis); decreased H^+ excretion (eg, renal failure, renal tubular acidosis, Fanconi syndrome); increased acid intake (eg, ion-exchange resins, salicylates, ammonium chloride, ethylene glycol, methanol); and increased loss of alkaline body fluids (eg, diarrhea, fistulas, aspiration of gastrointestinal contents, biliary drainage).	The pH of a standing sample decreases because of cellular metabolism. The correction of pH (measured at 37°C), based on the patient's temperature, is not clinically useful. See acid–base disturbances (Figure 9–1, Table 8–1). Simpson H. Interpretation of arterial blood gases: a clinical guide for nurses. Br J Nurs 2004;13:522. [PMID: 15215728] Whittier WL et al. Primer on clinical acid-base problem solving. Dis Mon 2004;50:122. [PMID: 15069420]

	Phosphorus		
Test/Range/Collection	Physiologic Basis	Interpretation	Comments
Phosphorus, serum or plasma 2.5–4.5 mg/dL [0.8–1.45 mmol/L] *Panic:* <1.0 mg/dL [<0.32 mmol] SST, green $ Avoid hemolysis.	The plasma concentration of inorganic phosphate is determined by parathyroid gland function, action of vitamin D, intestinal absorption, renal function, bone metabolism, and nutrition. Serum phosphorus concentrations have a circadian rhythm (highest level in late morning, lowest in evening) and are subject to rapid change secondary to environmental factors such as diet (carbohydrate), phosphate-binding antacids, and fluctuations in GH, insulin, and renal function. There is also a seasonal variation with maximum levels in May and June (low levels in winter). During first decade of menopause, values increase –0.2 mg/dL (–0.06 mmol/L). Bedrest causes increase up to 0.5 mg/dL (0.16 mmol/L). Ingestion of food may cause a transient decrease in blood levels. Low values are also seen during menstruation.	**Increased in:** Renal failure, calcific uremic arteriolopathy (calciphylaxis), tumor lysis syndrome, massive blood transfusion, hypoparathyroidism, sarcoidosis, neoplasms, adrenal insufficiency, acromegaly, hypervitaminosis D, osteolytic metastases to bone, leukemia, milk-alkali syndrome, healing bone fractures, pseudohypoparathyroidism, diabetes mellitus with ketosis, malignant hyperpyrexia, cirrhosis, lactic acidosis, respiratory acidosis. Drugs: phosphate infusions or enemas, anabolic steroids, ergocalciferol, furosemide, hydrochlorothiazide, clonidine, verapamil, potassium supplements, and others. Thrombocytosis may cause spurious elevation of serum phosphate, but plasma phosphate levels are normal.	Maintenance of a normal serum phosphorus level depends upon regulation of phosphorus reabsorption by the kidney. Most of this reabsorption (80%) occurs in the proximal tubule and is mediated by the sodium-phosphate cotransporter (NaPi-II). Parathyroid hormone, via a variety of intracellular signaling cascades leading to NaPi-IIa internalization and downregulation, is the main regulator of renal phosphate reabsorption. In renal insufficiency, phosphorus excretion declines and hyperphosphatemia develops. The body's homeostatic mechanisms cause secondary hyperparathyroidism and renal osteodystrophy. Shift of phosphorus from extracellular to intracellular compartments, decreased gastrointestinal absorption, and increased urinary losses, are the primary mechanisms of hypophosphatemia. Hypophosphatemia has been implicated as a cause of rhabdomyolysis, respiratory failure, hemolysis, and left ventricular dysfunction. Cirillo M et al. Ageing and changes in phosphate transport: clinical implications. J Nephrol 2010;23(Suppl 16):S152. [PMID: 21170873] Marks J et al. Phosphate homeostasis and the renal-gastro-intestinal axis. Am J Physiol Renal Physiol 2010;299:F285. [PMID: 20534868]

Phosphorus (*continued*)

Decreased in: Hyperparathyroidism, hypovitaminosis D (rickets, osteomalacia, malabsorption [steatorrhea], malnutrition, starvation or cachexia, refeeding syndrome, bone marrow transplantation, renal phosphate wasting due to autosomal dominant or X-linked dominant hypophosphatemic rickets, GH deficiency, chronic alcoholism, severe diarrhea, vomiting, nasogastric suction, acute pancreatitis, severe hypercalcemia (any cause) acute gout, osteoblastic metastases to bone, severe burns (diuretic phase), respiratory alkalosis, hyperalimentation with inadequate phosphate repletion, carbohydrate administration (eg, intravenous D_{50} W glucose bolus), renal tubular acidosis and other renal tubular defects, diabetic ketoacidosis (during recovery), acid-base disturbances, hypokalemia, pregnancy, hypothyroidism, hemodialysis. Drugs: acetazolamide, phosphate-binding antacids, anticonvulsants, β-adrenergic agonists, catecholamines, estrogens, isoniazid, oral contraceptives, prolonged use of thiazides, glucose infusion, insulin therapy, salicylates (toxicity).

	Platelet antibodies

Test/Range/Collection	Physiologic Basis	Interpretation	Comments
Platelet antibodies, whole blood, plasma/serum Negative Lavender, yellow, or SST (methodology-dependent) $$$$	Clinically significant platelet antibodies (platelet-associated IgG) include autoimmune platelet antibodies that cause idiopathic thrombocytopenic purpura (ITP), platelet-specific alloantibodies that cause neonatal alloimmune thrombocytopenia (NATP) and posttransfusion purpura (PTP), and HLA alloantibodies that are associated with refractoriness to platelet transfusions. Platelet-specific alloantibodies are most commonly directed at the human platelet antigen referred to as HPA-1a (also known as PlA1), while ITP autoantibodies typically target platelet glycoproteins IIb/IIIa and/or Ib/IX. Several methods with variable sensitivity and specificity are available, and no method detects all antibodies. A combination of a sensitive binding assay such as a direct platelet immunofluorescence test along with an antigen capture immunoassay is useful. Enzyme-linked immunosorbent assay (ELISA) kits are available that detect specific antibodies against platelet glycoproteins or HLA class I antigens.	**Positive in:** Chronic ITP (90–95%), autoimmune thyroid disease (51%), antiphospholipid syndrome, NATP, PTP. Testing serum/plasma for NATP should be performed using a maternal sample.	Routine testing for platelet antibodies is generally not recommended. In selected cases (eg, refractory ITP, NATP, PTP), the testing may be of value. An assay for platelet-bound antibody (direct) is more informative than detection of unbound antibodies in plasma or serum (indirect). For patients who have repeatedly failed to respond to random donor platelet transfusions, detection and characterization of the specific HLA antibody may permit HLA-matched and crossmatched platelet transfusion. McMillan R. Antiplatelet antibodies in chronic immune thrombocytopenia and their role in platelet destruction and defective platelet production. Hematol Oncol Clin North Am 2009;23:1163. [PMID: 19932426] Toltl LJ et al. Pathophysiology and management of chronic immune thrombocytopenia: focusing on what matters. Br J Haematol 2011;152:52. [PMID: 21083652]

Platelet count			
Platelet count, whole blood (Plt) 150–450 × 10³/mcL [× 10⁹/L] *Panic:* <25 × 10³/mcL [× 10⁹/L] Lavender $	Platelets are released from megakaryocytes in bone marrow and are important for normal hemostasis. Platelet counting is performed as part of the complete blood cell count (CBC) panel. It is typically obtained by automated hematology analyzer. An estimated platelet count may be obtained from blood smear by multiplying the number of platelets per 100 × oil immersion field by 10,000.	**Increased in:** Myeloproliferative disorders (polycythemia vera, chronic myeloid leukemia, essential thrombocythemia, myelofibrosis), some myelodysplastic disorders, acute blood loss, postsplenectomy, preeclampsia, reactive thrombocytosis secondary to inflammatory disorders, infection, tissue injury, iron deficiency, malignancies. **Decreased in:** Decreased production: bone marrow suppression or replacement/infiltration, myelodysplasia, chemotherapy, drugs, alcohol, infection (eg, HIV), congenital marrow failure (eg, Fanconi anemia, Wiskott-Aldrich syndrome, Thrombocytopenia with absent radius [TAR] syndrome, etc); increased destruction or excessive pooling: hypersplenism, DIC, TTP, platelet antibodies (idiopathic thrombocytopenic purpura, Evans' syndrome, posttransfusion purpura, neonatal isoimmune thrombocytopenia, drugs [eg, quinidine, cephalosporins, clopidogrel, HIT]).	Platelet counts are determined in patients with suspected bleeding disorders, purpura or petechiae, leukemia/lymphoma, or DIC, and in patients on chemotherapy, and to determine the response to platelet transfusions. There is little tendency to bleed until the platelet count falls below 20,000/mcL. Bleeding due to low platelet counts typically presents as petechiae, epistaxis, and gingival bleeding. For invasive procedures, platelet counts >50,000/mcL are desirable. HIV infection may result in both decreased platelet production and decreased platelet survival. Please also see platelet antibodies, heparin-associated antibody, and complete blood cell count entries, as well as the diagnostic algorithms for thrombocytopenia and thrombocytosis (Figures 9–25 & 9–26). Geddis AE. Megakaryopoiesis. Semin Hematol 2010;47:212. [PMID: 20620431] Valent J et al. Thrombocytopenia and platelet transfusions in patients with cancer. Cancer Treat Res 2011;157:251. [PMID: 21052961]

	Platelet function assay		
Test/Range/Collection	**Physiologic Basis**	**Interpretation**	**Comments**
Platelet function assay (PFA-100 closure time), blood

CEPI: 70–170 seconds

CADP: 50–110 seconds

(laboratory-specific)

Blue

$$

Specimen must be kept at room temperature and the test should be performed within 4 hours of collection. | The PFA (platelet function assay)-100 closure time (CT) measures the time taken for blood to block a membrane aperture coated with collagen and epinephrine (CEPI) or collagen and ADP (CADP). The test is a combined measure of platelet adhesion and aggregation. PFA-100 CT serves as an alternative to the bleeding time in assessing primary hemostasis.

Compared with bleeding time, the PFA-100 CT test is more reproducible, less invasive, rapid, and technically more appealing. | **Increased in:** Inherited or acquired abnormality of platelet function, von Willebrand disease (vWD), valvular heart disease, renal insufficiency, aspirin. **Increases in both CEPI CT and CADP CT:** Abnormal platelet function, vWD. **Increase in CEPI CT only:** Aspirin. | Normal PFA-100 CT can help exclude some severe platelet defects (eg, Glanzmann thrombasthenia and Bernard-Soulier syndrome) and moderate-severe vWD (eg, types 3, 2A, 2M, and severe type 1). It is less sensitive to mild platelet disorders such as primary secretion defects or dense granule deficiencies and mild type 1 vWD.

There is no evidence that a preoperative PFA-100 CT test can predict bleeding during a surgical procedure. The role of PFA-100 CT in therapeutic monitoring (eg, DDAVP and factor concentrates in vWD) also remains to be established.

Patients with thrombocytopenia (platelets <100,000/mcL) and/or anemia (hematocrit <28%) may exhibit a prolonged PFA-100 CT.

Favaloro EJ. Clinical utility of the PFA-100. Semin Thromb Hemost 2008;34:709. [PMID: 19214910]

Gadisseur A et al. Laboratory diagnosis and molecular classification of von Willebrand disease. Acta Haematol 2009;121:71. [PMID: 19506352] |

Porphobilinogen

Porphobilinogen, urine (PBG)		
Negative (<8.8 mmol/L or <11 mmol/24 hr) $$ Protect from light.	Porphyrias are characterized clinically by neurologic and cutaneous manifestations and chemically by overproduction of porphyrin and other precursors of heme production. PBG is a water-soluble precursor of heme whose urinary excretion is increased in symptomatic hepatic porphyrias, including acute intermittent prophyria (AIP) and other acute attack types of porphyrias associated with neurologic and/or psychiatric symptoms. PBG is detected qualitatively by a color reaction with Ehrlich reagent and confirmed by extraction into chloroform (Watson-Schwartz test).	**Positive in:** Acute intermittent porphyria, variegate porphyria, coproporphyria, hereditary coproporphyria. **Negative in:** 20–30% of patients with hepatic porphyria between attacks.	Positive qualitative urinary PBG tests should be followed up by quantitative measurements. Many laboratories report frequent false positives with the Watson–Schwartz test. A screening PBG test is insensitive, and a negative test does not rule out porphyria between attacks or in the carrier state. Specific porphyrias can be better defined by quantitative measurement of urine PBG, 5-aminolevulinic acid and total porphyrin levels and by measurement of erythrocyte PBG deaminase (rarely used). Puy H et al. Porphyrias. Lancet 2010;375:924. [PMID: 20226990] Siegesmund M et al. The acute hepatic porphyrias: current status and future challenges. Best Pract Res Gastroenterol 2010;24:593. [PMID: 20955962]

	Potassium		
Test/Range/Collection	**Physiologic Basis**	**Interpretation**	**Comments**
Potassium (K⁺), serum or plasma 3.5–5.0 meq/L [mmol/L] ***Panic:*** <3.0 or >6.0 meq/L SST, green $ Avoid hemolysis.	Potassium is predominantly an intracellular cation whose plasma level is regulated by renal excretion. Plasma potassium concentration determines neuromuscular irritability. Elevated or depressed potassium concentrations interfere with muscle contraction.	**Increased in:** Massive hemolysis, severe tissue damage, rhabdomyolysis, acidosis, dehydration, acute or chronic renal failure, Addison disease, renal tubular acidosis type IV (hyporeninemic hypoaldosteronism, (hyperkalemic) familial periodic paralysis, exercise (transient). Drugs: potassium salts, potassium-sparing diuretics (eg, spironolactone, triamterene, eplerenone), nonsteroidal anti-inflammatory drugs, β-blockers, ACE inhibitors, ACE-receptor blockers, high-dose trimethoprim-sulfamethoxazole. **Decreased in:** Low potassium intake, prolonged vomiting or diarrhea, renal tubular acidosis types I and II, hyperaldosteronism, Cushing syndrome, osmotic diuresis (eg, hyperglycemia), alka-losis, (hypokalemic) familial periodic paralysis, trauma (transient), subarachnoid hemorrhage, genetic hypokalemic salt-losing tubulopathies such as Gitelman syndrome (familial hypokalemia-hypocalciuria-hypomagnesemia). Drugs: adrenergic agents (isoproterenol), diuretics.	Spurious hyperkalemia can occur with hemolysis of sample, delayed separation of serum from erythrocytes, prolonged fist clenching during blood drawing, and prolonged tourniquet placement. Very high white blood cell or platelet counts may cause spurious elevation of serum potassium, but plasma potassium levels are normal. Walsh SB et al. Clinical hypokalemia and hyperkalemia at the bedside. J Nephrol 2010;23(Suppl 16):S105. [PMID: 21170866] Weir MR et al. Potassium homeostasis and renin-angiotensin-aldosterone system inhibitors. Clin J Am Soc Nephrol 2010;5:531. [PMID: 20150448]

Procalcitonin		
Procalcitonin (ProCT), serum or plasma <0.10 ng/mL [<0.10 mcg/L] SST, PST $$$$	Procalcitonin (ProCT) is a peptide precursor of calcitonin, produced by the parafollicular cells of the thyroid gland and by the neuro-endocrine cells of the lung and intestine. Increased production by lung, intestine, and other tissues occurs in response to inflammatory stimulus, especially bacterial. The serum values of ProCT correlate with the severity of sepsis; they recede with its improvement and worsen with exacerbation. Serum ProCT has become useful as a biomarker to assist in the diagnosis of sepsis, as well as related infectious or inflammatory conditions. Its half-life is 25–30 hours.	**Increased in:** Bacteremia (sensitivity 76%, specificity 70%), systemic inflammatory response syndrome (SIRS), sepsis, septic shock.	ProCT levels >2.00 ng/mL on the first day of ICU admission represent a high risk for progression to severe sepsis and/or septic shock. ProCT levels <0.50 ng/mL on admission represent a low risk for such progression. ProCT has also been proposed as a guide to antibiotic therapy in respiratory infections, ie, levels <0.1 ng/mL would indicate that antibiotics are not needed; levels > 0.5 ng/mL would indicate that antibiotics are needed. Further clinical investigation is needed to further validate its clinical utility in this regard. Antibodies have been developed that neutralize the harmful effects of ProCT, which could be therapeutic in sepsis. Becker KL et al. Procalcitonin in sepsis and systemic inflammation: a harmful biomarker and a therapeutic target. Br J Pharmacol 2010;159:253. [PMID: 20002097] Kopterides P et al. Procalcitonin-guided algorithms of antibiotic therapy in the intensive care unit: a systematic review and meta-analysis of randomized controlled trials. Crit Care Med 2010;38:2229. [PMID: 20729729] Schuetz P et al. Effect of procalcitonin-based guidelines vs standard guidelines on antibiotic use in lower respiratory infections: the ProHOSP randomized controlled trial. JAMA 2009;302:10590. [PMID: 19738090] Yealy DM et al. Measurement of serum procalcitonin: a step closer to tailored care of respiratory infections? JAMA 2009;302:1115. [PMID: 19738100]

Prolactin			
Test/Range/Collection	Physiologic Basis	Interpretation	Comments
Prolactin, serum or plasma (PRL) <25 ng/mL [mcg/L] SST, PPT, green $$$	Prolactin is a polypeptide hormone secreted by the anterior pituitary. It functions in the initiation and maintenance of lactation in the postpartum period. PRL secretion is inhibited by hypothalamic secretion of dopamine. Prolactin levels increase with renal failure, hypothyroidism, and drugs that are dopamine antagonists.	**Increased in:** Sleep, nursing, nipple stimulation (breast feeding), pregnancy, exercise, hypoglycemia, stress, hypothyroidism, pituitary tumors (prolactinomas and others), hypothalamic/pituitary stalk lesions, renal failure, cirrhosis. HIV infection, CHF, SLE, advanced multiple myeloma, Rathke's cyst. Drugs: phenothiazines, haloperidol, risperidone, reserpine, metoclopramide, methyldopa, estrogens, opiates, cimetidine. **Decreased in:** Drugs: levodopa.	Serum PRL is used primarily in work-up of suspected pituitary tumor (60% of pituitary adenomas secrete PRL). Clinical presentation is usually amenorrhea and galactorrhea in women and impotence in men. (See Amenorrhea algorithm, Figure 9–4.) In patients with macroadenoma, PRL is frequently >500 ng/mL; in microadenoma, PRL is usually >150 ng/mL. When there is a discrepancy between a very large pituitary tumor and a mildly elevated prolactin level, serial dilution of serum samples is recommended to eliminate an artifact that can occur with some immunometric assays leading to a falsely low prolactin value ("hook effect"). Screening for macroprolactin (dimeric or polymeric form) is suggested in investigation of asymptomatic hyperprolactinemic patients. Klibanski A. Clinical practice. Prolactinomas. N Engl J Med 2010;362:1219. [PMID: 20357284] Melmed S et al. Diagnosis and treatment of hyperprolactinemia: an Endocrine Society practice guideline. J Clin Endocrinol Metab 2011;96:273. [PMID: 21296991]

Prostate-specific antigen		
Prostate-specific antigen, total (PSA) 0–4 ng/mL [mcg/L] SST, red, PPT, lavender, green $$$	PSA is a glycoprotein produced by cells of the prostatic ductal epithelium and is present in the serum of all men. It is absent from the serum of women.	**Increased in:** Prostate carcinoma (sensitivity ~20%; specificity ~60–70% at a 4.0 ng/mL cutoff), biochemical recurrence after localized treatment, benign prostatic hypertrophy (BPH), prostatitis. **Decreased in:** Metastatic prostate carcinoma treated with antiandrogen therapy, postprostatectomy, 5α-reductase inhibitor therapy.	PSA is used both for the early detection of prostate cancer and as a tumor marker to assess response and monitor recurrence of treated prostate cancer. There is still no consensus on whether PSA measurement should be used as a screening test for early detection of prostate cancer. A decrease in mortality rates resulting from use for cancer screening is unproven, and the risks of early therapy are significant. As a result, the United States Preventive Services Task Force discourages use of the test for healthy men in all age groups. The PSA nadir (the lowest PSA level achieved after therapeutic intervention) appears to correlate with the likelihood of remaining disease-free. Three consecutive PSA rises are interpreted as an indicator of treatment (biochemical) failure. PSA is often increased in BPH, and the positive predictive value in healthy older men is low. Use of the free/total PSA ratio or the complexed PSA test and prostate volume can improve the diagnostic accuracy for prostate cancer. Using PSA velocity as a guide for biopsy in prostate cancer detection is not recommended. Carroll F et al. Prostate-Specific Antigen Best Practice Statement: 2009 Update. American Urological Association. http://www.auanet.org/content/guidelines-and-quality-care/clinical-guidelines/main-reports/psa09.pdf D'avan B et al. Prostate-specific antigen testing and prostate cancer screening. Prim Care 2010;37:441. [PMID: 20705192] Djulbegovic M et al. Screening for prostate cancer: systematic review and meta-analysis of randomized controlled trials. BMJ 2010;341:c4543. [PMID: 20843937] Yao S. et al. The science and art of prostate cancer screening. J Natl Cancer Inst 2011;103:450. [PMID: 21350220]

Test/Range/Collection	Physiologic Basis	Interpretation	Comments
Protein C, plasma 70–170% (functional) 65–150% (antigenic) Blue $$$ Transport to lab on ice. Plasma must be separated and frozen in a polypropylene tube within 2 hours.	Protein C is a vitamin K–dependent proenzyme synthesized in the liver. It is activated at the endothelial surface when thrombin binds to thrombomodulin. In the presence of its cofactor protein S, activated protein C (APC) inactivates Va and VIIIa, thereby impeding further thrombin generation. APC also has cytoprotective effects such as anti-inflammatory, anti-apoptotic, and endothelial barrier protection. The functional assay detects both quantitative (type I) and qualitative (type II) deficiency of protein C. The antigenic assay detects patients with quantitative protein C deficiency, but does not detect patients with qualitative abnormalities. Deficiency is inherited in an autosomal dominant fashion with incomplete penetrance or is acquired. Deficient patients may present with a hypercoagulable state, with recurrent thrombophlebitis or pulmonary embolism.	**Decreased in:** Congenital deficiency, liver disease, cirrhosis (13–25%), warfarin use (28–60%), vitamin K deficiency, DIC, thrombosis (acute). **Interfering factors:** Artifactually decreased functional protein C values may be seen in patients with abnormally elevated levels of factor VIII. Artifactually increased protein C values may be seen in patients on heparin therapy.	Homozygous deficiency of protein C (<1% activity) is associated with fatal neonatal purpura fulminans and massive venous thrombosis at birth. Heterozygous patients (1 in 200–300 of the population, with levels 25–50% of normal) may be at risk for venous thrombosis. Kindreds with dysfunctional protein C of normal quantity have been identified. Interpretation of an abnormally low protein C must be related to the clinical setting. Anticoagulant therapy, DIC, and liver disease must not be present. There is overlap between lower limits of normal values and values found in heterozygotes. Patients should be off oral anticoagulant therapy for 2 weeks for accurate measurement of functional protein C levels. See recommended testing for venous thrombosis (Figure 9–27). Khor B et al. Laboratory tests for protein C deficiency. Am J Hematol 2010;85:440. [PMID: 20309856] Soare AM et al. Deficiencies of proteins C, S and antithrombin and factor V Leiden and the risk of ischemic strokes. J Med Life 2010;3:235. [PMID: 20945813]

Protein C

Protein electrophoresis		
Protein electrophoresis, serum (SPEP) Adults: Albumin: 3.3–5.7 g/dL α_1: 0.1–0.4 g/dL α_2: 0.2–0.9 g/dL β_2: 0.7–1.5 g/dL γ: 0.5–1.4 g/dL SST $$	Electrophoresis of serum separates serum proteins into albumin, α_1, α_2, β_2, and γ fractions. Albumin is the principal serum protein (see Albumin, p. 56). The term *globulin* generally refers to the nonalbumin fraction of serum protein. The α_1 fraction contains α_1-antitrypsin (90%), α_1-lipoprotein, and α_1-acid glycoprotein. The α_2 fraction contains α_2-macroglobulin, haptoglobin, and ceruloplasmin. The β fraction contains transferrin, hemopexin, complement C3, and β-lipoproteins. The γ fraction contains immunoglobulins G, A, D, E, and M (see Immunoglobulins, p. 185). The conventional agarose gel and immunofixation electrophoresis (SPEP/IFE) are being replaced by automated capillary zone and immunosubtraction electrophoresis.	↑ α_1: inflammatory states (α_1-antiprotease), pregnancy. ↑ α_2: nephrotic syndrome, inflammatory states, oral contraceptives, corticosteroid therapy, hyperthyroidism. ↑ β: hyperlipidemia, hemoglobinemia, iron deficiency anemia. ↑ γ: polyclonal gammopathies (liver disease, cirrhosis [associated with β–γ "bridging"], chronic infections, autoimmune disease), plasma cell neoplasms including myeloma and monoclonal gammopathy of undetermined significance (MGUS), Waldenström macroglobulinemia, lymphoid malignancies). ↓ α_1: α_1-antiprotease deficiency. ↓ α_2: in vivo hemolysis, liver disease. ↓ β: hypo-β-lipoproteinemias. ↓ γ: immune deficiency.	Presence of "spikes" in α_2, β_2, γ regions necessitates the use of IFE (p. 184) to verify the presence of a monoclonal gammopathy. SPEP/IFE in combination with serum free light-chain (FLC) assay are highly sensitive for the detection of myeloma and related plasma cell neoplasms. If Bence Jones proteins (light chains) are suspected, UPEP followed by IFE needs to be done. Test is insensitive for detection of decreased levels of immunoglobulins and α_1-antitrypsin. Specific quantitation is required (see Immunoglobulins and α_1-Antitrypsin). If plasma is used, fibrinogen will be detected in the α–γ region. The acute-phase reactant protein pattern seen with acute illness, surgery, infarction, or trauma is characterized by an ↑ α_2 (haptoglobin) and ↑ α_1 (α_1-antitrypsin). Bossuyt X. Advances in serum protein electrophoresis. Adv Clin Chem 2006;42:43. [PMID: 17131624] Vavricka SR et al. Serum protein electrophoresis: an under-used but very useful test. Digestion 2009;79:203. [PMID: 19365122]

	Protein S		
Test/Range/Collection	**Physiologic Basis**	**Interpretation**	**Comments**
Protein S (total antigen), plasma 55–155% Blue $$$ Transport to lab on ice. Plasma must be separated and frozen in a polypropylene tube within 2 hours.	Protein S is a vitamin K-dependent glycoprotein, synthesized in the liver. It has an anticoagulant function and acts as the cofactor of activated protein C (APC), with which it forms a stoichiometric complex. This complex inactivates Va and VIIIa. There are two forms of protein S: free and bound. Free protein S represents about 40% of the total and is the functional form that acts as the cofactor for APC. Bound protein S, attached to C4b-binding protein, does not possess any anticoagulant activity. Deficiency is associated with recurrent venous thrombosis and/or thromboembolism before age 45.	**Decreased in:** Congenital protein S deficiency, liver disease, thrombosis (acute), warfarin therapy, DIC, vitamin K deficiency, nephrotic syndrome.	This immunoassay measures the total protein S antigen, not biologic activity of protein S. Functional protein S clotting assay (APC cofactor activity) and free protein S antigen immunoassay are available to differentiate subtypes of congenital protein S deficiency (type I: decreased antigen and functional levels; type II: decreased functional levels, but normal total and free antigen levels; type IIa or type III: decreased functional and free antigen levels, but normal total antigen levels). Ten Kate MK et al. Protein S deficiency: a clinical perspective. Haemophilia 2008;14:1222. [PMID: 18479427] Soare AM et al. Deficiencies of proteins C, S and antithrombin and factor V Leiden and the risk of ischemic strokes. J Med Life 2010;3:235. [PMID: 20945813]

Protein, total		
Protein, total, plasma or serum 6.0–8.0 g/dL [60–80 g/L] SST, green, PPT, lavender $ Avoid prolonged venous stasis during collection.	Plasma protein concentration is determined by nutritional state, hepatic function, renal function, hydration, and various disease states. Plasma protein concentration determines the colloidal osmotic pressure.	**Increased in:** Polyclonal or monoclonal gammopathies, marked dehydration. Drugs: anabolic steroids, androgens, corticosteroids, epinephrine. **Decreased in:** Protein-losing enteropathies, acute burns, nephrotic syndrome, severe dietary protein deficiency, chronic liver disease, malabsorption syndrome, agammaglobulinemia, cancer cachexia.	Serum total protein consists primarily of albumin and globulin. Serum globulin level is calculated as total protein minus albumin. Hypoproteinemia usually indicates hypoalbuminemia, because albumin is the major serum protein. Braamskamp MJ et al. Clinical practice: protein-losing enteropathy in children. Eur J Pediat 2010;169:1179. [PMID: 20571826] Hennessey DB et al. Preoperative hypoalbuminemia is an independent risk factor for the development of surgical site infection following gastrointestinal surgery: a multi-institutional study. Ann Surg 2010;252:325. [PMID: 20647925]

	Prothrombin time		
Test/Range/Collection	**Physiologic Basis**	**Interpretation**	**Comments**
Prothrombin time, PT, whole blood (PT) 11–15 seconds (laboratory specific) Blue $ Fill tube completely.	PT evaluates the extrinsic and common coagulation pathways. It is measured by adding calcium and tissue thromboplastin to a sample of citrated, platelet-poor plasma. The time required for fibrin clot formation is determined. It is most sensitive to deficiencies in the vitamin K-dependent clotting factors II, VII, and X. It is also sensitive to deficiency of factor V. It is less sensitive to fibrinogen deficiency and heparin. PT is the most commonly used test for monitoring warfarin therapy. In addition to results reported in seconds, the International Normalized Ratio (INR) is calculated. $INR = [Patient\ PT/Normal\ mean\ PT]^{ISI}$ Point-of-care PT/INR tests are increasingly being used for monitoring warfarin therapy.	**Increased in:** Warfarin, liver disease, DIC, vitamin K deficiency, hereditary deficiency in factors VII, X, V and II, fibrinogen abnormality (eg, hypofibrinogenemia, afibrinogenemia, dysfibrinogenemia), circulating anticoagulant affecting the PT system (rarely lupus anticoagulant), massive transfusion. **Decreased in:** Recombinant factor FVII (Novoseven) treatment.	Routine preoperative measurement of PT is unnecessary unless there is clinical history of a bleeding disorder (see Figure 9–7 and Table 8–7). The INR was introduced in the early 1980s to improve PT reporting and standardization. An International Sensitivity Index (ISI) is assigned to each thromboplastin by the reagent manufacture. The ISI is a measure of a reagent's responsiveness to low levels of vitamin K-dependent factors compared with the WHO International Reference Preparation. Despite the improvement with INR reporting, significant variation in INR results between laboratories persists. These differences in INR reflect local variables (eg, reagent and/or instrument system). A high-sensitivity, low ISI thromboplastin reagent is recommended to improve precision and accuracy of the INR. Warfarin therapeutic range is INR 2.0–3.0. Bleeding has been reported to be 3 × more common in patients with INRs of 3.0–4.5 than in patients with INRs of 2.0–3.0. Dempfle CE et al. Point of care coagulation tests in critically ill patients. Semin Thromb Hemost 2008;34:445. [PMID: 18956284] Osinbowale O et al. An algorithm for managing warfarin resistance. Cleve Clin J Med 2009;76:724. [PMID: 19952297] Perry DJ et al. Point-of-care testing in haemostasis. Br J Haematol 2010;150:501. [PMID: 20618331]

Q fever antibody		

Q fever antibody, serum		
<1:8 titer SST $$$ Submit paired sera, one collected within 1 week of illness and another 2–3 weeks later. Avoid hemolysis.	*Coxiella burnetii* is a rickettsial organism that is the causative organism for Q fever. Most likely mode of transmission is inhalation of aerosols from common reservoirs, sheep, and cattle. Tick bites (ixodid ticks) may also be a mode of transmission. Antibodies to the organism can be detected by the presence of agglutinins, by complement fixation (CF), by immunofluorescent antibody testing (IFA), or by enzyme-linked immunosorbent assay (ELISA). Agglutinin titers are found 5–8 days after infection. IgM can be detected at 7 days (IFA, ELISA) and may persist for up to 32 weeks (ELISA). IgG (IFA, ELISA) appears after 7 days and peaks at 3–4 weeks. Phase I and phase II antibodies are produced in response to the organism, phase II antibodies appearing first and phase I antibodies weeks to months later. Diagnosis of Q fever is usually confirmed by serologic findings of anti–phase II antigen IgM titers of ≥1:50 and IgG titers of ≥1:200. The finding of elevated levels of both IgM and IgA by ELISA has both high sensitivity and high specificity for acute Q fever. In chronic Q fever, phase I antibodies, especially IgG and IgA, are predominant.	**Increased in:** Acute or chronic Q fever (CF antibodies are present by the second week in 65% of cases and by the fourth week in 90%, acute and convalescent titers [immunofluorescent antibody testing, IFA, or enzyme-linked immunosorbent assay ELISA] detect infection with 89–100% sensitivity and 100% specificity), and recent vaccination for Q fever.	Clinical presentation is similar to that of severe influenza. Typically, there is no rash. Test acute and convalescent sera for evidence of current or recent *C. burnetii* infection. Occasionally, titers do not rise for 4–6 weeks, especially if antimicrobial therapy has been given. Initial testing may not be helpful; treatment should be based on clinical and other laboratory assessment. As with any serologic procedure, demonstration of seroconversion or a fourfold increase in titer between acute and convalescent sera suggests current or recent infection. Patients with Q fever have a high prevalence of antiphospholipid antibody (81%), especially as measured by lupus anticoagulant test or measurement of antibodies to cardiolipin. These tests may be useful in diagnosing patients presenting with fever alone. Antibodies to Q fever do not cross-react with other rickettsial antibodies; a rise in titer is considered diagnostic for recent infection in the absence of prior vaccination. If chronic disease (endocarditis) suspected, order phase I antibodies; if acute disease suspected, order phase II antibodies. Versalovic J et al (editors): *Manual of Clinical Microbiology*. 10th ed. ASM Press, 2011.

QuantiFERON-TB (Interferon-gamma releasing assay)

Test/Range/Collection	Physiologic Basis	Interpretation	Comments
QuantiFERON-TB (Interferon-gamma releasing assay), whole blood Negative Green top (must be delivered to test laboratory within 12 hr) or unique QFT-G blood collection tubes (Nil, TB Antigen, Mitogen) $$$	QuantiFERON-TB Gold (QFT-G) is an indirect test for *Mycobacterium tuberculosis* infection. It measures a cell-mediated immune response in infected persons. The T lymphocytes of infected persons are sensitized to *M. tuberculosis* proteins. When whole blood is incubated with the *M. tuberculosis* specific antigens used in the test, the T lymphocytes produce and secrete interferon-gamma (IFN-γ), which is measured via a sensitive enzyme-linked immunosorbent assay. The test does not distinguish between active tuberculosis disease and latent tuberculosis infection and is intended for use in conjunction with risk assessment, chest radiograph, and other medical and diagnostic evaluations. Compared with the conventional tuberculin skin test, QFT-G is a simpler and more accurate, specific, and convenient TB diagnostic tool.	**Positive:** Active *M. tuberculosis* infection, latent tuberculosis infection. **Negative:** No active or latent *M. tuberculosis* infection. **Indeterminate:** Test error or patient anergy.	QFT-G is highly specific; a positive test result is strongly predictive of *M. tuberculosis* infection. QFT-G test is completely unaffected by BCG vaccination status or by sensitization due to most nontuberculous mycobacteria, with the exception of *M. kansasii, M. marinum,* and *M. szulgai.* The ability of QFT-G to predict the risk of latent tuberculosis infection progression to active tuberculosis has not been determined. Risk may be different from that of those with a positive tuberculin skin test. Diel R et al. Evidence-based comparison of commercial interferon-gamma release assays for detecting TB: a meta-analysis. Chest 2010;137:952. [PMID: 20022968] Lalvani A et al. Interferon gamma release assays: principles and practice. Enferm Infecc Microbiol Clin 2010;28:245. [PMID: 19783328]

Rapid plasma reagin		
Rapid plasma reagin (RPR) serum Nonreactive SST $	Measures nontreponemal antibodies that are produced when *Treponema pallidum* interacts with host tissue. The card test is a flocculation test performed by using a cardiolipin–lecithin–cholesterol carbon-containing antigen reagent mixed on a card with the patient's serum. A positive test (presence of antibodies) is indicated when black carbon clumps produced by flocculation are seen by the naked eye.	**Increased in:** Syphilis: primary (78%), secondary (97%), symptomatic late (74%). Biologic false positives occur in a wide variety of conditions, including leprosy, malaria, intravenous drug abuse, aging, infectious mononucleosis, HIV infection (≤15%), autoimmune diseases (SLE, rheumatoid arthritis), pregnancy.	RPR is historically used as a screening test and in suspected primary and secondary syphilis. Because the test lacks specificity (false-positive rates 5–20%), positive tests should be confirmed with the specific treponemal antibody tests (FTA-ABS or TP-PA, p. 139 and 274). RPR titers can be used to follow serologic response to treatment. (See Table 8–24.) The incidence of syphilis has been on the rise and there is a high coinfection rate with HIV. A new syphilis testing algorithm using treponemal tests for screening and nontreponemal serologic tests for confirmation has been proposed. Seña AC et al. Novel *Treponema pallidum* serologic tests: a paradigm shift in syphilis screening for the 21st century. Clin Infect Dis 2010;51:700. [PMID: 20687840]

	Red blood cell count		
Test/Range/Collection	Physiologic Basis	Interpretation	Comments
Red blood cell count (RBC or erythrocyte count), whole blood Males: $4.3–6.0 \times 10^6$/mcL Females: $3.5–5.5 \times 10^6$/mcL [$\times 10^{12}$/L] Lavender $	Red blood cells (erythrocytes) are counted by automated instruments using electrical impedance or light scattering.	**Increased in:** Secondary polycythemia, hemoconcentration (dehydration), polycythemia vera. Spurious increase with increased white blood cells. **Decreased in:** Anemias. Spurious decrease with autoagglutination (eg, cold agglutinins).	In patients with cold agglutinins, the spurious lowering of the RBC count is disproportionately greater than the false elevation of MCV, so the hematocrit is falsely depressed and the MCH and MCHC are falsely elevated. Janus J et al. Evaluation of anemia in children. Am Fam Physician 2010;81:1462. [PMID: 20540485] Milcic TL. The complete blood count. Neonatal Netw 2010;29:109. [PMID: 20211833]

		Renin activity
Renin activity, plasma (PRA) Lavender $$	The renal juxtaglomerular apparatus generates renin, an enzyme that converts angiotensinogen to angiotensin I. The inactive angiotensin I is then converted to angiotensin II, which is a potent vasopressor. Renin activity is measured by the ability of patient's plasma to generate angiotensin I from substrate (angiotensinogen). Normal values depend on the patient's hydration, posture, and salt intake.	**Increased in:** Dehydration, some hypertensive states (eg, renal artery stenosis), edematous states (cirrhosis, nephrotic syndrome, CHF), hypokalemic states (gastrointestinal sodium and potassium loss, Bartter syndrome), adrenal insufficiency, chronic renal failure, left ventricular hypertrophy. Drugs: ACE inhibitors, estrogen, hydralazine, nifedipine, minoxidil, oral contraceptives. **Decreased in:** Hyporeninemic hypoaldosteronism, some hypertensive states (eg, primary aldosteronism, severe preeclampsia). Drugs: β-blockers, aspirin, clonidine, prazosin, reserpine, methyldopa, indomethacin.	The ratio of plasma aldosterone concentration to plasma renin activity is an effective screening test for primary aldosteronism (sensitivity 95%). It has a high negative predictive value even during antihypertensive therapy. Because of a low specificity of the ratio, autonomous aldosterone production must be confirmed by demonstration of high and autonomous secretion of aldosterone (using an aldosterone suppression test). (see Aldosterone, plasma, p. 58). Plasma renin activity is also useful in evaluation of hypoaldosteronism (low-sodium diet, patient standing). Tomaschitz A et al. Aldosterone to renin ratio—a reliable screening tool for primary aldosteronism? Horm Metab Res 2010;42:382. [PMID: 20225167] Viera AJ et al. Diagnosis of secondary hypertension: an age-based approach. Am Fam Physician 2010;82:1471. [PMID: 21166367]

Test/Range/Collection	Physiologic Basis	Interpretation	Comments
Reticulocyte count, whole blood $33–137 \times 10^3$/mcL [$\times 10^9$/L] Lavender $	Reticulocytes are young red blood cells that contain cytoplasmic RNA. A reticulocyte count measures how rapidly reticulocytes are produced by the bone marrow and then released into the bloodstream. Reticulocyte count reflects the erythropoietic activity of the bone marrow and is thus useful in both the diagnosis of anemias and in monitoring bone marrow response to therapy.	**Increased in:** Hemolytic anemia, blood loss (before development of iron deficiency), recovery from iron, B_{12} or folate deficiency, or from drug-induced anemia. **Decreased in:** Iron deficiency anemia, aplastic anemia, anemia of chronic disease, megaloblastic anemia, sideroblastic anemia, pure red cell aplasia, renal disease, bone marrow suppression or infiltration, myelodysplastic syndrome.	This test is indicated for the evaluation of anemia to distinguish hypoproliferative from hemolytic anemia or blood loss. See anemia evaluation (Figure 9–5; Tables 8–2 & 8–3). The old method of measuring reticulocytes (manual staining and counting) has poor reproducibility. It has been replaced by automated methods (eg, flow cytometry-based), which are more precise and provide absolute reticulocyte counts. Method-specific reference ranges must be used. Piva E et al. Automated reticulocyte counting: state of the art and clinical application in the evaluation of erythropoiesis. Clin Chem Lab Med 2010;48:1369. [PMID: 20666695]

Reticulocyte count

Rh(D) typing		
Rh typing, red cells (Rh) Red, lavender/pink $ Proper identification of specimen is critical.	The Rhesus blood group system is second in importance only to the ABO system for transfusion practice. Anti-Rh antibodies are the leading cause of hemolytic disease of the newborn and may also cause hemolytic transfusion reactions. Although there are other Rhesus antigens, only tests for the D antigen are performed routinely in pretransfusion testing because the D antigen is the most immunogenic. The terms Rh-positive and Rh-negative refer to the presence and absence of the D antigen on the red cell surface, respectively. Persons whose red cells lack D do not regularly have anti-D in their serum. Formation of anti-D almost always results from exposure through transfusion or pregnancy to red cells possessing the D antigen.	83% of US non-Hispanic whites are Rh(D)-positive, 17% negative; 93% of Hispanic-Americans are Rh(D)-positive 7% negative; 93% of African Americans are Rh(D)-positive. 7% negative; 98% of Asian Americans are Rh(D)-positive, 2% negative; 90% of North American Indians are Rh(D)-positive, 10% negative.	Of D-reactive persons receiving a single D-positive[+] blood unit, 50–75% will develop anti-D. The blood of all donors and recipients is therefore routinely tested for D, so that D-negative recipients can be given D-negative blood. Donor units must also be tested for a weak form of D antigen, previously called D^u, and must be labeled D-positive if "weak D" is detected. It is not required to test recipient blood specimen for weak D. *Technical Manual of the American Association of Blood Banks,* 17th ed. American Association of Blood Banks, 2011. Westhoff CM. The structure and function of Rh antigen complex. Semin Hematol 2007;44:42. [PMID: 17198846]

	Rheumatoid factor	
Test/Range/Collection	Physiologic Basis	Interpretation	Comments

Test/Range/Collection	Physiologic Basis	Interpretation	Comments
Rheumatoid factor, serum (RF) Negative (<1:16) SST $	RF consists of heterogeneous autoantibodies usually of the IgM class that react against the Fc region of human IgG. Most methods detect only IgM-class RF.	**Positive in:** Rheumatoid arthritis (75–90%), Sjögren syndrome (80–90%), scleroderma, dermatomyositis, SLE (30%), sarcoidosis, Waldenström macroglobulinemia, chronic infection. Drugs: methyldopa, others. Low-titers of RF (eg, ≤1:80) are questionable and can be found in healthy older patients (20%), in 1–4% of normal individuals, and in a variety of acute immune responses (eg, viral infections, including infectious mononucleosis and viral hepatitis), chronic bacterial infections (tuberculosis, leprosy, subacute infective endocarditis), and chronic active hepatitis.	Rheumatoid factor can be useful in differentiating rheumatoid arthritis from other chronic inflammatory arthritides. However, a positive RF test is only one of several criteria needed to make the diagnosis of rheumatoid arthritis. (See also Autoantibodies, Table 8–6.) RF must be ordered selectively because its predictive value is low (34%) if it is used as a screening test. The test has poor positive predictive value because of its lack of specificity. The subset of patients with seronegative rheumatic disease limits its sensitivity and negative predictive value. McInnes IB et al. State-of-the-art: rheumatoid arthritis. Ann Rheum Dis 2010;69:1898. [PMID: 20959326] Pincus T et al. Laboratory tests to assess patients with rheumatoid arthritis: advantages and limitations. Rheum Dis Clin North Am 2009;35:731. [PMID: 19962617]

Ribonucleoprotein antibody		
Ribonucleoprotein antibody, serum (RNP) Negative SST $$	This is an antibody to a ribonucleoprotein-extractable nuclear antigen. The presence of high-titer antibodies to U1-RNP are associated with mixed connective tissue disease (MCTD), and may also be present in systemic erythematosus (SLE) and systemic sclerosis.	**Increased in:** Scleroderma (20–30% sensitivity, low specificity), mixed connective tissue disease (MCTD) (95–100% sensitivity, low specificity), SLE (38–44%), Sjögren syndrome, rheumatoid arthritis (10%), discoid lupus (20–30%). Anti-RNP is present in 2.7% of patients with positive ANA.	A negative test essentially excludes MCTD. (See also Autoantibodies, Table 8–6.) Kattah NH et al. The U1-snRNP complex: structural properties relating to autoimmune pathogenesis in rheumatic diseases. Immunol Rev 2010;233:126. [PMID: 20192997] Keith MP et al. Anti-RNP immunity: implications for tissue injury and the pathogenesis of connective tissue disease. Autoimmun Rev 2007;6:232. [PMID: 17317614]

	Rubella antibody

Test/Range/Collection	Physiologic Basis	Interpretation	Comments
Rubella antibody, serum <1:8 titer SST $ For diagnosis of a recent infection, submit paired sera, one collected within 1 week of illness and another 2–4 weeks later.	Rubella (German measles) is a viral infection that causes fever, malaise, coryza, lymphadenopathy, fine maculopapular rash, and congenital birth defects when infection occurs in utero. Antibodies to rubella can be detected by hemagglutination inhibition, complement fixation, indirect hemagglutination, enzyme-linked immunosorbent assay (ELISA), or latex agglutination. Tests can detect IgG and IgM antibody. Titers usually appear as rash fades (1 week) and peak at 10–14 days for hemagglutination inhibition and 2–3 weeks for other techniques. Baseline titers may remain elevated for life. Serologic tests are used to determine the immune status of the individual, to diagnose postnatal rubella, and occasionally to support the diagnosis of rubella. IgM antibody disappears within 4–5 weeks; IgG antibody remains for life.	**Increased in:** Recent rubella infection, congenital rubella infection, previous rubella infection, or vaccination (immunity). Spuriously increased IgM antibody occurs in the presence of rheumatoid factor or cross-reacting antibodies to other viral infections or autoimmune illnesses.	Rubella titers of ≤1:8 indicate susceptibility and need for immunization to prevent infection during pregnancy. Titers of >1:32 indicate immunity from prior infection or vaccination. Demonstration of a 4-fold rise in titer between acute and convalescent sera may be indicative of a recent infection. Single titers, even >1:256, cannot be interpreted as evidence of recent infection, since they are more likely to indicate immune status. The recent resurgence of congenital rubella can largely be prevented with improved rubella testing and vaccination programs. Robinson JL et al. Prevention of congenital rubella syndrome: what makes sense in 2006? Epidemiol Rev 2006;28:81. [PMID: 16775038] Versalovic J et al (editors). *Manual of Clinical Microbiology,* 10th ed. ASM Press, 2011.

Russell viper venom time (dRVVT)		
Russell viper venom time (dilute, dRVVT), plasma 24–37 seconds (laboratory-specific) Blue $$	Russell viper venom is extracted from a pit viper (*Vipera russelli*), which causes a rapidly fatal syndrome of consumptive coagulopathy with hemorrhage, shock, rhabdomyolysis, and renal failure. Approximately 70% of the protein content of the venom is phospholipase A_2, which activates factor X in the presence of phospholipid, bypassing factor VII. dRVVT is used in detection of antiphospholipid antibodies (so-called lupus anticoagulant, LAC). It should be noted that the 'anticoagulant' detected *in vitro* may be associated with vascular thrombosis and pregnancy-related morbidity *in vivo*.	**Increased in:** Circulating lupus anticoagulants (LAC) (sensitivity 96%, specificity 5C–70%), severe fibrinogen deficiency (<50 mg/dL), deficiencies in prothrombin, factor V, factor X, and heparin therapy. **Normal in:** Factor VII deficiency and all intrinsic pathway deficiencies.	The test is sensitive to phospholipid, and if heparin is not present, a prolonged dRVVT may indicate the presence of LAC (antiphospholipid antibodies). Activated partial thromboplastin time (aPTT)–based hexagonal phase phospholipid test is also used for LAC detection. More than one antibody is associated with LAC activity. As examples, both anticardiolipin and antibodies to beta2-glycoprotein-I can have LAC activity. See Figure 9–22 for its use in evaluating isolated prolongation of PTT. Dembitzer FR et al. Lupus anticoagulant testing: performance and practices by North American clinical laboratories. Am J Clin Pathol 2010;134(5):764. [PMID: 20959659] Pengo V et al. Update of the guidelines for lupus anticoagulant detection. J Thromb Haemost 2009;7:1737. [PMID: 19624461]

	Salicylate		
Test/Range/Collection	**Physiologic Basis**	**Interpretation**	**Comments**
Salicylate, serum (aspirin) 20–30 mg/dL [200–300 mg/L] ***Panic:*** >35 mg/dL [> 350 mg/L] Red $$	At high concentrations, salicylate stimulates hyperventilation, uncouples oxidative phosphorylation, and impairs glucose and fatty acid metabolism. Salicylate toxicity is thus marked by respiratory alkalosis and metabolic acidosis.	**Increased in:** Acute or chronic salicylate intoxication.	The potential toxicity of salicylate levels after acute ingestion can be determined by using the salicylate toxicity nomogram (Figure 10–10). Nomograms have become less valid with the increasing popularity of enteric-coated slow-release aspirin preparations. Routine testing may not be required for fully conscious asymptomatic adult patients who deny ingesting salicylate. Acute toxicity can be readily diagnosed if an ingestion history is provided. O'Malley GF. Emergency department management of the salicylate-poisoned patient. Emerg Med Clin North Am 2007;25:333. [PMID: 17482023] Pearlman BL et al. Salicylate intoxication: a clinical review. Postgrad Med 2009;121:162. [PMID: 19641282]

Scleroderma-associated antibody		
Scleroderma-associated antibody (Scl-70 antibody), serum Negative SST $$	This antibody reacts with a nuclear antigen (DNA topoisomerase 1, or topo-I) that is responsible for the relaxation of super-coiled DNA.	**Increased in:** Scleroderma (systemic sclerosis), SLE (5%).	Scl-70 antibody is seen in 20–50% of patients with scleroderma and is considered diagnostic and specific for scleroderma if it is the only antibody present. Predictive value of a positive test is >95% for scleroderma. Scl-70 antibodies are associated with diffuse cutaneous scleroderma and a higher risk of severe interstitial lung disease. Low levels of Scl-70 antibody are also present in approximately 5% of patients with systemic lupus erythematosus. 50–70% of patients with limited scleroderma (CREST syndrome) have detectable anti-centromere antibody. (See also Autoantibodies, Table 8–6.) Czompoly T et al. Anti-topoisomerase I autoantibodies in systemic sclerosis. Autoimmun Rev 2009;8:692. [PMID: 19393194] Mahler M et al. Anti-Scl-70 (topo-I) in SLE: myth or reality? Autoimmun Rev 2010;9:756. [PMID: 20601198]

	Semen analysis		
Test/Range/Collection	**Physiologic Basis**	**Interpretation**	**Comments**
Semen analysis, ejaculate Sperm count: >20 × 10^6/mL [10^9/L] Motility score: >60% motile Volume: 2–5 mL Normal morphology: >60% $$$ Semen is collected in a urine container after masturbation following 3 days of abstinence from ejaculation. Specimen must be examined promptly.	Conventional semen analysis includes the determination of sperm count, semen volume, sperm motility (qualitative and quantitative), and sperm morphology. Sperm are viewed under the microscope for motility and morphology. In addition to sperm count, sperm morphology and motility may have the most predictive utility. Infertility can be associated with low counts or with sperm of abnormal morphology or decreased motility.	**Decreased in:** Primary or secondary testicular failure, cryptorchidism, following vasectomy, drugs.	A low sperm count should be confirmed by sending two other appropriately collected semen specimens for evaluation. The usefulness of conventional semen analysis parameters as predictors of fertility is somewhat limited. Therefore, alternative tests based on more functional aspects (sperm penetration, capacitation, acrosome reaction) have been developed. Flow cytometer-based Sperm Chromatin Structure Assay (SCSA) can provide an assessment of DNA integrity as another parameter of sperm quality. Frey KA. Male reproductive health and infertility. Prim Care 2010;37:643. [PMID: 20705204] Samplaski MK et al. New generation of diagnostic tests for infertility: review of specialized semen tests. Int J Urol 2010;17:839. [PMID: 20887631]

	Smith (anti-Sm) antibody	Smooth muscle antibodies
Smith (anti-Sm) antibody, serum Negative SST $$	This antibody to Smith antigen (an extractable nuclear antigen) is a marker antibody for SLE.	**Positive in:** SLE (30–40% sensitivity, 90–95% specificity).	A positive test substantially increases posttest probability of the diagnosis of SLE. Test rarely needed for the diagnosis of SLE. (See also Autoantibodies, Table 8–6.) Breda L et al. Laboratory tests in the diagnosis and follow-up of pediatric rheumatic diseases: an update. Semin Arthritis Rheum 2010;40:53. [PMID: 19246077]
Smooth muscle antibodies, serum Negative SST $$	Antibodies against smooth muscle proteins are found in patients with chronic active hepatitis and primary biliary cirrhosis.	**Positive in:** Autoimmune chronic active hepatitis (40–70%, predominantly IgG antibodies), lower titers in primary biliary cirrhosis (50% predominantly IgM antibodies), viral hepatitis, infectious mononucleosis, cryptogenic cirrhosis (28%), HIV infection, vitiligo (25%), endometriosis, Behçet disease (<2% of normal individuals).	The presence of high titers of smooth muscle antibodies (>1:80) is useful in distinguishing autoimmune chronic active hepatitis from other forms of hepatitis. Bogdanos DP et al. Autoantibodies and their antigens in autoimmune hepatitis. Semin Liver Dis 2009;29:241. [PMID: 19675997] Mieli-Vergani G et al. Autoimmune hepatitis in children: what is different from adult AIH? Semin Liver Dis 2009;29:297. [PMID: 19676002]

Sodium

Test/Range/Collection	Physiologic Basis	Interpretation	Comments
Sodium, serum or plasma (Na+) 135–145 meq/L [mmol/L] **Panic:** <125 or >155 meq/L SST, green $	Sodium is the predominant extracellular cation. The serum sodium level is primarily determined by the volume status of the individual. Hyponatremia can be divided into hypovolemia, euvolemia, and hypervolemia categories. (See Hyponatremia algorithm, Figure 9–16.) Sodium is commonly measured by ion-selective electrode.	**Increased in:** Dehydration (excessive sweating, severe vomiting, or diarrhea), polyuria (diabetes mellitus, diabetes insipidus), hyperaldosteronism, inadequate water intake (coma, hypothalamic disease). Drugs: steroids, licorice, oral contraceptives. **Decreased in:** CHF, cirrhosis, vomiting, diarrhea, exercise, excessive sweating (with replacement of water but not salt, eg, marathon running), salt-losing nephropathy, adrenal insufficiency, nephrotic syndrome, water intoxication, syndrome of inappropriate antidiuretic hormone (SIADH), AIDS. Drugs: thiazides, diuretics, ACE inhibitors, chlorpropamide, carbamazepine, antidepressants (selective serotonin reuptake inhibitors), antipsychotics.	Spurious hyponatremia may be produced by severe lipemia or hyperproteinemia if sodium analysis involves a dilution step. Many guidelines recommend a correction factor, whereby the serum sodium concentration decreases by 1.6 meq/L for every 100 mg/dL (5.56 mmol/L) rise in plasma glucose above normal, but there is evidence that the decrease may be greater when patients have more severe hyperglycemia (>400 mg/dL or 22.2 mmol/L) and/or volume depletion. One group has suggested that, when the serum glucose is >200 mg/dL, the serum sodium concentration decreases by at least 2.4 meq/L. Hyponatremia in a normovolemic patient with urine osmolality higher than serum (or plasma) osmolality suggests the possibility of SIADH, myxedema, hypopituitarism, or reset osmostat. Treatment of disorders of sodium balance relies on clinical assessment of the patient's extracellular fluid volume rather than the serum sodium. Ball SG. Hyponatremia. J R Coll Physicians Edinb 2010;40:240. [PMID: 21127769] Hillier TA et al. Hyponatremia: evaluating the correction factor for hyperglycemia. Am J Med. 1999;106(4):399. [PMID: 10225241] Nemerovski C et al. Treatment of hypervolemic or euvolemic hyponatremia associated with heart failure, cirrhosis, or the syndrome of inappropriate antidiuretic hormone with tolvaptan: a clinical review. Clin Ther 2010;32:1015. [PMID: 20637957] Vaidya C et al. Management of hyponatremia: providing treatment and avoiding harm. Cleve Clin J Med 2010;77:715. [PMID: 20889809]

Somatostatin		
Somatostatin, plasma <25 pg/mL [<25 ng/L] (laboratory-specific) Lavender $$$$ Specimen should be collected in pre-chilled lavender tube and refrigerated.	Somatostatin is a peptide hormone produced by the hypothalamus and digestive system (stomach, intestine, and pancreas). It has 2 active forms produced by alternative cleavage of a single preprotein, one of 14 amino acids, the other of 28 amino acids. Somatostatin is a physiologic regulator of islet cell and gastrointestinal functions and is an inhibitor of the release of many pituitary hormones including growth hormone, prolactin, and thyrotropin.	**Increased in:** Somatostatinoma and other somatostatin-producing neuroendocrine tumors.	Useful as a tumor marker for diagnosis and follow-up of somatostatinoma and other somatostatin-producing neuroendocrine tumors. Results obtained with different somatostatin assays can differ substantially. Serial measurements should therefore always be performed using the same assay. Öberg K. Pancreatic endocrine tumors. Semin Oncol 2010;37:594. [PMID: 21167379]

	SS-A/Ro antibody		
Test/Range/Collection	Physiologic Basis	Interpretation	Comments
SS-A/Ro antibody, serum Negative SST $$	Antibodies to Ro (SSA) cellular ribonucleoprotein complexes are found in connective tissue diseases such as Sjögren syndrome (SS), SLE, neonatal lupus (particularly with congenital heart block), rheumatoid arthritis (RA), and vasculitis. There are two types of anti-Ro/SSA antibodies, anti-SSA-52 kDa and anti-SSA-60 kDa, each specific for different antigens.	**Increased in:** Sjögren syndrome (60–70% sensitivity), low specificity), SLE (30–40%), RA (10%), subacute cutaneous lupus, vasculitis.	Useful in counseling women of childbearing age with known connective tissue disease, because a positive test is associated with a small but real risk of neonatal SLE and congenital heart block. The few (<10%) patients with SLE who do not have a positive ANA commonly have antibodies to SS-A. (See also Autoantibodies, Table 8–6.) Defendenti C et al. Clinical and laboratory aspects of Ro/SSA-52 autoantibodies. Autoimmun Rev 2011;10:150. [PMID: 20854935] Fauchais AL et al. Immunological profile in primary Sjögren syndrome: clinical significance, prognosis and long-term evolution to other auto-immune disease. Autoimmun Rev 2010;9:595. [PMID: 20457283] Hernandez-Molina G et al. The meaning of anti-Ro and anti-La antibodies in primary Sjögren's syndrome. Autoimmun Rev 2011;10:123 [PMID: 20833272] Lazzerini PE et al. Anti-Ro/SSA antibodies and cardiac arrhythmias in the adult: facts and hypotheses. Scand J Immunol 2010;72:213. [PMID: 20696018]

	SS-B/La antibody	T-cell receptor gene rearrangement
SS-B/La antibody, serum Negative SST $$	Antibodies to La (SSB) cellular ribonucleoprotein complexes are found in Sjögren syndrome and appear to be relatively more specific for Sjögren syndrome than are antibodies to SSA. They are quantitated by immunoassay.	**Increased in:** Sjögren syndrome (50% sensitivity, higher specificity than anti-SSA), SLE (10%).	Direct pathogenicity and usefulness of autoantibody test in predicting disease exacerbation not proven. (See also Autoantibodies, Table 8–6.) Fauchais AL et al. Immunological profile in primary Sjögren syndrome: clinical significance, prognosis and long-term evolution to other auto-immune disease. Autoimmun Rev 2010;9:595. [PMID: 20457283] Hernandez-Molina G et al. The meaning of anti-Ro and anti-La antibodies in primary Sjögren's syndrome. Autoimmun Rev 2011;10:123. [PMID: 20833272]
T-cell receptor (TCR) gene rearrangement, whole blood, bone marrow, frozen or paraffin-embedded tissue Lavender $$$$	In general, the percentage of T lymphocytes with identical T-cell receptors is very low; in malignancies, however, the clonal expansion of one population leads to a large number of cells with identical T-cell receptor gene rearrangement. T-cell clonality can be assessed by restriction fragment Southern blot hybridization or polymerase chain reaction (PCR).	**Positive in:** T-cell neoplasms such as T-cell prolymphocytic leukemia, Sézary syndrome, peripheral T-cell lymphoma (monoclonal T-cell proliferation).	The diagnostic sensitivity and specificity are heterogeneous and laboratory- and method-specific. Results of the test must always be interpreted in the context of morphologic and other relevant data (eg, flow cytometry), and should not be used alone for a diagnosis of malignancy. The test is primarily for initial diagnosis, but is also used to detect minimal residual disease. Garcia-Castillo H et al. Detection of clonal immunoglobulin and T-cell receptor gene recombination in hematological malignancies: monitoring minimal residual disease. Cardiovasc Hematol Disord Drug Targets 2009;9:124. [PMID: 19519371] Hodges E et al. T-cell receptor molecular diagnosis of T-cell lymphoma. Methods Mol Med 2005;115:197. [PMID: 15998969]

	Testosterone	
Test/Range/Collection	**Physiologic Basis**	**Interpretation**	**Comments**

Test/Range/Collection	Physiologic Basis	Interpretation	Comments
Testosterone, total, serum or plasma Males: 3.0–10.0 ng/mL [Males: 10–35 nmol/L] Females: 0.3–0.7 ng/mL [Females: 1.0–2.4 nmol/L] SST, green $$$	Testosterone is the principal male sex hormone, produced by the Leydig cells of the testes. Dehydroepiandrosterone (DHEA) is produced in the adrenal cortex, testes, and ovaries and is the main precursor for serum testosterone in women. In normal males after puberty, the testosterone level is twice as high as all androgens in females. In serum, it is largely bound to albumin (38%) and to a specific steroid hormone–binding globulin (SHBG) (60%), but it is the free hormone (2%) that is physiologically active. The total testosterone level measures both bound and free testosterone in the serum (by immunoassay). Free or bioavailable testosterone may be calculated or measured.	**Increased in:** Idiopathic sexual precocity (in boys, levels may be in adult range), adrenal hyperplasia (boys), adrenocortical tumors, trophoblastic disease during pregnancy, idiopathic hirsutism, virilizing ovarian tumors, arrhenoblastoma, virilizing luteoma, testicular feminization (normal or moderately elevated), cirrhosis (through increased SHBG), hyperthyroidism. Drugs: anticonvulsants, barbiturates, estrogens, oral contraceptives (through increased SHBG). **Decreased in:** Hypogonadism (primary and secondary), orchidectomy, Klinefelter syndrome, uremia, hemodialysis, hepatic insufficiency, ethanol [men]). Drugs: digoxin, spironolactone, acarbose.	The diagnosis of male hypogonadism is based on clinical symptoms and signs plus laboratory confirmation of low AM total serum testosterone levels on two different occasions. Levels <3.0 ng/mL should be treated. Free testosterone should be measured in symptomatic patients with normal total testosterone levels. Obtain serum luteinizing hormone and FSH levels to distinguish between primary (hypergonadotropic) and secondary (hypogonadotropic) hypogonadism. Hypogonadism associated with aging (andropause) may present a mixed picture, with low testosterone levels and low to low-normal gonadotropin levels. In men, there is a diurnal variation in serum testosterone with a 20% elevation in levels in the evenings. Schulman CC et al. Testosterone measurement in patients with prostate cancer. Eur Urol 2010;58:65. [PMID: 20434831] Vesper HW et al. Standardization of testosterone measurements in humans. J Steroid Biochem Mol Biol 2010;121:513. [PMID: 20302935]

Thrombin time

Thrombin time, plasma (TT)

17–23 seconds
(laboratory-specific)

Blue

$

The thrombin time (TT) is a clot-based assay that measures the conversion of fibrinogen to fibrin. The TT is therefore affected by the level of fibrinogen and the presence of thrombin inhibitor (eg, heparin) and/or fibrin degradation products (FDPs). Because it bypasses all other coagulation reactions, it is not influenced by deficiencies of other coagulation factors.

Increased in: Low fibrinogen (<50 mg/dL), abnormal fibrinogen (dysfibrinogenemia), increased FDPs (eg, DIC, heparin, fibrinolytic agents [streptokinase, urokinase, tissue plasminogen activator]), liver disease.

The TT is very sensitive to heparin and has been used to monitor unfractionated heparin therapy, although this use has declined.
Can be used to qualitatively assess anticoagulation status of patients receiving direct thrombin inhibitors (eg, dabigatran).
Heparin contamination is a common cause of an unexplained significantly prolonged TT. If suspected, heparin neutralization can be performed.
Functional fibrinogen assay has largely replaced TT for evaluating fibrinogen.
See evaluation for bleeding disorders (Figure 9–7 and Table 8–7).
Van Ryn J et al. Dabigatran etexilate—a novel, reversible, oral direct thrombin inhibitor: interpretation of coagulation assays and reversal of anticoagulation activity. Thromb Haemost 2010;103:1116. [PMID: 20352166]

Test/Range/Collection	Physiologic Basis	Interpretation	Comments
Thyroglobulin, serum or plasma (Tg) 3–42 ng/mL [mcg/L] SST, green $$$	Tg is a large protein specific to the thyroid gland from which thyroxine is synthesized and cleaved. Highly sensitive immunometric assays for Tg are available. Tg autoantibodies can interfere with the measurement of Tg.	**Increased in:** Hyperthyroidism, subacute thyroiditis, untreated thyroid carcinomas (except medullary carcinoma): follicular cancer (sensitivity 72%, specificity 81%), Hürthle cell cancer (sensitivity 56%, specificity 84%). **Decreased in:** Factitious hyperthyroidism, presence of thyroglobulin autoantibodies, after (>25 days) total thyroidectomy.	Follow-up of patients with differentiated thyroid cancers who are apparently disease-free after surgery and radioiodine therapy involves periodic measurement of serum Tg. Patients with detectable serum Tg during thyroid-stimulating hormone (TSH) suppression by thyroxine therapy or Tg that rises higher than 2 ng/mL after TSH stimulation are highly likely to harbor residual tumor. Undetectable serum Tg during TSH suppressive therapy does not exclude persistent disease. Therefore, serum Tg should be measured after TSH stimulation achieved either by thyroxine withdrawal or by administration of recombinant human TSH (rhTSH). Results are equivalent in detecting recurrent thyroid cancer, but use of rhTSH helps to prevent symptomatic hypothyroidism. Follow-up based on serial measurements of basal (ie, unstimulated) Tg may be superior to the single Tg measurement after TSH stimulation. Tg is typically measured together with Tg antibody. In patients with positive Tg Ab, the Tg level should be interpreted with caution. Sabet A et al. Postoperative management of differentiated thyroid cancer. Otolaryngol Clin North Am 2010;43:329. [PMID: 20510717] Zucchelli G et al. Serum Tg measurement in the follow-up of patients treated for differentiated thyroid cancer. Q J Nucl Med Mol Imaging 2009;53:482. [PMID: 19910901]

Thyroglobulin antibody	Thyroid peroxidase antibody
Thyroglobulin antibody, serum or plasma <1:10 (highly method-dependent) SST, green $$	Antibodies against thyroglobulin are produced in autoimmune diseases of the thyroid and other organs. Of the normal population, 10% has slightly elevated titers (especially women and the elderly).	**Increased in:** Hashimoto thyroiditis (>90%), thyroid carcinoma (45%), thyrotoxicosis, pernicious anemia (50%), SLE (20%), subacute thyroiditis, Graves disease. **Not increased in:** Multinodular goiter, thyroid adenomas, and some carcinomas.	The thyroid peroxidase antibody test is more sensitive than the thyroglobulin antibody test in autoimmune thyroid disease. (See Thyroperoxidase Antibody, below.) There is limited use for this test, ie, monitoring of patients with thyroid carcinoma after treatment. (See Thyroglobulin.) Shivaraj G et al. Thyroid function tests: a review. Eur Rev Med Pharmacol Sci 2009;13:341. [PMID: 19961039] Sinclair D. Clinical and laboratory aspects of thyroid autoantibodies. Ann Clin Biochem 2006;43:173. [PMID: 16704751]
Thyroid peroxidase antibody (TPO Ab), serum or plasma Negative SST, lavender, green $$	TPO is a membrane-bound glycoprotein. This enzyme mediates the oxidation of iodide ions and incorporation of iodine into tyrosine residues of thyroglobulin. Its synthesis is stimulated by thyroid-stimulating hormone (TSH). TPO is the major antigen involved in thyroid antibody–dependent cell-mediated cytotoxicity. TPO Ab can be measured by enzyme-linked immunosorbent assay (ELISA) or automated immunoassay.	**Increased in:** Hashimoto thyroiditis (>99%), idiopathic myxedema (>99%), Graves disease (75–85%), Addison disease (50%), and Riedel thyroiditis. Low titers are present in approximately 10% of normal individuals and patients with nonimmune thyroid disease.	TPO antibody is an antibody to the main autoantigenic component of microsomes and is a more sensitive and specific test than hemagglutination assays for microsomal antibodies in the diagnosis of autoimmune thyroid disease. TPO antibody testing alone is often sufficient to detect autoimmune thyroid disease. TPO antibody titers correlate with TSH levels; their presence may herald impending thyroid failure. See thyroid function tests and thyroid disorders (Table 8–26, Figures 9–14 and 9–17.) McLachlan SM et al. Thyroid peroxidase as an autoantigen. Thyroid 2007;17:939. [PMID: 17822378] Todd CH. Management of thyroid disorders in primary care: challenges and controversies. Postgrad Med J 2009;85:655. [PMID: 20075403]

Test/Range/Collection	Physiologic Basis	Interpretation	Comments
Thyroid-stimulating hormone	Thyroid-stimulating hormone, serum or plasma (TSH; thyrotropin)	TSH is an anterior pituitary hormone that stimulates the thyroid gland to produce thyroid hormones. Secretion is stimulated by thyrotropin-releasing hormone from the hypothalamus. There is negative feedback on TSH secretion by circulating thyroid hormone.	**Increased in:** Hypothyroidism, mild increases in recovery phase of acute illness, subclinical hypothyroidism. **Decreased in:** Hyperthyroidism, subclinical hyperthyroidism, acute medical or surgical illness (euthyroid sick syndrome), pituitary hypothyroidism. Drugs: dopamine, high-dose corticosteroids.	TSH assays are used for screening thyroid function, aiding the diagnosis of hyperthyroidism and hypothyroidism, and monitoring thyroid replacement therapy. The currently used TSH immunoassays are very sensitive, typically with functional sensitivity of $\leq$0.02 mIU/L. Measurement of serum TSH is the best initial laboratory test of thyroid function. It should be followed by measurement of free thyroxine (FT$_4$) if the TSH value is low and by measurement of anti-thyroperoxidase antibody (TPO Ab) if the TSH value is high. Most experts recommend against routine screening of asymptomatic patients, but screening is recommended for high-risk populations. See also Thyroid function tests and thyroid disorders (Table 8–26; Figures 9–14 and 9–17). Test is also useful for following patients taking anti-thyroid medication. Jones DD et al. Subclinical thyroid disease. Am J Med 2010;123:502. [PMID: 20569751] Shivaraj G et al. Thyroid function tests: a review. Eur Rev Med Pharmacol Sci 2009;13:341. [PMID: 19961039]. Todd CH. Management of thyroid disorders in primary care: challenges and controversies. Postgrad Med J 2009;85:655. [PMID: 20075403] Waise A et al. The upper limit of reference range for TSH should not be confused with a cut-off to define subclinical hypothyroidism. Ann Clin Biochem 2009;46:93. [PMID: 19164339]

0.35–3.0 mcIU/mL [mIU/L]

(assay-dependent)

SST, PPT, green

$$

Thyroid stimulating immunoglobulin

Thyroid stimulating immunoglobulin (TSI), serum		Positive in: Graves disease (adults, 80–90%; children, 50–60%), toxic multinodular goiter (15–20%), transient neonatal thyrotoxicosis.	Although TSI is a marker for Graves disease, the test is not necessary for its diagnosis in most cases. It is helpful in confirming subclinical disease in euthyroid patients presenting with exophthalmos.
Negative (TSI index <1.3, or <130% basal activity)	TSIs are autoimmune immuno-globulins (IgG type) that can bind to thyroid-stimulating hormone (TSH) receptors in the thyroid gland. TSIs mimic the action of TSH, causing excess secretion of thyroxine (T4) and triiodothyronine (T3). The level of the TSIs detected in this test is abnormally high in hyperthyroidism due to Graves disease. TSIs can cross the placental barrier, causing transient hyperthyroidism in the neonates of mothers with Graves disease.		Since none of the treatments for Graves disease are aimed at the underlying pathophysiologic mechanism, but rather ablate thyroid tissue or block thyroid hormone synthesis, TSI may be detectable after apparent cure.
SST, red			Pregnant women with history of Graves disease should be tested for TSI; if present, it may predict neonatal thyrotoxicosis.
$$$			Gestational thyrotoxicosis, which is due to a combination of hCG cross-reactivity (binding to the TSH receptor) and to transient changes in thyroid hormone protein binding, is not associated with TSI. Finding an elevated TSI in pregnancy suggests underlying Graves disease. Kamishian A et al. Different outcomes of neonatal thyroid function after Graves' disease in pregnancy: patient reports and literature review. J Pediatr Endocrinol Metab 2005;18:1357. [PMID: 16459661]
	TSIs are typically detected by a bioas-say measuring the ability of the patient's serum (or IgG) to stimulate cyclic AMP production in tissue cultures, using cell lines carrying the human TSH receptor.		Lytton SD et al. A novel TSI bioassay is a functional indicator of activity and severity of Graves orbitopathy. J Clin Endocrinol Metab 2010;95:2123. [PMID: 20237164]
	TSIs can also be detected by measur-ing the ability of patient's serum (or IgG) to inhibit binding of TSH to the solubilized TSH receptor in a bind-ing assay format. This test is often referred to as TSH receptor antibody test (TRAb test). The TSH-R antibody (TRAb) test is less expensive and has a shorter turnaround time; it can often be used instead of the TSI bioassay.		Quadbeck B et al. Binding, stimulating and blocking TSH-R antibodies to the thyrotropin receptor as predictors of relapse of Graves' disease after withdrawal of antithyroid treatment. Horm Metab Res 2005;37:745. [PMID: 16372228]
			Schott M et al. Relevance of TSH receptor stimulating and blocking autoantibody measurement for the prediction of relapse in Graves' disease. Horm Metab Res 2005;37:741. [PMID: 16372227]

Test/Range/Collection	Physiologic Basis	Interpretation	Comments
Thyroxine, total, serum or plasma (T$_4$) 5.0–11.0 mcg/dL [64–142 nmol/L] SST, PPT, green $	Total T$_4$ is a measure of thyroid gland secretion of T$_4$, bound and free, and thus is influenced by levels of thyroid hormone-binding proteins. Only free T$_4$ is biologically active.	**Increased in:** Hyperthyroidism, increased thyroid-binding globulin (TBG) (eg, pregnancy, drug). Drugs: amiodarone, high-dose β-blockers (especially propranolol). **Decreased in:** Hypothyroidism, low TBG due to illness or drugs, congenital absence of TBG. Drugs: phenytoin, carbamazepine, androgens.	Total T$_4$ should be interpreted with the TBG level, TSH and free T$_4$ measurements. Jones DD et al. Subclinical thyroid disease. Am J Med 2010;123:502. [PMID: 20569751] Todd CH. Management of thyroid disorders in primary care: challenges and controversies. Postgrad Med J 2009;85:655. [PMID: 20075403]
Thyroxine, free, serum or plasma (free T$_4$ or FT$_4$) 0.8–1.7 ng/dL (method-dependent) SST, PPT, green $$	FT$_4$ is a direct measure of the free T$_4$ hormone concentration (biologically available hormone). It can be measured by equilibrium dialysis/HPLC-mass spectrometry, although immunoassays are equally effective.	**Increased in:** Hyperthyroidism, nonthyroidal illness, especially psychiatric. Drugs: amiodarone, β-blockers (high-dose). **Decreased in:** Hypothyroidism, nonthyroidal illness. Drugs: phenytoin.	The free thyroxine is used along with sensitive TSH assays for detecting clinical hyperthyroidism and hypothyroidism. The TSH assay detects subclinical thyroid dysfunction (normal FT$_4$) and monitors levo-thyroxine treatment better, whereas the free thyroxine test detects central hypothyroidism and monitors rapidly changing function status better. Jones DD et al. Subclinical thyroid disease. Am J Med 2010;123:502. [PMID: 20569751] Kharlip J et al. Recent developments in hyperthyroidism. Lancet 2009;373:1930. [PMID: 19501730] Todd CH. Management of thyroid disorders in primary care: challenges and controversies. Postgrad Med J 2009;85:655. [PMID: 20075403]

Toxoplasma antibody		
Toxoplasma antibodies, serum or CSF (Toxo) IgG: <1:16 titer IgM: Infant <1:2 titer Adult <1:8 titer SST (serum) or CSF $$$ Submit paired sera, one collected within 1 week of illness and another 2–3 weeks later.	*Toxoplasma gondii* is an obligate intracellular protozoan that causes human infection via ingestion, transplacental transfer, blood products, or organ transplantation. Cats are the definitive hosts of *T. gondii* and pass oocysts in their feces. Human infection occurs through ingestion of sporulated oocysts or via the transplacental route. In the immunodeficient host (eg, HIV/AIDS), acute infection may progress to lethal meningoencephalitis, pneumonitis, or myocarditis. Chemoprophylaxis should be considered for patients who have a CD4 count <200/mcL. In acute primary infection, IgM antibodies develop 1–2 weeks after onset of illness, peak in 6–8 weeks, and then decline. IgG antibodies develop on a similar time-course but persist for years. In adult infection, the disease usually represents a reactivation, not a primary infection. Therefore, the IgM test is less useful. Approximately 30% of all US adults have antibodies to *T. gondii*.	**Increased in:** Acute or congenital toxoplasmosis (IgM), previous toxoplasma exposure (IgG), and false-positive (IgM) reactions (SLE, HIV infection, rheumatoid arthritis).	Single IgG titers of >1:256 are considered diagnostic of active infection; titers of >1:128 are suspicious. Titers of 1:16–1:64 may merely represent past exposure. If titers subsequently rise, they probably represent early disease. An IgM titer >1:16 is very important in the diagnosis of congenital toxoplasmosis. High titer IgG antibody results should prompt an IgM test. IgM, however, is generally not detected in adult AIDS patients because toxoplasmosis usually represents a reactivation. Some recommend ordering baseline toxoplasma IgG titers in all asymptomatic HIV-positive patients because a rising toxoplasma titer can help diagnose CNS toxoplasmosis in the future. Culture of the *T. gondii* organism is difficult, and most laboratories are not equipped for the procedure. (See also Brain abscess, Chapter 5.) Boothroyd JC. *Toxoplasma gondii:* 25 years and 25 major advances for the field. Int J Parasitol 2009;39:935. [PMID: 19630140] Nissapatorn V. Toxoplasmosis in HIV/AIDS: a living legacy. Southeast Asian J Trop Med Public Health 2009;40:1158. [PMID: 20578449]

Transferrin

Test/Range/Collection	Physiologic Basis	Interpretation	Comments
Transferrin (Tf), serum or plasma 200–400 mg/dL SST, PPT, green $	Transferrin is the major plasma transport protein for iron. Only a small amount of transferrin is required for normal homeostasis. The presence of moderate amounts of unsaturated transferrin may be important in control of infections and infestations by iron-requiring organisms. Immunochemical assays of transferrin are more accurate than chemical assays of total iron-binding capacity (TIBC). Assuming a molecular weight for transferrin of 89,000 daltons, 1 mg of transferrin binds 1.25 mcg of iron. Therefore, a serum transferrin level of 300 mg/dL is equal to a TIBC of 375 mcg/dL. The utility of TIBC in addition to serum iron is to calculate the percent saturation of transferrin: $$\% \text{ saturation of Tf} = \frac{\text{serum iron}}{\text{TIBC}} \times 100$$ In healthy state, about 33% of the circulating iron binding sites are occupied (interval: 20–50%). It is decreased in iron deficiency and increased in iron overload (eg, hemochromatosis).	**Increased in:** Pregnancy, oral contraceptives, iron deficiency. **Decreased in:** Inherited atransferrinemia (rare), disorders associated with inflammation or necrosis, chronic inflammation or malignancy, generalized malnutrition, nephrotic syndrome, iron overload states.	Indications for transferrin quantitation include screening for nutritional status and differential diagnosis of anemia. To control for effects of estrogens and acute-phase responses, other acute-phase reactant proteins should be assayed at the same time. Iron deficiency and iron overload are best diagnosed using assays of serum levels of iron, transferrin, transferrin saturation and ferritin in combination. Transferrin in CSF appears in its desialated form, the Tau protein (β_2-transferrin). This form can be identified electrophoretically by immunofixation with antitransferrin antibody. The clinical application for identification of the Tau protein is in the investigation of rhinorrhea or otorrhea suspected to be of CSF origin. Alexander J et al. HFE-associated hereditary hemochromatosis. Genet Med 2009;11:307. [PMID: 19444013] Bermjo F et al. A guide to diagnosis of iron deficiency and iron deficiency anemia in digestive diseases. World J Gastroenerol 2009;15:4638. [PMID: 19787826]

Transferrin receptor, soluble

| Transferrin receptor, soluble (sTfR), serum or plasma

Males: 2.2–5 mg/L

Females: 1.9–4.4 mg/L

(laboratory-specific)

SST or green

$$ | The transferrin receptor (TfR) is expressed on the surface of human cells that require iron and acts as an iron transporting molecule. The expression of TfR depends on the concentration of iron in the cellular cytoplasm. The concentration of soluble TfR (sTfR) has been reported to be proportional to the total amount of cell-associated TfR.

Measurement of sTfR is used as a surrogate marker of the status of body iron stores. | **Increased in:** Iron deficiency anemia, conditions of high red cell turnover (eg, hemolytic anemia). | The use of sTfR improves the clinical diagnosis of iron deficiency anemia, especially in the presence of coexisting chronic disease or gastrointestinal malignancies.

A patient with ferritin ≤10 mcg/L is considered to be iron deficient in all cases regardless of sTfR level. A patient with ferritin ≥220 mcg/L is not considered to be iron deficient. For ferritin values between 10 and 220 mcg/L, levels of sTfR may be used to identify iron-deficient patients.

When assessing iron deficiency, the combination of both ferritin and sTfR levels minimizes false positives due to hemolytic anemia that elevates sTfR and false negatives due to acute-phase elevation of ferritin.

Koulaouzidis A et al. Soluble transferrin receptors and iron deficiency, a step beyond ferritin. A systematic review. J Gastrointestin Liver Dis 2009;18:345. [PMID: 19795030] |

				Treponema pallidum

Test/Range/Collection	Physiologic Basis	Interpretation	Comments
Treponema pallidum antibody by TP-PA, serum Nonreactive SST $$	The TP-PA test measures specific antibody against *T. pallidum* in a patient's serum by agglutination of *T. pallidum* antigen-coated erythrocytes. Antibodies to nonpathogenic treponemes are first removed by binding to nonpathogenic treponemal antigens.	**Increased in:** Syphilis: primary (64–87%), secondary (96–100%), late latent (96–100%), tertiary (94–100%), infectious mononucleosis, collagen vascular diseases, hyperglobulinemia, and dysglobulinemia.	The test is historically used to confirm reactive nontreponemal serologic tests for syphilis (RPR or VDRL). New syphilis testing algorithm using treponemal tests for screening and nontreponemal serologic tests for confirmation has been proposed. Compared with FTA-ABS (p. 139), TP-PA is slightly less sensitive in early primary syphilis (See Table 8–24.) Because test usually remains positive for long periods of time regardless of therapy, it is not useful in assessing the effectiveness of therapy. In one study, 36 months after treatment of syphilis, 13% of patients had nonreactive TP-PA tests. The TP-PA, like the FTA-ABS, is not recommended for CSF specimens. VDRL is the preferred test for CSF. Daskalakis D. Syphilis: continuing public health and diagnostic challenges. Curr HIV/AIDS Rep 2008;5:72. [PMID: 18510892] Seña AC et al. Novel *Treponema pallidum* serologic tests: a paradigm shift in syphilis screening for the 21st century. Clin Infect Dis 2010;51:700. [PMID: 20687840]

Triglycerides		
Triglycerides, serum or plasma (TG) <165 mg/dL [<1.65 g/L] SST, green, PPT $ Fasting specimen required.	Dietary fat is hydrolyzed in the small intestine, absorbed and resynthesized by mucosal cells, and secreted into lacteals as chylomicrons. Triglycerides in the chylomicrons are cleared from the blood by tissue lipoprotein lipase. Endogenous triglyceride production occurs in the liver. These triglycerides are transported in association with β-lipoproteins in very-low-density lipoproteins (VLDL).	**Increased in:** Hypothyroidism, diabetes mellitus, nephrotic syndrome, chronic alcoholism (fatty liver), biliary tract obstruction, stress, familial lipoprotein lipase deficiency, familial dysbetalipoproteinemia, familial combined hyperlipidemia, obesity, the metabolic syndrome, viral hepatitis, cirrhosis, pancreatitis, chronic renal failure, gout, pregnancy, glycogen storage diseases types I, III, and VI, anorexia nervosa, dietary excess. Drugs: β-blockers, cholestyramine, corticosteroids, diazepam, diuretics, estrogens, oral contraceptives. **Decreased in:** Tangier disease (α-lipoprotein deficiency), hypo- and abetalipoproteinemia, malnutrition, malabsorption, parenchymal liver disease, hyperthyroidism, intestinal lymphangiectasia. Drugs: ascorbic acid, clofibrate, nicotinic acid, gemfibrozil.	If serum is clear, the serum triglyceride level is generally <350 mg/dL. Elevated triglycerides are now considered an independent risk factor for coronary artery disease and a major risk factor for acute pancreatitis, particularly when serum triglyceride levels are >1000 mg/dL. However, screening is not currently recommended. Triglycerides >1000 mg/dL can be seen when a primary lipid disorder is exacerbated by alcohol or fat intake or by corticosteroid or estrogen therapy. Jialal I et al. Management of hypertriglyceridemia in the diabetic patient. Curr Diab Rep 2010;10:316. [PMID: 20532703] Kistali P et al. Triglyceride level affecting shared susceptibility genes in metabolic syndrome and coronary artery disease. Curr Med Chem 2010;17:3533. [PMID: 20738247] Sarwar N et al. Triglycerides and coronary heart disease: have recent insights yielded conclusive answers? Curr Opin Lipidol 2009;20:275. [PMID: 19512922]

Test/Range/Collection	Physiologic Basis	Interpretation	Comments
Triiodothyronine, total, serum or plasma (T3) 95–190 ng/dL [1.5–2.9 nmol/L] SST, PPT, green $$	T3 is the primary active thyroid hormone. Approximately 80% of T3 is produced by extrathyroidal deiodination of T4 and the rest by thyroid gland. Total T3 is influenced by levels of thyroxine binding proteins.	**Increased in:** Hyperthyroidism (some), increased thyroid-binding globulin. **Decreased in:** Hypothyroidism, nonthyroidal illness, decreased thyroid-binding globulin. Drugs: amiodarone.	T3 may be increased in approximately 5% of hyperthyroid patients in whom free T4 is normal (T3 toxicosis). Therefore, test is indicated when hyperthyroidism is suspected and free T4 value is normal. Test is of no value in the diagnosis and treatment of primary hypothyroidism. Jones DD et al. Subclinical thyroid disease. Am J Med 2010;123:502. [PMID: 20569751] Kharlip J et al. Recent development in hyperthyroidism. Lancet 2009;373:1930. [PMID: 19501730] Padmanabhan H. Amiodarone and thyroid dysfunction. South Med J 2010;103:922. [PMID: 20689491]

Triiodothyronine

Troponin-I, cardiac

| Troponin-I, cardiac, plasma (cTnI) <0.05 ng/mL (method-dependent) PPT $$ | Troponin is the contractile regulatory protein of striated muscle. It contains three subunits: T, C, and I. Subunit I consists of three forms, which are found in slow-twitch skeletal muscle, fast-twitch skeletal muscle, and cardiac muscle, respectively. Troponin I is predominantly a structural protein and is released into the circulation after cellular necrosis. Cardiac troponin I is expressed only in cardiac muscle, and thus its presence in serum can distinguish between myocardial injury and skeletal muscle injury. cTnI is measured by immunometric assays using monoclonal antibodies. Between-method variation is 2- to 5-fold due to lack of calibration standard. Sensitive cTnI immunoassays with diagnostic thresholds of 0.02–0.05 ng/mL are routinely used. Although point-of-care cTnI assays are also used, they are less sensitive. | **Increased in:** Myocardial infarction (MI), cardiac trauma, cardiac surgery, myocardial damage following percutaneous transluminal coronary angioplasty, and other cardiac interventions, nonischemic dilated cardiomyopathy, acute and chronic heart failure, prolonged supraventricular tachycardia, acute dissection of the ascending aorta. Slight elevations (eg, <1.0 ng/mL) are sometimes noted in patients with recent aggravated unstable angina, muscular disorders, CNS disorders, HIV infection, chronic renal failure, cirrhosis, sepsis, lung diseases, and endocrine disorders.

Not increased in: Skeletal muscle disease (myopathy, myositis, dystrophy), external electrical cardioversion, noncardiac trauma or surgery, rhabdomyolysis, severe muscular exertion, chronic renal failure. | Cardiac troponin I is a more specific marker for MI than CK-MB and is the preferred marker for the diagnosis of MI. cTnI appears in serum approximately 4 hours after onset of chest pain, peaks at 8–12 hours, and persists for 5–7 days. This prolonged persistence gives it much greater sensitivity than CK-MB for diagnosis of MI beyond the first 36–48 hours. Given its utility in detection of acute coronary syndrome (ACS), the plasma troponin is important in the evaluation and stratification of patients with chest pain in the emergency room. Blood samples should be obtained for testing at hospital presentation and 6–9 hours later. With a clinical history suggestive of ACS, a cTnI level exceeding 0.05 ng/mL (method-dependent) on at least one occasion during the first 24 hours after the clinical event is indicative of myocardial necrosis consistent with MI.

In patients with suspected ACS, using a high-sensitivity cTnI assay (lowering the diagnostic threshold value) increases the diagnosis of MI and identifies patients at high risk of recurrent MI and death.

Mills NL et al. Implementation of a sensitive troponin I assay and risk of recurrent myocardial infarction and death in patients with suspected acute coronary syndrome. JAMA 2011;305:1210. [PMID: 21427373]

Morrow DA et al. NACB and laboratory medicine practice guidelines: clinical characteristics and utilization of biochemical markers in acute coronary syndrome. Clin Chem 2007;53:552. [PMID: 17384331] |

Test/Range/Collection	Physiologic Basis	Interpretation	Comments
Tularemia agglutinins, serum <1:80 titer SST $$	*Francisella tularensis* is an organism of wild rodents (rabbits and hares) that infects humans (eg, trappers and skinners) via contact with animal tissues, by the bite of certain ticks and flies, and by consumption of undercooked meat or contaminated water. Agglutinating antibodies appear in 10–14 days and peak in 5–10 weeks. A 4-fold rise in titers is typically needed to prove acute infection. Titers decrease over years.	**Increased in:** Tularemia; cross-reaction with brucella antigens and proteus OX-19 antigen (but at lower titers).	Single titers of >1:160 are indicative of infection. Maximum titers are >1:1280. A history of exposure to rabbits, ticks, dogs, cats, or skunks is suggestive of, but not a requirement for, the diagnosis. The most common presentation is a single area of painful lymphadenopathy with low-grade fever. Initial treatment should be empiric. Culture of the organism is difficult, requiring special media, and hazardous to laboratory personnel. Serologic tests are the mainstay of diagnosis. Ellis J et al. Tularemia. Clin Microbiol Rev 2002;15:631. [PMID: 12364373] Versalovic J et al (editors); *Manual of Clinical Microbiology.* 10th ed. ASM Press, 2011.

Tularemia agglutinins

Type and crossmatch			
Type and crossmatch (T/C), serum and red cells (type and cross) Red or lavender/pink $$ Specimen label must be signed by the person drawing the blood. A second "check" specimen is needed at some hospitals. The number of RBC units required must be specified.	A type and crossmatch involves ABO and Rh typing, antibody screen, and crossmatch. (Compare with Type and screen, below.) If the recipient's serum contains a clinically significant RBC alloantibody by antibody screen or by history, the antibody is then identified and RBC units negative for the corresponding antigen are selected. A crossmatch testing recipient serum (or plasma) against donor cells is also performed using anti-human globulin (AHG) to detect recipient antibodies to donor red cells (Coombs crossmatch). If no clinically significant antibodies are detected in current screen and there is no record of previous detection of such antibodies, only a method to detect ABO incompatibility, such as an immediate-spin or computer crossmatch, is required.	See Type and screen below.	A type and screen is adequate preparation for operative procedures unlikely to require transfusion. Unnecessary type and crossmatch orders reduce blood availability and add to labor and reagent costs. A preordering system should be in place, indicating the number of units of blood likely to be needed for each operative procedure. Genotyping is a powerful adjunct to serologic testing and in the future could enable electronic selection of units with antigen matched to recipients at multiple blood group loci and could therefore improve transfusion outcomes. Sandler SG et al. Historic milestones in the evolution of the crossmatch. Immunohematol 2009;25:147. [PMID: 20406021] *Technical Manual of the American Association of Blood Banks,* 16th ed. American Association of Blood Banks, 2008.

Test/Range/Collection	Physiologic Basis	Interpretation	Comments
Type and screen			**Type and screen**
Type and screen (T/S), serum and red cells	Type and screen includes ABO and Rh typing and antibody screen. (Compare with Type and cross-match, above.)	A negative antibody screen implies that a recipient can receive uncrossmatched type-specific blood with minimal risk.	Type and screen is indicated for patients undergoing operative procedures unlikely to require transfusion. However, in the absence of preoperative indications, routine preoperative blood type and screen testing
Red or lavender/pink	This is a procedure in which the patients blood sample is tested for ABO, Rh(D), and unexpected	If the recipient's serum contains a clinically significant alloantibody by antibody screen, a crossmatch	is not cost-effective and may be eliminated for some procedures, such as laparoscopic cholecystectomy, expected vaginal delivery, and vaginal hysterectomy.
$$	antibodies, then stored in the transfusion service for future crossmatch if a unit is needed for	is required if transfusion is needed.	*Technical Manual of the American Association of Blood Banks,* 16th ed. American Association of Blood Banks, 2008.
Specimen label must be signed by the person drawing the blood.	transfusion.		
A second "check" specimen is needed at some hospitals.			

Uric acid		
Uric acid, serum or plasma Males: 2.4–7.4 mg/dL [Males: 140–440 mcmol/L] Females 1.4–5.8 mg/dL [Females: 80–350 mcmol/L] SST, PPT, green $	Uric acid is an end product of nucleoprotein metabolism and is excreted by the kidney. An increase in serum uric acid concentration occurs with increased nucleoprotein synthesis or catabolism (blood dyscrasias, therapy of leukemia) or decreased renal uric acid excretion (eg, thiazide diuretic therapy or renal failure).	**Increased in:** Renal failure, gout, myeloproliferative disorders (leukemia, lymphoma, myeloma, polycythemia vera), psoriasis, glycogen storage disease (type I), Lesch-Nyhan syndrome (X-linked hypoxanthine-guanine phosphoribosyltransferase deficiency), lead nephropathy, hypertensive diseases of pregnancy (preeclampsia and eclampsia), menopause, syndrome X (obesity, insulin resistance, hypertension, hyperuricemia dyslipidemia). Drugs: antimetabolite and chemotherapeutic agents, diuretics, ethanol, nicotinic acid, salicylates (low-dose), theophylline. **Decreased in:** Syndrome of inappropriate antidiuretic hormone (SIADH), xanthine oxidase deficiency, low-purine diet, Fanconi syndrome, neoplastic disease (various, causing increased renal excretion), liver disease. Drugs: salicylates (high-dose), allopurinol or febuxostat (xanthine oxidase inhibitors) or uricase.	Sex, age, and renal function affect uric acid levels. The incidence of hyperuricemia is greater in some ethnic groups (eg, Filipinos) than others (whites). Gout with elevated uric acid levels is an independent risk factor for heart disease. Serum uric acid is a poor predictor of maternal and fetal complications in women with preeclampsia. Dalbeth N et al. Hyperuricaemia and gout: state of the art and future perspectives. Ann Rheum Dis 2010;69:1738. [PMID: 20858623] Jinnah HA et al. Attenuated variants of Lesch-Nyhan disease. Brain 2010;133:671. [PMID: 20176575] Schlesinger N, et al. Serum urate during acute gout. J Rheumatol 2009;36:1287. [PMID: 19369457]

Test/Range/Collection	Physiologic Basis	Interpretation	Comments
	Vanillylmandelic acid		
Vanillylmandelic acid, urine (VMA) 2–7 mg/24 hr [10–35 mcmol/d] Urine bottle containing hydrochloric acid $$ Collect 24-hour urine.	Catecholamines secreted in excess by pheochromocytomas are metabolized by the enzymes monoamine oxidase and catechol-*O*-methyltransferase to VMA, which is excreted in urine.	**Increased in:** Pheochromocytoma (64% sensitivity, 95% specificity), neuroblastoma, ganglioneuroma, generalized anxiety. **Decreased in:** Drugs: monoamine oxidase inhibitors.	Because of its low sensitivity, test is no longer recommended for the diagnosis of pheochromocytoma. A urine or plasma free metanephrine level is the recommended test. (See also Figure 9–20.) The ratio of urinary VMA to urinary creatinine (VMA/Cr) is of diagnostic and prognostic significance in neuroblastoma. Aydin GB et al. The prognostic significance of vanillylmandellic acid in neuroblastoma. Pediatr Hematol Oncol 2010;27:435. [PMID: 20578806] Barron J. Pheochromocytoma: diagnostic challenges for biochemical screening and diagnosis. J Clin Pathol 2010;63:669. [PMID: 20547690] Maris JM. Recent advances in neuroblastoma. N Engl J Med 2010;362:2202. [PMID: 20558371]
	VDRL test, serum		
Venereal Disease Research Laboratory test, serum (VDRL) Nonreactive SST $	This syphilis test measures nontreponemal antibodies that are produced when *Treponema pallidum* interacts with host tissues. The VDRL usually becomes reactive at a titer of >1:32 within 1–3 weeks after the genital chancre appears.	**Increased in:** Syphilis: primary (59–87%), secondary (100%), late latent (79–91%), tertiary (37–94%), collagen vascular diseases (rheumatoid arthritis, SLE), infections (mononucleosis, leprosy, malaria), pregnancy, drug abuse.	VDRL has historically been used as a syphilis screening test and in suspected cases of primary and secondary syphilis. Positive tests should be confirmed with specific treponemal tests (FTA-ABS or TP-PA). The VDRL has sensitivity and specificity similar to the rapid plasma reagin (RPR) (See Table 8–24.). New syphilis testing algorithm using treponemal tests for screening and nontreponemal serologic tests for confirmation has been proposed. Karp G et al. Syphilis and HIV co-infection. Eur J Intern Med 2009;20:9. [PMID: 19237085] Seña AC et al. Novel *Treponema pallidum* serologic tests: a paradigm shift in syphilis screening for the 21st century. Clin Infect Dis 2010;51:700. [PMID: 20687840]

VDRL test, CSF		
Venereal Disease Research Laboratory test, CSF (VDRL) Nonreactive $$ Deliver in a clean plastic or glass tube.	The CSF VDRL test measures nontreponemal antibodies that develop in the CSF when *Treponema pallidum* interacts with the central nervous system.	**Increased in:** Tertiary neurosyphilis (10–27%).	The quantitative CSF VDRL is the test of choice for CNS syphilis. Because the sensitivity of CSF VDRL is very low, a negative test does not rule out neurosyphilis. Clinical features, CSF white cell count, and CSF protein should be used together to make the diagnosis (see CSF profiles, Table 8–8). Because the specificity of the CSF VDRL test is high, a positive test confirms the presence of neurosyphilis. Patients being screened for neurosyphilis with CSF VDRL testing should have a positive serum RPR, VDRL, FTA-ABS, TP-PA test, or other evidence of infection. Repeat testing may be indicated in HIV-infected patients in whom neurosyphilis is suspected. Ghanem KG. Neurosyphilis: a historical perspective and review. CNS Neurosci Ther 2010;16:e157. [PMID: 20626434] Sefia AC et al. Novel *Treponema pallidum* serologic tests: a paradigm shift in syphilis screening for the 21st century. Clin Infect Dis 2010;51:700. [PMID: 20687840]

Test/Range/Collection	Physiologic Basis	Interpretation	Comments
Vitamin B$_{12}$, serum or plasma 170–820 pg/mL [121–600 pmol/L] SST, red, green $$ Serum vitamin B$_{12}$ specimens should be frozen if not analyzed immediately.	Vitamin B$_{12}$ is a necessary cofactor for three important biochemical processes: conversion of methylmalonyl-CoA to succinyl-CoA and methylation of homocysteine to methionine and demethylation of methyltetrahydrofolate to tetrahydrofolate (THF). All vitamin B$_{12}$ comes from ingestion of foods of animal origin. Vitamin B$_{12}$ in serum is protein bound; 70% to transcobalamin I (TC I) and 30% to transcobalamin II (TC II). The B$_{12}$ bound to TC II is physiologically active; that bound to TC I is not.	**Increased in:** Leukemia (acute myelocytic, chronic myelocytic, chronic lymphocytic, monocytic, marked leukocytosis, polycythemia vera. (Increased B$_{12}$ levels are not diagnostically useful.) **Decreased in:** Pernicious anemia, gastrectomy, gastric carcinoma, malabsorption (sprue, celiac disease, steatorrhea, regional enteritis, fistulas, bowel resection, ileal disease, *Diphyllobothrium latum* [fish tapeworm] infestation, small bowel bacterial overgrowth), pregnancy, dietary deficiency, HIV infection (with or without malabsorption), chronic high-flux hemodialysis, Alzheimer disease, drugs (eg, omeprazole, metformin, carbamazepine).	The previously used Schilling test is no longer used for evaluating pernicious anemia. New testing algorithms have been developed using B$_{12}$, methylmalonic acid (MMA), intrinsic factor antibodies, parietal cell autoantibodies, and serum gastrin measurements. Different methods (chemiluminescence immunoassay, radioimmunoassay, etc) are available for B$_{12}$ measurement. Test results are very variable. In general, serum B$_{12}$ <170 pg/mL is consistent with deficiency, 170–300 pg/mL is borderline insufficiency, and >300 pg/mL is adequate. Low serum B$_{12}$ levels warrant treatment; intermediate levels should be followed by repeated serum tests or by urine methylmalonic acid tests (see Methylmalonic acid, p. 213) as well as by serum homocysteine levels. Neurologic disorders caused by low serum B$_{12}$ level can occur in the absence of macrocytic anemia or pancytopenia. Den Elzen WP et al. Subnormal vitamin B$_{12}$ concentrations and anemia in older people: a systematic review. BMC Geriatr 2010;10:42. [PMID: 20573208] Lahner E et al. Pernicious anemia: new insights from a gastroenterologic point of view. World J Gastroenterol 2009;15:5121. [PMID: 19891010]

Vitamin D, 25-hydroxy		
Vitamin D, 25-hydroxy, serum or plasma (25[OH]D) 20–50 ng/mL [50–125 nmol/L] SST or green $$$	The vitamin D system functions to maintain serum calcium levels. Vitamin D is a fat-soluble steroid hormone. Two molecular forms exist: D_3 (cholecalciferol), synthesized in the epidermis, and D_2 (ergocalciferol), derived from plant sources. To become active, both need to be further metabolized. Two sequential hydroxylations occur: in the liver to 25(OH)D and then, in the kidney, to 1,25[OH]$_2$D. Besides consequences for bone health, vitamin D deficiency reportedly is associated with a number of conditions such as cardiovascular disease, autoimmunity and cancer; however, evidence-based cause-and-effect relationships have not been established.	**Increased in:** Heavy milk drinkers (up to 64 ng/mL), vitamin D intoxication, sun exposure. **Decreased in:** Dietary deficiency, malabsorption, rickets, osteomalacia, biliary and portal cirrhosis, nephrotic syndrome, renal failure, inadequate sun exposure, advanced age (>70), primary hyperparathyroidism. Drugs: phenytoin, phenobarbital.	Serum or plasma total 25(OH)D is an integrated marker of vitamin D status, incorporating endogenous synthesis from solar exposure, dietary intake, fortified products and/or supplements. There is no universal or strong evidence-based consensus on the appropriate level of 25(OH)D level. However, according to a 2011 US Institute of Medicine Report, a 25(OH)D level of 20–30 ng/mL is all that is needed for bone and general health, and nearly everyone (97.5%) in the general population is in that range. A 25(OH)D level above 30 ng/mL has not been consistently associated with increased health benefits, and, in fact, risks have been identified for outcomes at levels above 50 ng/mL. Routine screening for vitamin D deficiency is not necessary. Patients with the following conditions should be considered for testing: osteoporosis, osteomalacia, malabsorption, liver disease, pancreatic insufficiency, chronic kidney disease, COPD, bariatric surgery, cancer, bedridden or home-bound, obesity, taking anticonvulsants or long-term glucocorticoids, atraumatic fractures, elderly (>70 years old), and chronic inflammatory conditions.

Vitamin D, 25-hydroxy (*continued*)

Test/Range/Collection	Physiologic Basis	Interpretation	Comments
			Vitamin D toxicity can occur after taking excessive doses of vitamin D, a condition that is manifested by hypercalcemia, hyperphosphatemia, soft tissue calcification, and renal failure. Holick MF et al. Evaluation, treatment, and prevention of vitamin D deficiency: an Endocrine Society Clinical Practice Guideline. J Clin Endocrinol Metab. 2011;96:1911. [PMID: 21646368] Kennel KA et al. Vitamin D deficiency in adults: when to test and how to treat. Mayo Clin Proc. 2010;85:752. [PMID: 20675513] Ross AC et al. The 2011 report on dietary reference intakes for calcium and vitamin D from the Institute of Medicine: what clinicians need to know. J Clin Endocrinol Metab. 2011;96:53. [PMID: 21118827] Souberbielle JC et al. Vitamin D and musculoskeletal health, cardiovascular disease, autoimmunity and cancer: recommendations for clinical practice. Autoimmun Rev. 2010;9:709. [PMID: 20601202]

Vitamin D, 1,25-dihydroxy

Vitamin D, 1,25-dihydroxy, serum or plasma (1,25(OH)$_2$D) 20–76 pg/mL SST or green $$$$	1,25-Dihydroxy vitamin D is the most active form of vitamin D, and is the primary regulator of calcium and phosphorus homeostasis. The main actions of vitamin D are the acceleration of calcium and phosphate absorption in the intestine and stimulation of bone resorption.	**Increased in:** Primary hyper-parathyroidism, idiopathic hypercalciuria, sarcoidosis, some lymphomas, 1,25(OH)$_2$D-resistant rickets, normal growth (children), pregnancy, lactation, vitamin D toxicity. **Decreased in:** Chronic renal failure, anephric patients, hypoparathyroidism, pseudohy-poparathyroidism, 1-α-hydroxy-lase deficiency, postmenopausal osteoporosis.

Test is rarely needed.

Measurement of 1,25(OH)$_2$D is only useful in distinguishing 1-α-hydroxylase deficiency from 1,25(OH)$_2$D-resistant rickets or in monitoring vitamin D status of patients with chronic renal failure.

Test is not useful for assessment of vitamin D intoxication because of efficient feedback regulation of 1,25(OH)$_2$D synthesis.

Parathyroid tissue expresses the vitamin D receptor, and it is thought that circulating 1,25(OH)$_2$D participates in the regulation of parathyroid cell proliferation, differentiation, and secretion. Primary hyperparathyroidism is usually associated with increased plasma 1,25(OH)$_2$D.

Alizadeh Naderi AS et al. Hereditary disorders of renal phosphate wasting. Nat Rev Nephrol 2010;6:657. [PMID: 20924400]

Kalantar-Zadeh K et al. Kidney bone disease and mortality in CKD: revisiting the role of vitamin D, calcimimetics, alkaline phosphatase, and minerals. Kidney Int Suppl 2010;117:S10. [PMID: 20671739]

	von Willebrand factor	
Test/Range/Collection	**Physiologic Basis**	**Interpretation**	**Comments**

Test/Range/Collection	Physiologic Basis	Interpretation	Comments
von Willebrand factor (vWF), plasma Blue Antigen (vWFAg by enzyme-linked immuno-sorbent assay [ELISA]) Activity (ristocetin cofactor) 50–180% $$$	vWF is an endothelium-derived multimeric plasma protein with two important functions in hemostasis: (1) promoting platelet adhesion at the site of injury; and (2) transporting and stabilizing factor VIII in plasma. von Willebrand disease (vWD) is caused by hereditary quantitative (types 1 and 3) or qualitative (types 2A, 2B, 2M, 2N) defects of the vWF. Acquired vWD can occur but is rare.	**Increased in:** Inflammatory states (acute-phase reactant). **Decreased in:** Hereditary or acquired vWD: type 1, decreased antigen and activity levels; type 3, undetectable antigen and activity; type 2, antigen level may be normal, but activity is impaired (normal activity in 2B).	In vWD, the platelet count and morphology are generally normal, and the bleeding time is usually prolonged (markedly prolonged by aspirin). The PTT may not be prolonged if factor VIII coagulant level is >30%. Diagnosis of vWD is suggested by bleeding symptoms and family history. Initial tests for vWD (bleeding time or PFA-100 CT, platelet count, PTT) are typically followed by the diagnostic tests: vWF antigen and activity. Further tests may be necessary to distinguish the subtypes of vWD, such as vWF multimer analysis, factor VIII assay, vWF propeptide to vWF antigen ratio, platelet aggregation studies, etc (low-dose ristocetin). Castaman G et al. von Willebrand's disease diagnosis and laboratory issues. Haemophilia 2010;16(Suppl):67. [PMID: 20590859] Torres R et al. Laboratory testing for von Willebrand disease: toward a mechanism-based classification. Clin Lab Med 2009;29:193. [PMID: 19665675]

White blood cell count and differential			
White blood cell (WBC) count and differential, blood Reference ranges are age- and laboratory-specific Adult ranges: WBC 4.5–11.0 × 10³/mcL; differential: segmented neutrophils 50–70%; band neutrophils 0–5%; lymphocytes 20–40%; monocytes 2–6%; eosinophils 1–4%; basophils 0–1%. **Panic:** WBC <1.5 × 10³/mcL and/or ANC <0.5 × 10³/mcL Lavender $	The WBC count and differential determine the total number of white blood cells as well as the percentage and absolute number of each type of white cell in a blood sample. It is typically generated by an automated laboratory hematology analyzer as part of the CBC panel. The basic principles used for WBC count and differential are instrument-dependent (eg, Beckman Coulter, Siemens, Abbott, Sysmex). If indicated, manual differential is also performed by examining a blood smear under a microscope.	**Increased in:** Acute infections, inflammatory disorders, acute and chronic leukemias, myeloproliferative disorders, solid tumor (paraneoplastic reaction), circulating lymphoma, tissue injury/necrosis, G-CSF stimulation, various drugs, corticosteroids, allergies, hypersensitivity reactions, stress, smoking. **Decreased in:** Infections, constitutional and acquired myeloid hypoplasia, myelosuppression (eg, chemotherapy, radiation, various drugs), myelodysplasia, collagen vascular diseases, hypersplenism, cyclic neutropenia, autoimmune neutropenia, alcoholism.	There are five types of white cells, each with different functions: neutrophils, lymphocytes, monocytes, eosinophils, and basophils. Absolute counts for individual cell populations can be calculated from a combination of the WBC count and the percentage of each cell type from the differential. It is important to perform a manual differential in certain conditions such as presence of blasts, immature granulocytes, nucleated red blood cells, leukemia or lymphoma cells, plasma cells, or myelodysplasia. Briggs C. Quality counts: new parameters in blood cell counting. Int J Lab Hematol 2009;31:277. [PMID: 19452619] Granger JM et al. Etiology and outcome of extreme leukocytosis in 758 nonhematologic cancer patients: a retrospective, single-institution study. Cancer 2009;115:3919. [PMID: 19551882] Milcic TL. The complete blood count. Neonatal New 2010;29:109. [PMID: 20211833]

4

Therapeutic Drug Monitoring and Pharmacogenetic Testing: Principles and Test Interpretation

Diana Nicoll, MD, PhD, MPA, and Chuanyi Mark Lu, MD

UNDERLYING ASSUMPTIONS

The basic assumptions underlying therapeutic drug monitoring (Table 4–1) are that drug metabolism varies from patient to patient and that the plasma level of a drug is more closely related to the drug's therapeutic effect or toxicity than is the dosage.

The basic principle underlying pharmacogenetics testing (Table 4–2) is that the identification of genetic factors that influence drug absorption, metabolism, or action at the target level may allow for individualized therapy and thereby help optimize drug efficacy and minimize drug toxicity.

INDICATIONS FOR DRUG MONITORING

Drugs with **a narrow therapeutic index** (where therapeutic drug levels do not differ greatly from levels associated with serious toxicity) should be monitored. *Example:* Lithium.

Patients who have **impaired clearance of a drug with a narrow therapeutic index** are candidates for drug monitoring. The clearance mechanism of the drug involved must be known. *Example:* Patients with renal failure have decreased clearance of gentamicin and therefore are at a higher risk for gentamicin toxicity.

Drugs whose **toxicity is difficult to distinguish from a patient's underlying disease** may require monitoring. *Example:* Theophylline in patients with chronic obstructive pulmonary disease.

Drugs whose efficacy is **difficult to establish clinically** may require monitoring of plasma levels. *Example:* Phenytoin.

SITUATIONS IN WHICH DRUG MONITORING MAY NOT BE USEFUL

Drugs that can be given in extremely high doses before toxicity is apparent are not candidates for monitoring. *Example:* Penicillin.

If better means of assessing drug effects are available, drug level monitoring may not be appropriate. *Example:* Warfarin is typically monitored by prothrombin time and International Normalized Ratio (INR) determinations, not by serum levels.

Drug level monitoring to assess compliance is limited by the inability to distinguish noncompliance from rapid metabolism without direct inpatient scrutiny of drug administration.

Drug toxicity cannot be diagnosed with drug levels alone; it is a clinical diagnosis. Drug levels within the usual therapeutic range do not rule out drug toxicity in a given patient. *Example:* Digoxin, where other physiologic variables (eg, hypokalemia) affect drug toxicity.

In summary, therapeutic drug monitoring may be useful to guide dosage adjustment of certain drugs in certain patients. Patient compliance is essential if drug monitoring data are to be correctly interpreted.

OTHER INFORMATION REQUIRED FOR EFFECTIVE DRUG MONITORING

Reliability of the Analytic Method

The analytic **sensitivity** of the drug monitoring method must be adequate. For some drugs, plasma levels are in the nanogram per milliliter range. *Example:* Tricyclic antidepressants, digoxin.

The **specificity** of the method must be known, because the drug's metabolites or other drugs may interfere. Interference by metabolites, which may or may not be pharmacologically active, is of particular concern in immunologic assay methods using antibodies to the parent drug.

The **precision** of the method must be known to assess whether changes in levels are caused by method imprecision or by clinical changes.

Reliability of the Therapeutic Range

Establishing the therapeutic range for a drug requires a reliable clinical assessment of its therapeutic and toxic effects, together with plasma drug level measurements by a particular analytic method. In practice, as newer, more specific analytic methods are introduced, the therapeutic ranges for those methods are estimated by comparing the old and new methodologies—without clinical correlation.

PHARMACOKINETIC PARAMETERS

Five pharmacokinetic parameters that are important in therapeutic drug monitoring include:

1. *Bioavailability.* The bioavailability of a drug depends in part on its formulation. A drug that is significantly metabolized as it first passes through the liver exhibits a marked "first-pass effect," reducing the effective oral absorption of the drug. A reduction in this first-pass effect (eg, because of decreased hepatic blood flow in heart failure) could cause a clinically significant increase in effective oral drug absorption.

2. *Volume of distribution and distribution phases.* The volume of distribution of a drug determines the plasma concentration reached after a loading dose. The distribution phase is the time taken for a drug to distribute from the plasma to the periphery. Drug levels drawn before completion of a long distribution phase may not reflect levels of pharmacologically active drug at sites of action. *Examples:* Digoxin, lithium.

3. *Clearance.* Clearance is either renal or nonrenal (usually hepatic). Whereas changes in renal clearance can be predicted on the basis of serum creatinine or creatinine clearance, there is no routine liver function test for assessment of hepatic drug metabolism. For most therapeutic drugs measured, clearance is independent of plasma drug concentration, so that a change in dose is reflected in a similar change in plasma level. If, however, clearance is dose dependent, dosage adjustments produce disproportionately large changes in plasma levels and must be made cautiously. *Example:* Phenytoin.

4. *Half-life.* The half-life of a drug depends on its volume of distribution and its clearance and determines the time taken to reach a steady state level. In three or four half-lives, the drug level will be 87.5–93.75% of the way to steady state. Patients with decreased drug clearance and therefore increased drug half-lives will take longer to reach a higher steady-state level. In general, because non–steady-state drug levels are potentially misleading and can be difficult to interpret, it is recommended that most clinical monitoring be done at steady state.

5. *Protein binding of drugs.* All routine drug level analysis involves assessment of both protein-bound and free drug. However, pharmacologic activity depends on only the free drug level. Changes in protein binding (eg, in uremia or hypoalbuminemia) may significantly affect interpretation of reported levels for drugs that are highly protein-bound. *Example:* Phenytoin.

In cases in which the ratio of free to total measured drug level is increased, the usual therapeutic range based on total drug level does not apply.

Drug Interactions

For patients receiving several medications, the possibility of drug interactions affecting drug elimination must be considered. *Example:* Quinidine, verapamil, and amiodarone decrease digoxin clearance.

Time to Draw Levels

In general, the specimen should be drawn after steady state is reached (at least three or four half-lives after a dosage adjustment) and just before the next dose (trough level).

Peak and trough levels may be indicated to evaluate the dosage of drugs whose half-lives are much shorter than the dosing interval. *Example:* Gentamicin.

GENETIC INFLUENCES ON THERAPEUTIC DRUG RESPONSE

Genetic influences on drug response can be divided into four categories:

1. *Altered pharmacokinetics, ie, drug absorption, distribution, tissue localization, biotransformation, and excretion.* Examples include genetic polymorphisms in cytochrome P450 oxidase (CYP), thiopurine s-methyltransferase (TPMT) enzyme, and uridine diphosphate glucuronosyltransferase (UGT) enzyme.

2. *Altered pharmacodynamics, ie, the effect of a drug at its therapeutic target and at other non-target sites.* Genetic variations can modulate drug response by affecting the drug target itself or one of the downstream components in the target's mechanistic pathway. An example is the effect of polymorphisms in the gene encoding the vitamin K epoxide reductase complex (VKORC1) on response to the oral anticoagulant, warfarin.

3. *Effect on idiosyncratic drug reactions.* An idiosyncratic reaction is an adverse drug reaction (ADR) that cannot be anticipated based on the known drug target. An example is the association of HLA-B*5701 with a hypersensitivity reaction to the antiretroviral nucleoside analog, abacavir.

4. *Effect on disease pathogenesis, ie, certain genetic variations can influence a disease pathogenesis by altering the disease severity or the response to specific therapy.* For example, vemurafenib, an inhibitor of kinase B-Raf, significantly improves survival in patients with unresectable or metastatic melanoma with the V600E mutation in the *BRAF* gene.

CLINICAL USE OF PHARMACOGENETIC TESTING

Pharmacogenetic testing may help in the selection of certain drugs and their dosages. However, integration of pharmacogenetic testing into clinical care has been generally slow and prospective randomized trials have not yet demonstrated improved clinical outcomes in cases in which drug therapy and specific dosage have been selected based on genotyping results.

Table 4–2 lists drugs for which genetic testing has been suggested.

TABLE 4-1. THERAPEUTIC DRUG MONITORING. [1]

Drug	Effective Concentrations	Half-Life (hours)	Dosage Adjustments	Comments
Amikacin	**Conventional dosing:** Peak: 20–30 mg/L; trough: <10 mg/L **High dose once daily:** Peak: 60 mg/L; trough: undetectable	2–3; ↑ in uremia	↓ in renal dysfunction	Concomitant kanamycin or tobramycin therapy may give falsely elevated amikacin results by immunoassay.
Amitriptyline	95–250 ng/mL	9–25		Drug is highly protein-bound. Patient-specific decrease in protein binding may invalidate quoted therapeutic reference interval for effective concentration.
Carbamazepine	4–12 mg/L	10–15		Induces its own metabolism. Metabolite 10,11-epoxide exhibits 13% cross-reactivity by immunoassay. *Adverse reactions:* skin reactions, myelosuppression.
Cyclosporine	100–300 mcg/L (ng/mL) whole blood	6–12	↓ in renal dysfunction, liver disease	Cyclosporine is lipid-soluble (20% bound to leukocytes; 40% to erythrocytes; 40% in plasma, highly bound to lipoproteins); the binding is temperature-dependent in vitro and concentration-dependent *in vivo.* HPLC and LC-tandem mass spectrometry methods are highly specific for parent drug and considered the gold standard assays. Monoclonal fluorescence polarization immunoassay (FPIA) and monoclonal chemiluminescence immunoassay also measure cyclosporine reliably; polyclonal immunoassays are less specific owing to cross-reaction with drug metabolites. Anticonvulsants and rifampin increase metabolism. Erythromycin, ketoconazole, and calcium channel blockers decrease metabolism. The main adverse reaction is concentration-related nephrotoxicity.

Desipramine	100–250 ng/mL	13–23		Drug is highly protein-bound. Patient-specific decrease in protein binding may invalidate quoted therapeutic reference interval for effective concentration.
Digoxin	CHF: 0.5–0.9 ng/mL Atrial fibrillation: 0.5–2 ng/mL	42; ↑ in uremia, CHF	↓ in renal dysfunction, CHF, hypothyroidism; ↑ in hyperthyroidism	Bioavailability of digoxin tablets is 50–90%. Specimen must not be drawn within 4 hours of an intravenous dose or 6 hours of an oral dose. Dialysis does not remove a significant amount. Hypokalemia potentiates toxicity. Digitalis toxicity is a clinical and *not* a laboratory diagnosis. Digibind (digoxin-specific antibody) therapy of digoxin overdose can interfere with measurement of digoxin levels depending on the digoxin assay. Elimination reduced by amiodarone, quinidine, and verapamil.
Ethosuximide	40–100 mg/L	Child: 30 Adult: 50		Levels used primarily to assess clinical response and compliance. Toxicity is rare and does not correlate well with plasma concentrations.
Gentamicin	**Conventional dosing:** Peak: 4–8 mg/L; trough: <2 mg/L **High dose once daily:** Peak: 20 mg/L: trough: undetectable	2–3; ↑ in uremia (7.3 during dialysis)	↓ in renal dysfunction	Draw peak specimen (conventional dosing) 30 minutes after end of 30- to 60-min infusion. Draw trough just before next dose. In uremic patients, some penicillins (eg, carbenicillin, ticarcillin, piperacillin) may decrease gentamicin half-life from 46 hours to 22 hours, posing a risk of reduced antibacterial efficacy. The main adverse reactions are CNS, otic, and renal toxicities.
Imipramine	180–350 ng/mL	10–16		Drug is highly protein-bound. Patient-specific decrease in protein binding may invalidate quoted therapeutic reference interval for effective concentration.
Lidocaine	1–5 mg/L	1.8; unchanged in uremia, CHF; ↑ in cirrhosis	↓ in CHF, liver disease	Levels increased with cimetidine therapy. CNS toxicity common in the elderly.

(continued)

TABLE 4–1. THERAPEUTIC DRUG MONITORING.[1] *(CONTINUED)*

Drug	Effective Concentrations	Half-Life (hours)	Dosage Adjustments	Comments
Lithium	0.5–1.5 mmol/L	22; ↑ in uremia	↓ in renal dysfunction	Thiazides and loop diuretics may increase serum lithium levels.
Methotrexate		3–10 low dose; 8–15 high dose; ↑ in uremia	↓ in renal dysfunction	Therapeutic concentrations depend on the treatment protocol (low versus high dose) and time of specimen collection. 7-Hydroxymethotrexate cross-reacts 1.5% in immunoassay. To minimize toxicity, leucovorin or glucarpidase should be continued if methotrexate level is >0.1 mcmol/L at 48 hours after start of therapy. Methotrexate >1 mcmol/L at >48 hours requires an increase in rescue therapy.
Nortriptyline	50–140 ng/mL	18–44		Drug is highly protein-bound. Patient-specific decrease in protein binding may invalidate quoted therapeutic reference interval for effective concentration.
Phenobarbital	10–40 mg/L	Child: 37–73 Adult: 53–140 ↑ in cirrhosis	↓ in liver disease	Metabolized primarily by the hepatic microsomal enzyme system. Many drug-drug interactions.
Phenytoin	10–20 mg/L; 5–10 mg/L in uremia and severe hypoalbuminemia	Dose/concentration-dependent		Drug metabolite cross-reacts in immunoassays; the cross-reactivity may be of significance only in the presence of advanced chronic kidney disease. Metabolism is capacity-limited. Increase dose cautiously when level approaches therapeutic reference interval, since new steady-state level may be disproportionately higher. Drug is very highly protein-bound; protein binding is decreased in uremia and hypoalbuminemia. Free drug level (pharmacologically active fraction) may be indicated in certain clinical circumstances.

Drug	Therapeutic range	Half-life (h)	Factors affecting	Comments
Sirolimus	Trough: 4–12 ng/mL when used in combination with cyclosporine A; 12–20 ng/mL if used alone	62	↓ in liver dysfunction and with drugs inhibiting CYP3A4 activity	Sirolimus is an immunosuppressant used in combination with cyclosporine and corticosteroids for prophylaxis of organ rejection after kidney transplantation. It has also been used in liver and heart transplantation. When used in combination with cyclosporine, careful monitoring of kidney function is required. Once the initial dose titration is complete, monitoring sirolimus trough concentrations weekly for the first month and every 2 weeks for the second month appears to be appropriate. The optimal time for specimen collection is 24 hours after the previous dose or 0.5 to 1 hour before the next dose (trough level).
Tacrolimus	Trough: 8–12 ng/mL	8.7–11.3	↓ in liver dysfunction and with drugs inhibiting CYP3A4 activity	Tacrolimus is used for prophylaxis of organ rejection in adult patients undergoing liver or kidney transplantation and in pediatric patients undergoing liver transplantation. It has also been used to prevent rejection in heart, small bowel, and allogeneic bone marrow transplant patients and to treat autoimmune diseases. Antacid or sucralfate administration should be separated from tacrolimus by at least 2 hours. The optimal time for specimen collection is 12 hours after the previous dose or 0.5 to 1 hour before the next dose (trough level).
Theophylline	5–15 mg/L	9	↓ in CHF, cirrhosis, and with cimetidine	Caffeine cross-reacts 10%. Elimination is increased by 1.5–2 times in smokers. 1,3-Dimethyl uric acid metabolite increased in uremia and, because of cross-reactivity, may cause an apparent slight increase in serum theophylline.
Tobramycin	**Conventional dosing:** Peak: 5–10 mg/L; trough: <2 mg/L **High dose once daily:** Peak: 20 mg/L; trough: undetectable	2–3; ↑ in uremia	↓ in renal dysfunction	Tobramycin, kanamycin, and amikacin may cross-react in immunoassay. Some antibiotics may decrease tobramycin half-life in uremic patients, causing reduced antibacterial efficacy.

(continued)

TABLE 4–1. THERAPEUTIC DRUG MONITORING. [1] *(CONTINUED)*

Drug	Effective Concentrations	Half-Life (hours)	Dosage Adjustments	Comments
Valproic acid	50–100 mg/L	Child: 6–8 Adult: 10–12		Significant fraction of the drug is protein-bound *in vivo* (concentration-dependent). Decreased binding in uremia and cirrhosis.
Vancomycin	Trough: 10–20 mg/L	6; ↑ in uremia	↓ in renal dysfunction	Ototoxicity in uremic patients may lead to irreversible deafness. Keep peak level <40–50 mg/L to avoid severe toxicity.

[1] Serum from plain red-top tube is typically used for therapeutic drug monitoring except for cyclosporine, which requires whole blood sample in a lavender (EDTA) tube. In general, the specimen should be drawn just before the next dose (trough).
↑, increased; ↓, decreased; CYP, cytochrome P450; HPLC, high-performance liquid chromatography; CHF, congestive heart failure; CNS, central nervous system.

TABLE 4–2. SELECTED PHARMACOGENETIC TESTS: CLINICAL RELEVANCE.[1]

Pharmacogenetic Biomarker	Selected Variants (Mutant Allele, Enzyme Activity)	Allele Frequency	Drugs	Clinical Relevance
Cytochrome P450 (CYP) 2C9 variants	2C9*2 (430C>T, ↓) 2C9*3 (1075A>C, ↓↓)	2C9*2 and 2C9*3 are present in 9–20% of whites, 1–3% of blacks, and <1% of Asians	Warfarin (Coumadin)	Hepatic CYP2C9 is responsible for the metabolic inactivation and clearance of the anticoagulant warfarin. Patients carrying 2C9*2 or 2C9*3 (or both) (heterozygote, homozygote, or compound heterozygote) require reduced maintenance dose to reach a therapeutic INR. Although INR remains the standard for monitoring warfarin therapy, CYP2C9 genotyping can be an important aid to dosing strategy for warfarin-naïve patients, particularly whites.
CYP 2C19 variants	2C19*2(681G>A, none) 2C19*3(636G>A, none) 2C19*4(1A>G, none) 2C19*5(1297C>T, none)	The mutant variants are present in 12–25% of Asians, and 2–7% of whites and blacks	Clopidogrel (Plavix)	Clopidogrel, an antiplatelet drug, must be metabolized in the liver by CYP isoenzymes, principally CYP2C19, to become active. When treated with clopidogrel at recommended dosage, patients who metabolize the drug poorly exhibit higher rates of cardiovascular events than those of patients with normal CYP2C19 function. Alternative drug or intervention strategies should be considered for patients identified as poor metabolizers. CYP 2C19*17 carrier status (25% of whites) is associated with increased enzyme activity and an increased risk of bleeding.
HLA-B*1502 allele	HLA-B*1502	10–15% of Asians; 1–2% of whites	Carbamazepine (Tegretol, Epitol)	Carbamazepine is associated with serious or even fatal idiosyncratic skin reactions, eg, Stevens-Johnson syndrome and toxic epidermal necrolysis. The reactions are significantly more common in patients who carry the HLA-B*1502 allele. This allele occurs almost exclusively in patients with ancestry across broad areas of Asia, including South Asian Indians. HLA-B*1502 genotyping may be useful for risk stratification in patients of Asian descent. Patients carrying the HLA-B*1502 allele should not be given carbamazepine unless the expected benefit clearly outweighs the increased risk of serious skin reactions.

(continued)

TABLE 4-2. SELECTED PHARMACOGENETIC TESTS: CLINICAL RELEVANCE.[1] (CONTINUED)

Pharmacogenetic Biomarker	Selected Variants (Mutant Allele, Enzyme Activity)	Allele Frequency	Drugs	Clinical Relevance
HLA-B*B5701 allele	HLA-B*5701	6–8% of whites and 1–2% of blacks and East Asians	Abacavir (Ziagen)	Abacavir is a nucleoside analog reverse transcriptase inhibitor used for HIV treatment. The major treatment-limiting toxicity for abacavir use is drug hypersensitivity, occurring in 5–8% of recipients within 6 weeks of commencing therapy. There is an established association between carriage of the HLA-B*5701 allele and abacavir hypersensitivity reactions. HLA-B*5701-positive patients should not be prescribed abacavir or an abacavir-containing regimen.
Thiopurine methyltransferase (TPMT) variants	TPMT*2 (238G>C, ↓) TPMT*3A (460G>A and 719A>G, ↓↓) TPMT*3B (460G>A, ↓) TPMT*3C (719A>G, ↓)	About 10–12% of whites and blacks have reduced enzyme activity because they are heterozygous for one of the mutant alleles. About 1 in 300 whites is homozygous for a mutant allele.	Azathioprine (AZA), 6-mercaptopurine (6-MP)	AZA is a prodrug that is metabolized to 6-MP, which is then further metabolized to active 6-thioguanine (6-TG) and inactive 6-methylmercaptopurine (6-MMP) by hypoxanthine phosphoribosyltransferase and TPMT, respectively. Variation in the TPMT gene can result in functional inactivation of the enzyme and an increased risk of life-threatening 6-TG-associated myelosuppression. TPMT genotyping before instituting AZA or 6-MP can help prevent toxicity by identifying individuals with low or absent TPMT enzyme activity. Patients with homozygous or compound heterozygous mutant alleles ("poor metabolizers") should not be given AZA or 6-MP, whereas heterozygotes with a single mutant allele should be treated with lower doses.

Uridine diphospho-glucurono-syltransferase 1A1 (UGT 1A1) variants	UGT1A1*28 (7 TA repeats in promoter, ↓)	Homozygosity in 9–23% of whites, blacks, and in 1–2% of east Asians.	Irinotecan (Camptosar)	Irinotecan is used in the treatment of metastatic colorectal cancer. It is metabolized to active SN-38, a topoisomerase I inhibitor. SN-38 is further glucuronidated to inactive SN-38G by UGT1A1 and excreted. Heterozygous and homozygous UGT1A1*28 genotypes show a 25% and 70% decrease in the enzyme activity, respectively. The presence of the UGT1A1*28 allele is a risk factor for adverse drug reactions (eg, neutropenia, severe diarrhea). Testing for the allele can prevent drug toxicity at high doses of irinotecan.
Vitamin K epoxide reductase complex (VKORC1) variants	VKORC1 (−1639G>A)	The homozygous (−1639G>A) allele (−1639AA genotype) is present in approximately 15% of whites and 80% of Chinese.	Warfarin (Coumadin)	The primary therapeutic target of the anticoagulant warfarin is VKOR. Polymorphisms in the VKOR encoding gene (VKORC1) explain about 30% of the phenotypic variability in drug effect. Patients carrying the VKORC1 (−1639G>A) allele require a lower warfarin maintenance dose to reach a therapeutic INR.
BRAF gene	BRAF V600E mutation	40–60% of advanced melanomas	Vemurafenib (Zelboraf)	Activating mutations in BRAF (a serine–threonine protein kinase) are present in 40–60% of advanced melanomas, with 80–90% of the mutations being the substitution of glutamic acid for valine at amino acid 600 (V600E mutation), which is associated with a more aggressive clinical course. Vemurafenib, a potent inhibitor of the mutant BRAF, has a high level of therapeutic activity against advanced melanomas containing the V600E mutation.

[1]Testing of these genetic biomarkers before instituting drug therapy is now recommended per US Food and Drug Administration-approved drug labels. Note, however, that these tests are not yet mandated as standard practice.

↓, decreased; ↓↓, markedly decreased; >, single wild-type to variant nucleotide switch at the specific gene location; CYP, cytochrome P450 oxidase.

REFERENCES

NIH Pharmacogenetics Research Network. Pharmacogenomics Knowledge Base. http://www.pharmgkb.org

Winter ME. *Basic Clinical Pharmacokinetics,* 5th ed. Lippincott Williams & Wilkins, 2009.

5

Microbiology: Test Selection

Barbara Haller, MD, PhD

HOW TO USE THIS SECTION

This section displays information about clinically important infectious diseases in tabular form. Included in these tables are the *Organisms* involved in the disease/syndrome listed; *Specimens/Diagnostic Tests* that are useful in the evaluation; and *Comments* regarding the tests and diagnoses discussed. Topics are listed by body area/organ system: Central Nervous System, Eye, Ear, Sinus, Upper Airway, Lung, Heart and Vessels, Abdomen, Genitourinary, Bone, Joint, Muscle, Skin, and Blood.

Thereafter is a short section on emerging and re-emerging pathogens (viral and bacterial) and antibiotic resistance in bacterial pathogens.

Organisms

This column lists organisms that are known to cause the stated illness. Scientific names are abbreviated according to common usage (eg, *Streptococcus pneumoniae* as *S. pneumoniae* or pneumococcus) if appropriate. Specific age or risk groups are listed in order of increasing age or frequency (eg, Infant, Child, Adult, HIV).

When bacteria are listed, Gram stain characteristics follow the organism name in parentheses—eg, "*S. pneumoniae* (GPDC)." The following abbreviations are used:

AFB	Acid-fast bacilli	**GPC**	Gram-positive cocci
GPDC	Gram-positive diplococci	**GPCB**	Gram-positive coccobacilli
GPR	Gram-positive rods	**GVCB**	Gram-variable coccobacilli
GNC	Gram-negative cocci	**GNDC**	Gram-negative diplococci
GNCB	Gram-negative coccobacilli	**GNR**	Gram-negative rods

When known, the frequency of the specific organism's involvement in the disease process is also provided in parentheses—eg, "*S. pneumoniae* (GPDC) (50%)."

Specimen Collection/Diagnostic Tests

This column describes the collection of specimens, laboratory processing, useful radiographic procedures, and other diagnostic tests. Culture or test sensitivities with respect to the diagnosis in question are placed in parentheses immediately following the test when known—eg, "Gram stain (60%)." Pertinent serologic tests are also listed. Keep in mind that few infections can be identified by definitive diagnostic tests and that clinical judgment is critical to making difficult diagnoses when test results are equivocal.

Comments

This column includes general information about the utility of the tests and may include information about patient management. Appropriate general references are also listed.

Syndrome Name/Body Area

In the last two columns, the syndrome name and body area are placed perpendicular to the rest of the table to allow for quick referencing.

Organization

The table comprising the bulk of this chapter appears in two parts. The first table (Part I) is organized by body area and concerns common infections with established pathogens or infectious agents. The second table (Part II) concerns emerging (new) and re-emerging viral and bacterial pathogens and antibiotic resistance in bacterial pathogens.

PART I. COMMON INFECTIONS WITH ESTABLISHED PATHOGENS/INFECTIOUS AGENTS.

	CENTRAL NERVOUS SYSTEM	
	Brain abscess	
Organism	Specimen/Diagnostic Tests	Comments
Brain abscess		
Often polymicrobial (14–28% of cases)	Blood for bacterial and fungal cultures.	Occurs in patients with otitis media and
	Brain abscess aspirate for Gram stain (82%),	sinusitis; cyanotic congenital heart disease
Child: anaerobes (40%), aerobic and anaerobic viridans	bacterial (88%), AFB fungal cultures, and	and right-to-left shunting (eg, tetralogy of
streptococci (GPC in chains), S. aureus (GPC).	cytology.	Fallot) or arteriovenous vascular abnor-
S. pneumoniae (GPDC), S. pyogenes (GPC in chains);		malities of the lung (eg, Osler-Weber-
less common: Enterobacteriaceae (GNR), P. aeruginosa	Lumbar puncture is dangerous and contrain-	Rendu).
(GNR), H. influenzae (GNCB), N. meningitidis (GNDC).	dicated.	
Adults: Viridans streptococci (anaerobic streptococci,	Sources of infection in the ears, sinuses,	Mortality 8–25%.
S. milleri (70%).	lungs, or bloodstream should be sought for	Most toxoplasmosis abscesses are multiple
	culture when brain abscess is found.	and are seen on MRI in the basal ganglia,
Enterobacteriaceae (GNR) (23–33%), S. aureus (GPC) (10–	CT scan and MRI are the most valuable imag-	parietal and frontal lobes (ring-enhancing
15%), N. meningitidis, Listeria sp. anaerobes (20–40%)	ing procedures (see Chapter 6) and can guide	lesions with contrast on CT scan).
including bacteroides (GNR), prevotella (GNR), fusobac-	brain biopsy if a specimen is needed.	Stereotactic CT-guided aspiration of
terium (GNR), eubacterium (GPR), and propionibacterium	Serum toxoplasma antibody in HIV-infected	abscess material facilitates microbiologic
(GPR), and more rarely S. pneumoniae, Rhodococcus sp.,	patients may not be positive at initiation	diagnosis.
actinomyces (GPR), nocardia (GPR),	of presumptive therapy. If negative or if no	Hicks CW et al. Identifying and managing intracra-
Group B streptococci (GPC in chains), nocardia (GPR),	response to empiric therapy, biopsy may be	nial complications of sinusitis in children: a retro-
T. solium (cysticerci), Entamoeba	needed to rule out lymphoma, fungal infec-	spective series. Pediatr Infect Dis J 2011;30:222.
histolytica, Schistosoma sp. and fungi (1%).	tion, or tuberculosis. Biopsy material should	[PMID: 21416657]
	be sent for toxoplasma antigen (detected by	Prasad KN et al. Analysis of microbial etiology and
Immunocompromised: T. gondii, Cryptococcus neofor-	direct fluorescent antibody, DFA).	mortality in patients with brain abscess. J Infect
mans, nocardia (GPR), Listeria sp. (GPR), mycobacteria	Detection of toxoplasma DNA in blood or CSF	2006;53:221. [PMID: 16436297]
(AFB), Aspergillus sp., C. albicans, coccidioides,	samples by PCR techniques is now available	Shachor-Meyouhas Y et al. Brain abscess in
Zygomycetes (mucor, rhizopus), E. histolytica.	from specialized or reference laboratories.	children—epidemiology, predisposing factors
Posttraumatic: S. aureus (GPC), viridans streptococci (GPC	PCR for toxoplasma is not useful once	and management in the modern medicine era.
in chains), Enterobacteriaceae (GNR), coagulase-negative	therapy has been started. A positive PCR	Acta Paediatr 2010;99:1163. [PMID: 20222876]
staphylococci (GPC), Propionibacterium acnes (GPR).	result must be interpreted in the context of	
	the clinical presentation.	
	(See also Toxoplasma antibody, Chapter 3.)	

	CENTRAL NERVOUS SYSTEM
	Encephalitis

Organism	Specimen/Diagnostic Tests	Comments
Encephalitis Arboviruses (California encephalitis group, St. Louis encephalitis, eastern and western equine encephalitis, West Nile virus, Japanese encephalitis virus in summer and fall), enteroviruses (coxsackie, echo, polio), HSV (10–20%), *Bartonella henselae*, lymphocytic choriomeningitis virus, tick-borne encephalitis virus, measles, rubella, VZV, rabies (Central and South America, India, Africa), Nipah virus (Malaysia), Chikungunya virus (India and Nepal), Creutzfeldt-Jakob. Immunocompromised: CMV, VZV, EBV, West Nile virus, JC virus, HIV, *Toxoplasma gondii*.	CSF for pressure (elevated), cell count (WBCs elevated but variable [10–2000/mcL], mostly lymphocytes), protein (elevated, especially IgG fraction), glucose (normal), RBCs (suggestive of herpesvirus or other necrotizing virus). Repeat examination of CSF after 24 hours often useful. (See CSF [enteroviruses, HSV-2, mumps] profiles, Table 8–8). CSF cultures for viruses or bacteria (low yield). CSF PCR for CMV (33%), HSV (99%), VZV, EBV, JC virus, enterovirus, and West Nile virus. Identification of HSV DNA in CSF by PCR techniques is now the definitive diagnostic test. HSV DNA by PCR may not be detectable early in course of illness. Stool culture for enterovirus (2–5 days), which is frequently shed for weeks (especially in children) or in late illness. For rabies, direct fluorescent antibody staining of skin biopsy from nape of neck (50% positive in first week) or RT-PCR on CSF or saliva. Single serum for *Bartonella* (cat-scratch disease) IgM and IgG. Test single serum for West Nile virus IgM antibody or CSF IgM antibody, or PCR of serum or CSF. Paired sera for arboviruses and other viruses should be drawn immediately (acute specimen) and after 1–3 weeks of illness (convalescent specimen). Urine PCR and/or serum PCR are options for diagnosis of enteroviruses.	All patients with suspected encephalitis should undergo MRI with gadolinium (most sensitive) unless contraindicated. CT scan with contrast less sensitive (50% sensitive). Temporal lobe lesions are suggestive of herpes simplex encephalitis. Polyradiculopathy is highly suggestive of CMV in AIDS. Consult with laboratory regarding availability of serological tests. Baringer JR. Herpes simplex infections of the nervous system. Neurol Clin 2008;26:657. [PMID: 18657720] Hayes EB et al. West Nile virus: epidemiology and clinical features of an emerging epidemic in the United States. Annu Rev Med 2006;57:181. [PMID: 16409144] Long SS. Encephalitis diagnosis and management in the real world. Adv Exp Med Biol 2011;697:153. [PMID: 21120725]

CENTRAL NERVOUS SYSTEM		
Aseptic meningitis		

Aseptic meningitis

Acute: Enteroviruses (coxsackie, echo, polio) (90%), mumps, HSV, HIV (primary HIV seroconversion), VZV, lymphocytic choriomeningitis virus, adenovirus, parainfluenza virus 3, West Nile virus, St. Louis encephalitis virus and California group encephalitis viruses (rare).

Recurrent benign lymphocytic meningitis: HSV-2 (Mollaret meningitis).

CSF for pressure (elevated), cell count (WBCs 10–100/mcL, polomorphonuclear neutrophils (PMN nearly, lymphocytes later), protein (normal or slightly elevated), and glucose (normal). On repeat CSF after 24–28 hours, an increase in lymphocytes is seen. (See CSF profiles, Table 8–8.)

CSF viral culture can be negative despite active viral infection. Enteroviruses can be isolated from the CSF in the first few days after onset (positive in 40–80%) but only rarely after the first week.

Detection of enteroviral RNA, HSV DNA, or VZV DNA in CSF by PCR from specialized or reference laboratories.

Paired sera (acute and convalescent) for antibody titers: mumps, West Nile virus, and VZV.

Consult with laboratory regarding availability of diagnostic tests for other viruses.

CT or MRI of head should be performed before lumbar puncture to evaluate for mass lesions or hydrocephalus if focal neurologic signs or papilledema are present.

Aseptic meningitis is acute meningeal inflammation in the absence of pyogenic bacteria or fungi. Diagnosis is usually made by examination of the CSF, PCR of CSF, or serologic assays and by ruling out other infectious causes of acute mental status changes or seizures (eg, toxoplasmosis, Lyme disease, neurosyphilis, tuberculosis, Rocky Mountain spotted fever, ehrlichiosis, fungal infection, and parasitic infection). Consider noninfectious causes such as nonsteroidal anti-inflammatory drugs and other medications.

Enteroviral aseptic meningitis is rare after age 40. 10–30% of patients with primary genital HSV-2 infection can have stiff neck, headache, and photophobia suggestive of recurrent meningitis.

Irani DN. Aseptic meningitis and viral myelitis. Neurol Clin 2008;26:635. [PMID: 18657719]

Lee BE et al. Aseptic meningitis. Curr Opin Infect Dis 2007;20:272. [PMID: 17471037]

Poulikakos PJ et al. A case of recurrent benign lymphocytic (Mollaret's) meningitis and review of the literature. J Infect Public Health 2010;3:192. [PMID: 21126724]

	CENTRAL NERVOUS SYSTEM
	Bacterial meningitis

Organism	Specimen/Diagnostic Tests	Comments
Bacterial meningitis Neonate: Group B streptococci (GPC) (70%), *L. monocytogenes* (GPR) (20%), *S. pneumoniae* (GPC) (10%), *E. coli* (GNR) and *Klebsiella sp* (GNR) (1%), and other streptococci. Infant: *S. pneumoniae* (GPC) (47%), *N. meningitidis* (GNDC) (30%), group B streptococci (GPC) (18%), *Listeria monocytogenes* (GPR), *H. influenzae* (GNCB) (5%). Child: *N. meningitidis* (60%), *S. pneumoniae* (25%), *H. influenzae* (8%), and other streptococci. Adult: *S. pneumoniae* (60%), *N. meningitidis* (20%), *L. monocytogenes* (6%), group B streptococci (4%), other *Hemophilus* sp. and staphylococci (1%), *Ehrlichia chaffeensis* (rare). Postneurosurgical: *S. aureus* (GPC), *S. pneumoniae*, *P. acnes* (GPR), coagulase-negative staphylococci (GPC), pseudomonas (GNR), *E. coli* (GNR), other Enterobacteriaceae, *Acinetobacter* (GNR). Alcoholic patients and the elderly: In addition to the adult organisms, Enterobacteriaceae, pseudomonas, *H. influenzae*.	CSF for pressure (>180 mm H_2O), cell count (WBCs 5000–20,000/mcL, >50% PMNs), protein (150–500 mg/dL), glucose (low <40 mg/dL). (See CSF profiles, Table 8–8.) CSF for Gram stain of cytocentrifuged material (positive in 70–80%). CSF culture for bacteria (positive in 70–85%). Blood culture positive in 40–60% of patients with pneumococcal, meningococcal, and *H. influenzae* meningitis. CSF antigen tests are no longer considered useful because of their low sensitivity and false-positive results.	The first priority in the care of the patient with suspected acute meningitis is therapy, then diagnosis. Start antimicrobial agents based on Gram stain, or if no bacteria are seen, start empiric antibiotics immediately based on patient age and any underlying disease process. Adjunctive dexamethasone therapy has proved beneficial, especially for pneumococcal meningitis. If lumbar puncture is performed, administer antimicrobial therapy with dexamethasone immediately after CSF collection. The mortality rate for pneumococcal meningitis is about 20%, with 25–50% of patients having long-term neurologic complications. With recurrent *N. meningitidis* meningitis, suspect a terminal complement component deficiency. With other recurrent bacterial meningitides, suspect a CSF leak; *S. pneumoniae* is most likely pathogen. Therapy usually includes a 3rd generation cephalosporin plus vancomycin until culture results return. This will cover the most common pathogens as well as *H. influenzae*. Add ampicillin if *L. monocytogenes* is suspected. Therapy can be narrowed once the pathogen is identified and susceptibility results are determined. For *S. pneumoniae*, there has been an increase in prevalence of penicillin- and cephalosporin-resistant strains, so susceptibility testing of pneumococcal strains is very important to guide therapy. Bamberger DM. Diagnosis, initial management, and prevention of meningitis. Am Fam Physician 2010;82:1491. [PMID: 21166369] Brouwer MC et al. Epidemiology, diagnosis, and antimicrobial treatment of acute bacterial meningitis. Clin Microbiol Rev 2010;23:467. [PMID: 20610819] Kim KS. Acute bacterial meningitis in infants and children. Lancet Infect Dis 2010;10:32–42. [PMID: 20129147] Nudelman Y et al. Bacterial meningitis: epidemiology, pathogenesis and management update. Drugs 2009;69:2577. [PMID: 19943708]

CENTRAL NERVOUS SYSTEM
Fungal meningitis

Fungal meningitis		
C. neoformans (spherical, budding yeast), *C. immitis* (spherules), *H. capsulatum.* Immunocompromised: *Aspergillus* sp, *Pseudallescheria boydii*, *Candida* sp. sporothrix, blastomyces.	CSF for pressure (normal or elevated), cell count (WBCs 50–1000/mcL, mostly lymphocytes), protein (elevated), and glucose (normal or decreased). Serum cryptococcal antigen (CrAg) test (latex agglutination) for *C. neoformans* (>90% sensitive and specific). (This test can be performed on CSF specimens). For other fungi, collect at least 5 mL of CSF for fungal culture. Initial cultures are positive in 40% of coccidioides cases and 27–65% of histoplasma cases. Repeat cultures are frequently needed. Cultures of blood, bone marrow, skin lesions, or other involved organs, if clinically indicated. CSF India ink preparation for cryptococcus is not recommended. Cytospin Gram stain procedure concentrates CSF and can demonstrate round, budding yeast. Serum coccidioidal serology is a serum immunodiffusion test for antibodies against the organism (75–95%). CSF serologic testing is rarely necessary. (See Coccidioides serology, Chapter 3.) Complement fixation tests for coccidioides or histoplasma antibodies are available from reference laboratories or public health department laboratories (see Chapter 3) and can give titers that can be used to follow treatment. Histoplasma antigen can be detected in urine (90%), blood (70%), or CSF (61%) in cases of histoplasma meningitis.	The clinical presentation of fungal meningitis in non-immunocompromised and immunocompromised patients is that of an indolent chronic meningitis. Before AIDS, cryptococcal meningitis was seen both in patients with cellular immunologic deficiencies and in patients who lacked obvious defects (about 50%). In AIDs patients, cryptococcus is the most common cause of meningitis and may present with normal CSF findings. Titer of CSF CrAg can be used to monitor therapeutic success (falling titer) or failure (unchanged or rising titer) or to predict relapse during suppressive therapy (rising titer) in immunocompetent patients, though not in patients with AIDS. Ginsberg L et al. Chronic and recurrent meningitis. Pract Neurol 2008;8:348. [PMID: 19015295] Honda H et al. Central nervous system infections: meningitis and brain abscess. Infect Dis Clin North Am 2009;23:609. [PMID: 19665086] Li SS et al. Cryptococcus. Proc Am Thorac Soc 2010;7:186. [PMID: 20463247] Wheat LJ et al. Diagnosis and management of central nervous system histoplasmosis. Clin Infect Dis 2005;40:844. [PMID: 15736018] Williams PL. Coccidioidal meningitis. Ann N Y Acad Sci 2007;1111:377. [PMID: 17363442]

Organism	Specimen/Diagnostic Tests	Comments
Spirochetal meningitis/neurologic diseases *B. burgdorferi* (neuroborreliosis), *T. pallidum* (neurosyphilis), leptospira, other borreliae	**Neuroborreliosis:** CSF for pressure (normal or elevated), cell count (WBCs elevated, mostly lymphocytes), protein (may be elevated), and glucose (normal). Serum and CSF for serologic testing for antibody by ELISA or IFA. False-positive borderline or positive results. CSF serology for anti-*B. burgdorferi* IgM (90%). PCR is very specific for detecting *Borrelia* DNA, but sensitivity is variable owing to stage of disease and type of body fluid tested. (See Lyme disease serologies, Chapter 3.) **Acute syphilitic meningitis:** CSF for pressure (elevated), cell count (WBCs 25–2000/mcL, mostly lymphocytes), protein (elevated), and glucose (normal or low). (See CSF profiles, Table 8–8.) Serum VDRL. (See VDRL, serum, Chapter 3.) CSF VDRL is the preferred test (see Chapter 3), but is only 66% sensitive for acute syphilitic meningitis. **Neurosyphilis:** CSF for pressure (normal), cell count (WBCs normal or slightly increased, mostly lymphocytes), protein (normal or elevated), glucose (normal), and positive CSF VDRL. Serum RPR or VDRL with confirmatory FTA-ABS, or TP PA testing should be done with a positive serum result before CSF VDRL is performed. Traditionally, nontreponemal serologic tests (RPR or VDRL) are used as screening tests for detection of syphilis. Because of the lack of specificity for these tests, positive screening tests must be confirmed with FTA-ABS or TP PA treponemal-specific assays. A new syphilis testing algorithm using treponemal tests for screening followed by a nontreponemal serology test has been proposed. **Leptospirosis:** CSF cell count (WBCs <500/mcL, mostly monocytes), protein (slightly elevated), and glucose (normal). Urine for dark-field examination of sediment to detect leptospira organisms. Blood and CSF dark-field examination positive only in acute phase prior to meningitis. Serum for serology for IgM by EIA (93% specificity) and ELISA.	Neurosyphilis is a late stage of infection and can present with meningovascular (hemiparesis, seizures, aphasia), parenchymal (general paresis, tabes dorsalis), or asymptomatic (latent) disease. In HIV-infected patients, neurosyphilis can present in secondary syphilis. Because there is no single highly sensitive or specific test for neurosyphilis, the diagnosis must depend on a combination of clinical and laboratory data. Therapy of suspected neurosyphilis should not be withheld on the basis of a negative CSF VDRL if clinical suspicion is high. In HIV neurosyphilis, treatment failures may be common. Lyme disease can present as a lymphocytic meningitis, facial palsy, or painful radiculitis. Leptospirosis follows exposure to urine of infected rodents, small animals, or livestock. Kent ME et al. Reexamining syphilis: an update on epidemiology, clinical manifestations, and management. Ann Pharmacother 2008;42:226. [PMID: 18212261] O'Connell S. Lyme borreliosis: current issues in diagnosis and management. Curr Opin Infect Dis 2010;23:231. [PMID: 20407371] Sena AC et al. Novel *Treponema pallidum* serologic tests: a paradigm shift in syphilis screening for the 21st century. Clin Infect Dis 2010;51:700. [PMID: 20687840] Stoner BP. Current controversies in the management of adult syphilis. Clin Infect Dis 2007;44 (Suppl 3):S130. [PMID: 17342666] Toyokawa T et al. Diagnosis of acute leptospirosis. Expert Rev Anti Infect Ther 2011;9:111. [PMID: 21171882] Victoriano AF et al. Leptospirosis in the Asia Pacific region. BMC Infect Dis 2009;9:147. [PMID: 19732423]

CENTRAL NERVOUS SYSTEM
Parasitic meningoencephalitis

Parasitic meningo-encephalitis

T. gondii, Naegleria fowleri, T. solium (cysticerci),
Acanthamoeba (granulomatous amebic encephalitis
GAE), *Balamuthia* sp. (GAE),
Angiostrongylus (eosinophilic meningoencephalitis),
Trypanosoma sp.

CSF for pressure (normal or elevated), cell
count (WBCs 100–1000/mcL, chiefly
monocytes, lymphocytes), protein (elevated),
glucose (normal to low). Serum serology to
detect antibodies for *T. gondii, E. chaffeensis,
A. phagocytophilum.*

Toxoplasmosis: CT or MRI of brain, serology, Giemsa-stained touch prep of brain
tissue, CSF PCR.

Naegleria: CSF wet mount for amebic tro-
phozoites, or hematoxylin and eosin stain of
brain tissue. Serologic tests not helpful.

Cysticercosis: Characteristic findings on
CT and MRI are diagnostic. Serology is less
sensitive.

Balamuthia: Culture not helpful. Indirect
immunofluorescence or PCR of brain tissue
to detect organism.

Angiostrongyliasis: CSF pressure (normal
or elevated), cell count (WBC eosinophilic
pleocytosis), protein (elevated), glucose
(normal). CSF wet mount, ELISA serology.

Trypanosomiasis: Blood-Giemsa stain
on thick and thin smears. CSF wet mount.
Serologic tests by ELISA, IFA have 93–98%
sensitivity and 99% specificity in acute
stages. Serologic tests may be negative in
chronic stages.

Naegleria follows exposure to warm, fresh, and
polluted water (eg, swimming pools, sewers,
fresh-water lakes).

Pereira-Chioccola VL et al. *Toxoplasma gondii* infection
and cerebral toxoplasmosis in HIV-infected patients.
Future Microbiol 2009;4:1363. [PMID: 19995194]

Ramirez-Avila L et al. Eosinophilic meningitis due to
Angiostrongylus and *Gnathostoma* species. Clin Infect
Dis 2009;48:322. [PMID: 19123863]

Visvesvara GS. Amebic meningoencephalitides and kera-
titis: challenges in diagnosis and treatment. Curr Opin
Infect Dis 2010;23:590. [PMID: 20802332]

	CENTRAL NERVOUS SYSTEM
	Tuberculous meningitis

Organism	Specimen/Diagnostic Tests	Comments
Tuberculous meningitis *M. tuberculosis* (MTb),	CSF for pressure (elevated), cell count (WBCs 100–500/mcL, PMNs early, lymphocytes later), protein (elevated), glucose (decreased). (See CSF profiles, Table 8–8.) CSF for AFB stain. Stain is positive in only 30%; culture may be negative in 15–25% of cases. Cytocentrifugation and repeat smears increase yield. CSF for AFB culture (positive in <70%). Repeated sampling of the CSF during the first week of therapy is recommended; ideally, 3 or 4 specimens of 5–10 mL each should be obtained (87% yield with 4 specimens). CSF PCR available but sensitivity of most assays is low (50%). Positive CSF PCR is helpful with appropriate clinical picture, but negative PCR does not rule out tuberculous meningitis. DNA hybridization probes are available for rapid identification of mycobacteria from culture.	Tuberculous meningitis is usually secondary to rupture of a subependymal tubercle from pulmonary focus or may be a consequence of miliary tuberculosis rather than blood-borne invasion. Because CSF stain and culture are not sensitive for tuberculous meningitis, diagnosis and treatment should be based on a combination of clinical and microbiologic data. Evidence of inactive or active extrameningeal tuberculosis, especially pulmonary, is seen in 75% of patients. Garg RK. Tuberculous meningitis. Acta Neurol Scand 2010;122:75. [PMID: 20055767] Garg RK et al. Tuberculous meningitis in patients infected with human immunodeficiency virus. J Neurol 2011;258:3. [PMID: 20848123] Thwaites GE et al. Update on tuberculosis of the central nervous system: pathogenesis, diagnosis, and treatment. Clin Chest Med 2009;30:745. [PMID: 19925964]

EYE	
Conjunctivitis	

Conjunctivitis

Neonate (ophthalmia neonatorum): *C. trachomatis* (15–50%), *N. gonorrhoeae* (GNDC), HSV.

Children and adults: adenovirus, staphylococci (GPC), HSV, *H. influenzae* (GNCB), *S. pneumoniae* (GPDC), *S. pyogenes* (GPC), VZV, *N. gonorrhoeae* (GNDC), *M. lacunata* (GNCB), *M. catarrhalis*, *Bartonella* sp. (Parinaud oculoglandular syndrome).

Adult inclusion conjunctivitis/trachoma: *C. trachomatis*.

Acute hemorrhagic conjunctivitis (acute epidemic keratoconjunctivitis): enterovirus, coxsackievirus.

Conjunctival Gram stain is especially useful if gonococcal infection is suspected.

Bacterial culture for severe cases (routine bacterial culture) or suspected gonococcal infection.

Conjunctival scrapings or smears by direct immunofluorescent monoclonal antibody staining for *C. trachomatis*.

Cell culture for chlamydia.

Detection of chlamydial DNA on ocular swabs by PCR techniques may be available in research laboratories.

Ocular HSV and VZV PCR may be available in reference laboratories.

The causes of conjunctivitis change with the season. Adenovirus occurs mainly in the fall, *H. influenzae* in the winter.

Gonococcal conjunctivitis is an ophthalmologic emergency.

Cultures are usually unnecessary unless chlamydia or gonorrhea is suspected or the case is severe.

Consider noninfectious causes (eg, allergy, contact lens deposits, trauma).

Hu VH et al. Epidemiology and control of trachoma: systematic review. Trop Med Int Health 2010;15:673. [PMID: 20374566]

O'Brien TP et al. Acute conjunctivitis: truth and misconceptions. Curr Med Res Opin 2009;25:1953. [PMID: 19552618]

	EYE
	Keratitis

Organism	Specimen/Diagnostic Tests	Comments
Keratitis Bacteria: *P. aeruginosa* (GNR), staphylococci (GPC), *S. pneumoniae* (GPDC), *Haemophilus* sp. (GNCB), *Moraxella* sp. Virus: HSV (dendritic pattern on fluorescein slit-lamp examination), VZV. Contact lens: Acanthamoeba, Enterobacteri-aceae (GNR). Fungus: Candida, fusarium, aspergillus, rhodotorula, other filamentous fungi. Parasite: *O. volvulus* (river blindness), microsporidia (HIV).	Corneal scrapings for Gram stain, KOH, and culture. Routine bacterial culture is used for most bacterial causes, viral culture for herpes, and special media for acanthamoeba (can be detected with trichrome or Giemsa stain of smears). Treatment depends on Gram stain appearance and culture. Corneal biopsy may be needed if initial cultures are negative. Ocular viral DFA for HSV and VZV.	Prompt ophthalmologic consultation is mandatory. Acanthamoeba infection occurs in soft contact (extended-wear) lens wearers and may resemble HSV infection on fluorescein examination (dendritic ["branching"] ulcer). Bacterial keratitis is usually caused by contact lens use or trauma. Fungal (ie, *Fusarium* sp.) keratitis is usually caused by trauma. Increased resistance noted among all bacterial isolates (eg, coagulase-negative staphylococci) to ciprofloxa-cin (20–38%) and cefazolin (19–40%). Resistance to bacitracin, trimethoprim-sulfamethoxazole and vancomycin remains unchanged. Ahearn DG et al. *Fusarium* keratitis and contact lens wear: facts and speculations. Med Mycol 2008;46:397. [PMID: 18608899] Chang DC et al; *Fusarium* Keratitis Investigation Team. Multistate outbreak of *Fusarium* keratitis associated with use of a contact lens solution. JAMA 2006;296:953. [PMID: 16926355] Cronau H et al. Diagnosis and management of red eye in primary care. Am Fam Physician 2010;81:137. [PMID: 20082509] Joslin CE et al. Epidemiological characteristics of a Chicago-area Acanthamoeba keratitis outbreak. Am J Ophthalmol 2006;142:212. [PMID: 16876498]

EYE
Endophthalmitis

Endophthalmitis

Spontaneous or postoperative:
Coagulase-negative staphylococci (70%) (GPC), *S. aureus* (10%) (GPC), viridans group streptococci (5%) (GPC in chains), *S. pneumoniae* (5%) (GPC), gram-negative rods (6%) (eg, *E. coli*, *Klebsiella* sp., *Pseudomonas* sp.), and other gram-positive organisms (4%) (eg, group B streptococci, *Listeria* sp.).

Trauma: *Bacillus* sp. (GPR), fungi, coagulase negative staphylococci (GPC), streptococci (GPC), and gram-negative rods.

Postfiltering bleb created to control glaucoma: Viridans group streptococci (57%) (GPC in chains), *S. pneumoniae* (GPDC), *H. influenzae* (GNCB), *M. catarrhalis* (GNCB), *S. aureus* (GPC), *S. epidermidis* (GPC), enterococci (GPC), gram-negative rods.

IV drug abuse: Add *Bacillus cereus*.

Culture material from anterior chamber, vitreous cavity, and wound abscess for bacteria, mycobacteria, and fungi. Traumatic and postoperative cases should have aqueous and vitreous aspiration for culture and smear (55%).

Conjunctival cultures are inadequate and misleading.

Endophthalmitis refers to bacterial or fungal infections and is an inflammatory process of the ocular cavity and adjacent structures. Rapid diagnosis is critical, because vision may be compromised.

Bacterial endophthalmitis usually occurs as a consequence of ocular surgery (cataract surgery). 75% within first postoperative week. Prophylactic antibiotics are of unproven benefit, though topical antibiotics are widely used.

Also consider retinitis in immunocompromised patients, caused by CMV, HSV, VZV, and toxoplasma (retinochoroiditis), which is diagnosed by retinal examination.

Maguire JI. Postoperative endophthalmitis: optimal management and the role and timing of vitrectomy surgery. (Lond) 2008;22:1290. [PMID: 18356929]

Schwartz SG et al. Endophthalmitis after intravitreal injections. Expert Opin Pharmacother 2009;10:2119. [PMID: 19586422]

EAR		
Otitis media		
Organism	**Specimen/Diagnostic Tests**	**Comments**
Otitis media Infant, child, and adult: *S. pneumoniae* (23%) (GPDC), *H. influenzae* (36%) (GNCB), *M. catarrhalis* (3%) (GNDC), *S. aureus* (GPC), *S. pyogenes* (GPC in chains), viruses (eg, respiratory syncytial virus [RSV], influenza virus, rhinovirus, enteroviruses, human metapneumovirus), *M. pneumoniae, C. trachomatis* or *pneumoniae,* anaerobes, fungi (eg, *Blastomyces dermatitidis, Candida* sp., *Aspergillus* sp.). Neonate: Same as above plus Enterobacteriaceae (GNR), group B streptococcus (GPC). Endotracheal intubation: *Pseudomonas* sp. (GNR), *Klebsiella* (GNR), Enterobacteriaceae (GNR). Chronic: *P. aeruginosa* (GNR), anaerobes, *M. tuberculosis* (AFB).	Tympanocentesis aspirate for Gram stain and bacterial culture in the patient who has a toxic appearance. Otherwise, microbiologic studies of effusions are so consistent that empiric treatment is acceptable. CSF examination if clinically indicated. Nasopharyngeal swab may be substituted for tympanocentesis. Blood culture in the toxic patient.	Peak incidence of otitis media occurs in the first 3 years of life, especially between 6 and 24 months of age. In neonates, predisposing factors include cleft palate, hypotonia, mental retardation (Down syndrome). Tympanocentesis is indicated if the patient fails to improve after 48 hours or develops fever. It may hasten resolution and decrease sterile effusion. Persistent middle ear effusion may require placement of ventilating or tympanostomy tubes. Bullous myringitis suggests mycoplasma. Emerging antibiotic resistance should be considered in choice of empiric antibiotic therapy. There is emerging resistance of *S. pneumoniae* to macrolides, to erythromycin and to penicillin, so appropriate therapy should rely on local antibiograms. *M. catarrhalis* organisms (~33–50%) produce β-lactamase (90%), as do *H. influenzae* organisms (~33–50%). This lessens usefulness of amoxicillin, the usual drug of choice. Coker TR et al. Diagnosis, microbial epidemiology, and antibiotic treatment of acute otitis media in children: a systematic review. JAMA 2010;304:2161. [PMID: 21081729] Vergison A et al. Otitis media and its consequences: beyond the earache. Lancet Infect Dis 2010;10:195. [PMID: 20185098] Wald ER. Acute otitis media and acute bacterial sinusitis. Clin Infect Dis 2011;52(Suppl 4):S277. [PMID: 21460285]

EAR
Otitis externa

Otitis externa

Acute localized: *S. aureus* (15%) (GPC), anaerobes (32%), *S. pyogenes* (GPC in chains), *H. influenzae*, other gram-positive cocci.
"Swimmer's ear": *Pseudomonas* sp. (40%) (GNR), fungi (6%) (eg, *Aspergillus* sp., *Candida* sp.).
Chronic: Usually secondary to seborrhea or eczema.
Diabetes mellitus, AIDS ("malignant otitis externa"): *P. aeruginosa* (GNR), *Aspergillus* sp., *Candida* sp.
Furuncle of external canal: *S. aureus*.

Ear drainage for Gram stain and bacterial culture, especially in malignant otitis externa.
CT or MRI can aid in diagnosis by demonstrating cortical bone erosion or meningeal enhancement.

Infection of the external auditory canal is similar to infection of skin and soft tissue elsewhere.
If malignant otitis externa is present, exclusion of associated osteomyelitis and surgical drainage may be required.
Carfrae MJ et al. Malignant otitis externa. Otolaryngol Clin North Am 2008;41:537. [PMID: 18435997]
Kaushik V et al. Interventions for acute otitis externa. Cochrane Database Syst Rev 2010;(1):CD004740. [PMID: 20091565]
Rosenfeld RM et al; American Academy of Otolaryngology–Head and Neck Surgery Foundation. Clinical practice guideline: acute otitis externa. Otolaryngol Head Neck Surg 2006;134(4 Suppl):S4. [PMID: 16638473]

	SINUS	
	Sinusitis	
Organism	**Specimen/Diagnostic Tests**	**Comments**
Sinusitis Acute: *S. pneumoniae* (GPDC) (20–43%), *H. influenzae* (GNCB) (21–35%), *M. catarrhalis* (GNDC) (2–10%), other streptococci (3–9%) (GPC), anaerobes (1–9%), viruses (4%) (adenovirus, influenza, parainfluenza), *S. aureus* (GPC) (1–8%). Chronic (child): Viridans and anaerobic streptococci (GPC in chains) (23%), *S. aureus* (19%), *S. pneumoniae, H. influenzae, M. catarrhalis, P. aeruginosa* (GNR) in cystic fibrosis. Chronic (adult): Coagulase-negative staphylococci (GPC) (36%), *S. aureus* (GPC) (25%), viridans streptococci (GPC in chains) (8%), corynebacteria (GPR) (5%), anaerobes (6%), including *Bacteroides* sp., *Prevotella* sp. (GNR), peptostreptococcus (GPC), *Fusobacterium* sp. (GNR). Hospitalized with nasogastric tube or nasotracheal intubation: Enterobacteriaceae (GNR), *Pseudomonas* sp. (GNR). Fungal: Zygomycetes (rhizopus), aspergillus, *P. boydii*, other dematiaceous mold. Immunocompromised: *P. aeruginosa* (GNR), CMV, *Aspergillus* sp. and other filamentous fungi plus microsporidia, *Cryptosporidium parvum*, Acanthamoeba in HIV-infected patients.	Clinical diagnosis. Nasal aspirate for bacterial culture is not usually helpful due to respiratory flora contamination of aerobes and anaerobes. Maxillary sinus aspirate for bacterial culture may be helpful in severe or atypical cases.	Diagnosis and treatment of sinusitis are usually based on clinical and radiologic features. Microbiologic studies can be helpful in severe or atypical cases. Sinus CT scan (or MRI) is better than plain x-ray for diagnosing sinusitis, particularly if sphenoid sinusitis is suspected. However, sinus CT scans should be interpreted cautiously, because abnormalities are also seen in patients with the common cold. Acute and chronic sinusitis occur frequently in HIV-infected patients, may be recurrent or refractory, and may involve multiple sinuses (especially when the CD4 cell count is <200/mcL). Acute sinusitis often results from bacterial superinfection following viral upper respiratory infection. Mehtens JM et al. Acute sinusitis. Adolesc Med State Art Rev 2010;21:187. [PMID: 21047024] Orlandi RR et al. Fungus and chronic rhinosinusitis: weighing the evidence. Otolaryngol Head Neck Surg 2010;143:611. [PMID: 20974327] Ryan MW. Evaluation and management of the patient with "sinus." Med Clin North Am 2010;94:881. [PMID: 20736100] Wang X et al. Chronic rhinosinusitis. Adv Otorhinolaryngol 2011;70:114. [PMID: 21358193]

UPPER AIRWAY
Pharyngitis

Pharyngitis

Exudative: *S. pyogenes* (GPC) (15–30%), viruses (rhinovirus, coronavirus, adenovirus) (30%), group C and G streptococci (GPC) (5%), herpes simplex virus (HSV) (4%), parainfluenza and influenza virus A and B (2–4%), Epstein-Barr virus (mononucleosis) (1%), HIV (1%) *N. gonorrhoeae* (GNDC) (1%), *C. diphtheriae* (GPR) (≤1%), *Arcanobacterium hemolyticum* (GPR) (≤1%) *M. pneumoniae, C. pneumoniae.*

Membranous: *C. diphtheriae* (GPR), *C. pseudodiphtheriticum* (GPR), HSV, Epstein-Barr virus.

Throat swab for culture. Place in sterile tube or transport medium. If *N. gonorrhoeae* is suspected, use chocolate agar or Thayer-Martin media. If *C. diphtheriae* is suspected, use Tinsdale or blood agar. Throat swabs are routinely cultured for group A streptococcus only. If other organisms are suspected, this must be stated.

Throat culture has about 70–90% sensitivity and 95% specificity for group A streptococcus.

"Rapid" tests for group A streptococcus can speed diagnosis and aid in the treatment of family members. However, false-negative results may lead to underdiagnosis and failure to treat. Back-up throat cultures are recommended so group A streptococcus is not missed. Sequelae of group A streptococcus infection can be severe such as rheumatic fever, post-streptococcal glomerulonephritis.

Controversy exists over how to evaluate patients with sore throat, although some authors suggest culturing all patients and then treating only those with positive cultures.

Most laboratories only report group A streptococcus from throat culture.

In patients with compatible histories, be sure to consider pharyngeal abscess or epiglottitis, both of which may be life-threatening.

Complications include pharyngeal abscess and Lemierre syndrome (infection with *Fusobacterium* sp.), which can progress to sepsis and multi-organ failure.

Chan TV. The patient with sore throat. Med Clin North Am 2010;94:923. [PMID: 20736104]
Wessels MR. Clinical practice. Streptococcal pharyngitis. N Engl J Med 2011;364:648. [PMID: 21323542]

UPPER AIRWAY
Laryngitis

Organism	Specimen/Diagnostic Tests	Comments
Laryngitis Virus (90%) (influenza, rhinovirus, adenovirus, parainfluenza, Epstein-Barr virus), *S. pyogenes* (GPC) (10%), *M. catarrhalis* (GNDC), *H. influenzae* (GNCB), *M. tuberculosis*, fungus (cryptococcosis, histoplasmosis). Immunocompromised: *Candida* sp., CMV, HSV.	Diagnosis is made by clinical picture of upper respiratory infection with hoarseness.	Laryngitis usually occurs with common cold or influenzal syndromes. Fungal laryngeal infections occur most commonly in immunocompromised patients (AIDS, cancer, organ transplants, corticosteroid therapy, diabetes mellitus). Chronic laryngitis is associated with one or more chronic irritants such as gastric acid, chronic sinusitis, chronic alcohol use, inhaled toxins. Feierabend RH et al. Hoarseness in adults. Am Fam Physician 2009;80:363. [PMID: 19678604] Mau T. Diagnostic evaluation and management of hoarseness. Med Clin North Am 2010;94:945. [PMID: 20736105]

UPPER AIRWAY

Laryngotracheobronchitis

Laryngotracheobronchitis		
Infant/child: RSV (50–75%) (bronchiolitis), adenovirus, parainfluenza virus (HPIV types 1, 2, 3) (80%) (croup), *B. pertussis* (GNCB) (whooping cough), other viruses, including rhinovirus, coronavirus, influenza, bocavirus, human metapneumovirus. Adolescent/adult: Usually viruses, *M. pneumoniae*, *C. pneumoniae*, *B. pertussis*. Chronic adult: *S. pneumoniae* (GPDC), *H. influenzae* (GNCB), *M. catarrhalis* (GNDC), *Klebsiella* (GNR), other Enterobacteriaceae (GNR), viruses (eg, influenza), aspergillus (allergic bronchopulmonary aspergillosis). Chronic obstructive airway disease: Viral (25–50%), *S. pneumoniae* (GPC), *H. influenzae* (GNCB), *S. aureus* (GPC), Enterobacteriaceae (GNR), anaerobes (<10%).	Nasopharyngeal aspirate or swab for respiratory virus DFA, for viral culture (rarely indicated), and for PCR for *B. pertussis*. PCR for pertussis is test of choice; culture and DFA are less sensitive. Cellular examination of early morning sputum will show many PMNs in chronic bronchitis. Sputum Gram stain and culture for ill adults. In chronic bronchitis, mixed flora are usually seen with oral flora or colonized *H. influenzae* or *S. pneumoniae* on culture. Paired sera for mycoplasmal antibody assays can help make a diagnosis retrospectively in infants and children but are not clinically useful except for seriously ill patients.	Chronic bronchitis is diagnosed when sputum is coughed up on most days for at least 3 consecutive months for more than 2 successive years. Bacterial infections are usually secondary infections of initial viral or mycoplasma induced inflammation. Airway endoscopy can aid in the diagnosis of bacterial tracheitis in children. Cornia PB et al. Does this coughing adolescent or adult patient have pertussis? JAMA 2010;304:890. [PMID: 20736473] Everard ML. Acute bronchiolitis and croup. Pediatr Clin North Am 2009;56:119. [PMID: 19135584] Sobol SE et al. Epiglottitis and croup. Otolaryngol Clin North Am 2008;41:551. [PMID: 18435998]

	UPPER AIRWAY
	Epiglottitis

Organism	Specimen/Diagnostic Tests	Comments
Epiglottitis Child: *H. influenzae* type B (GNCB), *H. parainfluenzae* (GCNB), *S. pneumoniae* (GPC), *S. aureus* (GPC), other streptococci (groups A, B, C) Adult: *S. pyogenes* (GPC), *S. pneumoniae* (GPC), *Klebsiella* sp. (GNR), *H. influenzae* (GNCB), *Pseudomonas* sp. (GNR), HSV, viruses (parainfluenza and influenza). HIV: *Candida* (fungi) and *Pseudomonas* sp. (GNR).	Blood for bacterial culture: positive in 50–100% of children with *H. influenzae*. Lateral neck x-ray may show an enlarged epiglottis but has a low sensitivity (31%).	Acute epiglottitis is a rapidly moving cellulitis of the epiglottis and represents an airway emergency. Epiglottitis can be confused with croup, a viral infection of gradual onset that affects infants and causes inspiratory and expiratory stridor. Airway management is the primary concern, and an endotracheal tube should be placed or tracheostomy performed as soon as the diagnosis of epiglottitis is made in children. A tracheostomy set should be at the bedside for adults. Alcaide ML et al. Pharyngitis and epiglottitis. Infect Dis Clin North Am 2007;21:449. Erratum in: Infect Dis Clin North Am 2007;21:847. [PMID: 17561078] Al-Qudah M et al. Acute adult supraglottitis: current management and treatment. South Med J 2010;103:800. [PMID: 20622745]

LUNG
Community-acquired pneumonia

Community-acquired pneumonia

Neonate: *E. coli* (GNR), group A or B streptococcus (GPC), *S. aureus* (GPC), *Pseudomonas* sp (GNR), *C. trachomatis*.

Infant/child (<5 years): Virus, *S. pneumoniae* (GPC), *H. influenzae* (GNCB), *S. aureus*.

Age 5–40 years: Virus, *M. pneumoniae*, *C. pneumoniae* (formerly known as TWAR strain), *C. psittaci*, *S. pneumoniae*, *Legionella* sp.

Age >40 without other disease: *S. pneumoniae* (GPDC), *H. influenzae* (GNCB), *S. aureus* (GPC), *M. catarrhalis* (GNDC), *C. pneumoniae*, *Legionella* sp. (GNR), *S. pyogenes* (GPC), *K. pneumoniae* (GNR), Enterobacteriaceae (GNR), viruses (eg, influenza).

Cystic fibrosis: *P. aruginosa* (GNR), *Burkholderia cepacia*.

Elderly: *S. pneumoniae* (GPDC), *H. influenzae* (GNCB), *S. aureus* (GPC), Enterobacteriaceae (GNR), *M. catarrhalis* (GNDC), group B streptococcus (GPC), *legionella* (GNR), nocardia (GPR), influenza.

Aspiration: *S. pneumoniae* (GPDC), *K. pneumoniae* (GNR), Enterobacteriaceae (GNR), *Bacteroides* sp. and other oral anaerobes.

Fungal: *H. capsulatum*, *C. immitis*, *B. dermatitidis*

Exposure to birthing animals, sheep: *C. burnetii* (Q fever), rabbits: *F. tularensis* (tularemia), deer mice: hantavirus, birds: *C. psittaci*.

Sputum for Gram stain desirable; culture, if empiric therapy fails or patient is seriously ill. An adequate specimen should have <10 epithelial cells and >25 PMNs per low-power field. Special sputum cultures for legionella are available. *Legionella* urine antigen test is 70–80% sensitive, but only detects *Legionella pneumophila* serogroup 1 (90% of cases of Legionaire disease), so test may be falsely negative.

Blood for bacterial cultures (2 sets): obtain before antibiotic treatment, especially in ill patients.

Pleural fluid for bacterial culture if significant effusion is present.

Bronchoalveolar lavage or brushings for bacterial, fungal, and viral antigen tests and AFB culture in immunocompromised patients and atypical cases.

Paired sera for *M. pneumoniae* EIA testing can diagnose infection retrospectively.

Serologic tests for Q fever and for hantavirus (IgM and IgG) are available. Culture of respiratory specimens for *C. pneumoniae*, *C. psittaci* strains.

Other special techniques (bronchoscopy with telescoping plugged catheter and protected brush, transtracheal aspiration, transthoracic fine-needle aspiration, or, rarely, open-lung biopsy) can be used to obtain specimens for culture in severe cases, in immunocompromised patients, or in cases with negative conventional cultures and progression despite empiric antibiotic therapy.

About 60% of cases of community-acquired pneumonia have an identifiable microbial cause. Pneumatoceles suggest *S. aureus* but are also reported with pneumococcus, group A streptococcus, *H influenzae*, and Enterobacteriaceae (in neonates).

An "atypical pneumonia" presentation (diffuse pattern on chest x-ray with lack of organisms on Gram stain of sputum) should raise suspicion of mycoplasma, legionella, or chlamydial infection. Consider hantavirus pulmonary syndrome if pulmonary symptoms follow afebrile illness.

Aspiration pneumonias are most commonly associated with stroke, alcoholism, drug abuse, sedation, and periodontal disease.

Brar NK et al. Management of community-acquired pneumonia: a review and update. Ther Adv Respir Dis 2011;5:61. [PMID: 20935033]

Butt S et al. Treatment of community-acquired pneumonia in an ambulatory setting. Am J Med 2011;124:297. [PMID: 21435417]

Janssens JP. Pneumonia in the elderly (geriatric) population. Curr Opin Pulm Med 2005;11:226. [PMID: 15818184]

	LUNG
	Anaerobic pneumonia

Organism	Specimen/Diagnostic Tests	Comments
Anaerobic pneumonia/lung abscess Usually polymicrobial: Anaerobes: *Bacteroides* sp. (15% *B. fragilis*), *Peptostreptococcus*, *Prevotella* sp., *Porphyromonas* sp., *Fusobacterium* sp., micro-aerophilic streptococcus, veillonella, and facultative anaerobes; *S. aureus, P. aeruginosa, S. pneumoniae* (rare), *Klebsiella* (rare), *H. influenzae* type B, legionella, nocardia, actinomyces, fungi, parasites.	Sputum Gram stain and culture for anaerobes are of little value because of contaminating oral flora. Bronchoalveolar sampling (brush or aspirate or biopsy) for Gram stain and culture will usually make an accurate diagnosis. Percutaneous transthoracic needle aspiration may be useful for culture and for cytology to demonstrate coexistence of an underlying carcinoma. Blood cultures are usually negative (80%).	Aspiration is the most important underlying cause of lung abscess. Without clear-cut risk factors such as alcoholism, coma, or seizures, bronchoscopy is often performed to rule out neoplasm. Brook I. Anaerobic pulmonary infections in children. Pediatr Emerg Care 2004;20:636. [PMID: 15599270] Hogan MJ et al. Interventional radiology treatment of empyema and lung abscesses. Paediatr Respir Rev 2008;9:77. [PMID: 18513667] Patradoon-Ho P et al. Lung abscess in children. Paediatr Respir Rev 2007;8:77. [PMID: 17419981] Puligandla PS et al. Respiratory infections: pneumonia, lung abscess, and empyema. Semin Pediatr Surg 2008;17:42. [PMID: 18581141]

LUNG		
Hospital-acquired pneumonia		
Hospital-acquired pneumonia *P. aeruginosa* (GNR), *Klebsiella* (GNR), *S. aureus* (GPC), *Acinetobacter* (GNR), Enterobacteriaceae (GNR), *S. pneumoniae* (GPDC), *H. influenzae* (GNCB), influenza virus, RSV, parainfluenza virus, adenovirus, oral anaerobes, *S. maltophilia* (GNR), *B. cepacia* (GNR). Mendelson syndrome (see Comments): No organisms initially, then pseudomonas, Enterobacteriaceae, *S. aureus*, *S. pneumoniae*.	Sputum Gram stain and culture for bacteria (aerobic and anaerobic) and fungus (if suspected). Blood cultures for bacteria are often negative (80%). Endotracheal aspirate or bronchoalveolar sample for bacterial and fungal culture in selected patients. Ventilator-associated pneumonia (VAP) is difficult to diagnose. Suspect VAP in patient with fever, leukocytosis, purulent respiratory secretions or a progressive radiographic pulmonary infiltrate.	Most cases are related to aspiration. Hospital-acquired aspiration pneumonia is associated with intubation and the use of broad-spectrum antibiotics. A strong association between aspiration pneumonia and swallowing dysfunction is demonstrable by videofluoroscopy. Mendelson syndrome is due to acute aspiration of gastric contents (eg, during anesthesia or drowning). Hospital-acquired pneumonia is the second most common nosocomial infection, accounting for 25% of all ICU infections. Moreover, there has been a dramatic increase in multidrug-resistant bacteria. Jones RN. Microbial etiologies of hospital-acquired bacterial pneumonia and ventilator-associated bacterial pneumonia. Clin Infect Dis 2010;51(Suppl 1):S81. [PMID: 20597676] Torres A et al. Treatment guidelines and outcomes of hospital-acquired and ventilator-associated pneumonia. Clin Infect Dis 2010;51(Suppl 1):S48. Erratum in: Clin Infect Dis 2010;51(9):1114. [PMID: 20597672] Wall RJ et al. Evidence-based algorithms for diagnosing and treating ventilator-associated pneumonia. J Hosp Med 2008;3:409. [PMID: 18951395]

	LUNG
	Pneumonia in immunocompromised host

Organism	Specimen/Diagnostic Tests	Comments
Pneumonia in the immunocompromised host Child with HIV infection: Lymphoid interstitial pneumonia (LIP). AIDS: *M. avium* (31%), CMV (13%), *P. jiroveci* (13%), *H. capsulatum* (7%), *S. pneumoniae* (GPDC), *H. influenzae* (GPC), Enterobacteriaceae (GNR), *P. aeruginosa* (GNR), *C. neoformans, M. tuberculosis* (AFB), other mycobacteria, *C. immitis, P. marneffei, Rhodococcus equi* (GPR). Neutropenic: *S. aureus* (GPC), *Pseudomonas* sp. (GNR), *Klebsiella* sp., enterobacter (GNR), *Bacteroides* sp. and other oral anaerobes, legionella, candida, aspergillus, mucor. Transplant recipients: CMV (60–70%), *P. aeruginosa* (GNR), *S. aureus* (GPC), *S. pneumoniae* (GPDC), legionella (GNR), RSV, influenza virus, *P. jiroveci*, aspergillus, *P. boydii,* nocardia, strongyloides.	Expectorated sputum for Gram stain and bacterial culture, if purulent. AFB and fungal cultures of respiratory specimens. Sputum induction or bronchiolar lavage for Giemsa or methenamine silver staining or DFA for *P. jiroveci* trophozoites or cysts; for mycobacterial, fungal staining and culture, for legionella culture, and for CMV culture. Nasal washings or swab for viral respiratory direct fluorescent antibody (DFA) and viral culture. Urine for legionella and histoplasma antigen test. Blood for CMV quantitative PCR, or fungal galactomannan antigen test or beta-D-glucan assay for transplant patients. Blood, respiratory specimen, or bone marrow fungal culture for histoplasmosis (positive in 50%), coccidioidomycosis (positive in 30%). Blood culture for bacteria. Blood cultures are more frequently positive in HIV-infected patients with bacterial pneumonia and often are the only source where a specific organism is identified; bacteremic patients have higher mortality rates. Histoplasma urine antigen positive in 90% of AIDS patients with disseminated histoplasmosis. Immunodiffusion is useful for screening for antibodies, and complement fixation for antibody titers for suspected histoplasmosis or coccidioidomycosis. Serum cryptococcal antigen or culture of respiratory specimens when pulmonary cryptococcosis is suspected. Serum lactate dehydrogenase (LDH) levels are elevated in 63% and hypoxemia with exercise (Pa_{O_2} <75 mm Hg) occurs in 57% of PCP cases.	In pneumocystis pneumonia (PCP), the sensitivities of the various diagnostic tests are: sputum induction 80% (in experienced labs), bronchoscopy with lavage 90–97%, transbronchial biopsy 94–97%. In PCP, chest x-ray may show interstitial (36%) or alveolar (25%) infiltrates or may be normal (39%), particularly if leukopenia is present. Recurrent episodes of bacterial pneumonia are common. Kaposi sarcoma of the lung is a common neoplastic process that can imitate infection in homosexual and African HIV-infected patients. Carmona EM et al. Update on the diagnosis and treatment of *Pneumocystis* pneumonia. Ther Adv Respir Dis 2011;5:41. [PMID: 20736243] Catherinot E et al. *Pneumocystis jiroveci* pneumonia. Infect Dis Clin North Am 2010;24:107. [PMID: 20171548] Kasperbauer SH et al. Diagnosis and treatment of infections due to *Mycobacterium avium* complex. Semin Respir Crit Care Med 2008;29:569. [PMID: 18810690] Maddedu G et al. Pneumococcal pneumonia: clinical features, diagnosis and management in HIV-infected and HIV noninfected patients. Curr Opin Pulm Med 2009;15:236. [PMID: 19399965] Shirley RM et al. Cryptococcal lung disease. Curr Opin Pulm Med 2009;15:254. [PMID: 19352182]

LUNG
Mycobacterial pneumonia

Mycobacterial pneumonia

M. tuberculosis (MTb, AFB, acid-fast beaded rods), *M. kansasii, M. avium-intracellulare* complex (MAC), other mycobacteria. (*M. abscessus, M. xenopi, M. fortuitum, M. chelonei*).

Sputum for acid-fast bacilli (AFB; stain and culture. First morning samples are best, and at least three samples are required. Culture systems detect mycobacterial growth in as little as several days to 8 weeks

Bronchoalveolar lavage for AFB stain and culture or gastric washings for AFB culture can be used if sputum tests are negative or unable to obtain sputum (children).

Sputum for amplification assays to detect MTb available for confirmation of smear positive (99%), less sensitive for smear negative (75%). Once AFB has been detected on solid media or in broth culture, nucleic acid hybridization probes or high-performance liquid chromatography can be used to identify the mycobacterial species.

CT- or ultrasound-guided transthoracic fine-needle aspiration cytology can be used if clinical or radiographic features are nonspecific or if malignancy is suspected.

Blood culture for MTb (15%) or MAC.

Pleural fluid culture for MTb (25%).

AFB found on sputum stain do not necessarily make the diagnosis of tuberculosis, because they could represent nonpathogenic mycobacteria.

Tuberculosis is very common in HIV-infected patients, in whom the chest x-ray appearance may be atypical and occasionally (4%) may mimic PCP (especially in patients with CD4 cell counts <200/mcL).

Consider HIV testing if MTb is diagnosed.

Delayed diagnosis of pulmonary tuberculosis is common (up to 20% of cases), especially among patients who are older or who do not have respiratory symptoms.

In any patient with suspected tuberculosis, respiratory isolation is required.

Araújo-Filho JA et al. Extensively drug-resistant tuberculosis: a case report and literature review. Braz J Infect Dis 2008;12:447. [PMID: 19219288]

Schlossberg D. Acute tuberculosis. Infect Dis Clin North Am 2010;24:139. [PMID: 20171549]

Zuckerman JM. Prevention of health care-acquired pneumonia and transmission of *Mycobacterium tuberculosis* in health care settings. Infect Dis Clin North Am 2011;25:117. [PMID: 21315997]

	LUNG	
	Empyema	
Organism	**Specimen/Diagnostic Tests**	**Comments**
Empyema Neonate: *E. coli* (GNR), group A or B streptococcus (GPC), *S. aureus* (GPC), *Pseudomonas* sp. (GNR). Infant/child (<5 years): *S. aureus* (60%) (GPC), *S. pneumoniae* (27%) (GPC), *H. influenzae* (GNCB), anaerobes. Child (>5 years)/adult, acute: *S. pneumoniae* (GPC), group A streptococcus (GPC), *S. aureus* (GPC), *H. influenzae* (GNCB), legionella, coagulase-negative staphylococci, viridans streptococci (GPC in chains). Child (>5 years)/adult, chronic: Anaerobic streptococci, *Bacteroides* sp., *Prevotella* sp., *Porphyromonas* sp., *Fusobacterium* sp. (anaerobes 36–76%), Enterobacteriaceae, *E. coli, Klebsiella pneumoniae, M. tuberculosis, Actinomyces* sp.	Pleural fluid for cell count (WBCs 25,000–100,000/mcL, mostly PMNs), protein >50% of serum), glucose (<serum, often very low), pH (<7.20), LDH (>60% of serum). (See Pleural fluid profiles, Table 8–18.) Blood cultures for bacteria. Sputum for Gram stain and bacterial culture. Special culture can also be performed for legionella when suspected. Pleural fluid for Gram stain and bacterial culture (aerobic and anaerobic).	Chest tube drainage is paramount. The clinical presentation of empyema is nonspecific. Chest CT with contrast is helpful in demonstrating pleural fluid accumulations due to mediastinal or subdiaphragmatic processes and can identify loculated effusions, bronchopleural fistulae, and lung abscesses. 40–60% of empyemas develop following pneumonia. About 25% of cases result from trauma or surgery. Bronchoscopy is indicated when the infection is unexplained. Occasionally, multiple thoracenteses may be needed to diagnose empyema. Clark J. Microbiology and management of pleural empyema. Adv Exp Med Biol 2009;634:61. [PMID: 19280849] Lee SF et al. Thoracic empyema: current opinions in medical and surgical management. Curr Opin Pulm Med 2010;16:194. [PMID: 20224409]

HEART AND VESSELS

Pericarditis

Viruses: Enteroviruses (coxsackie A and B, echovirus), influenza, Epstein-Barr, HSV, mumps, HIV, CMV, varicella-zoster, rubella, hepatitis B.

Bacteria: *S. aureus* (GPC), *S. pneumoniae* (GPC), mycoplasma, *S. pyogenes* (GPC), Enterobacteriaceae (GNR), *N. meningitidis* (GNDC), *N. gonorrhoeae* (GDNC), *Haemophilus* sp., anaerobic bacteria, mycobacteria (HIV and AIDS).

Fungi: *Aspergillus* sp., *Candida* sp., histoplasma, coccidioides, blastomyces, cryptococcus (immunocompromised).

Parasites: *E. histolytica, T. gondii, Schistosoma* sp.

In acute pericarditis, specific bacterial diagnosis is made in only 19%.

Pericardial fluid aspirate for Gram stain and bacterial culture (aerobic and anaerobic). In acute pericarditis, only 54% have pericardial effusions.

Virus isolation from stool or throat can be attempted, but frequently fails to identify the pathogenic agent. PCR may be available in reference laboratories.

Surgical pericardial drainage with biopsy of pericardium for culture (22%) and histologic examination.

Acute and convalescent sera can be tested for antibodies (coxsackie B viruses and other enteroviruses and mycoplasma).

Viral pericarditis is usually diagnosed clinically (precordial pain, muffled heart sounds, pericardial friction rub, cardiomegaly). The diagnosis is rarely aided by microbiologic tests.

CT and MRI may demonstrate pericardial thickening.

Bacterial pericarditis is usually secondary to surgery, immunosuppression (including HIV), esophageal rupture, endocarditis with ruptured ring abscess, extension from lung abscess, aspiration pneumonia or empyema, or sepsis with pericarditis.

Hidron A et al. Cardiac involvement with parasitic infections. Clin Microbiol Rev 2010;23:324. [PMID: 20375355]

Khandaker MH et al. Pericardial disease: diagnosis and management. Mayo Clin Proc 2010;85:572. [PMID: 20511488]

Parikh SV et al. Purulent pericarditis: report of 2 cases and review of the literature. Medicine (Baltimore) 2009;88:52. [PMID: 19352300]

HEART AND VESSELS
Tuberculous pericarditis

Organism	Specimen/Diagnostic Tests	Comments
Tuberculous pericarditis *Mycobacterium tuberculosis* (MTb). MAC, *M. kansasii* (acid-fast beaded rods).	PPD skin testing or interferon-gamma release assays should be performed (negative in a sizable minority). The interferon gamma release assays are unaffected by BCG vaccination. Pericardial fluid obtained by needle aspiration can show AFB by smear (rare) or culture (low yield). Pericardial biopsy for culture and histologic examination for granulomatous inflammation has highest diagnostic yield. Pericardial fluid may show markedly elevated levels of adenosine deaminase. Pericardial fluid for cell count, protein (elevated), PMN (elevated leukocytes).	Major cause of heart disease in Africa and in patients with AIDS. Spread from nearby caseous mediastinal lymph nodes or pleurisy is the most common route of infection. Acutely, serofibrinous pericardial effusion develops with substernal pain, fever, and friction rub. Tamponade may occur. Tuberculosis accounts for 4% of cases of acute pericarditis, 7% of cases of cardiac tamponade, and 6% of cases of constrictive pericarditis. One-third to one-half of patients develop constrictive pericarditis despite drug therapy. Constrictive pericarditis can occur 2–4 years after acute infection. Metaxas EI et al. Tuberculous pericarditis: three cases and brief review. Monaldi Arch Chest Dis 2010;73:44. [PMID: 20499793] Syed FF et al. A modern approach to tuberculous pericarditis. Prog Cardiovasc Dis 2007;50:218. [PMID: 17976506]

HEART AND VESSELS		
Infectious myocarditis		
Infectious myocarditis Viruses: Enteroviruses (especially coxsackie A and B), Epstein-Barr, adenovirus, influenza virus, HIV, CMV. Bacteria: *Borrelia burgdorferi* (Lyme disease), scrub typhus, *Rickettsia rickettsii* (Rocky Mountain spotted fever), *Coxiella burnetii* (Q fever), *Mycoplasma pneumoniae*, *Chlamydophila pneumoniae*, *C. diphtheriae* (GPR). Parasites: *Trichinella spiralis* (trichinosis), *Trypanosoma cruzi* (Chagas disease), *T. gondii*.	Endomyocardial biopsy for pathologic examination, PCR, and culture in selected cases. Indium-111 antimyosin antibody imaging is more sensitive than endomyocardial biopsy. MRI techniques are improving. Stool or throat swab for enterovirus culture. Acute and convalescent sera for coxsackie B, *M. pneumoniae*, *C. pneumoniae*, scrub typhus, *R rickettsii*, *C. burnetii*; toxoplasma. Serum for antibodies against HIV, *B. burgdorferi*.	In most cases, no definitive cause is established. Viruses are most important infectious causes in U.S. and western Europe. Acute infectious myocarditis should be suspected in a patient with dynamically evolving changes in ECG, echocardiography, and serum CK levels and symptoms of an infection. The value of endomyocardial biopsy in such cases has not been established. In contrast, an endomyocardial biopsy is needed to diagnose lymphocytic inflammatory response with necrosis or giant cell myocarditis. The incidence of myocarditis in AIDS may be as high as 46%. Many patients with acute myocarditis progress to dilated cardiomyopathy. Andréoletti L et al. Viral causes of human myocarditis. Arch Cardiovasc Dis 2009;102:559. [PMID: 19664576] Blauwet LA et al. Myocarditis. Prog Cardiovasc Dis 2010;52:274. [PMID: 20109598] Durani Y et al. Myocarditis and pericarditis in children. Pediatr Clin North Am 2010;57:1281. [PMID: 21111118] Kühl U et al. Viral myocarditis: diagnosis, aetiology and management. Drugs 2009;69:1287. [PMID: 19563449] Schultz JC et al. Diagnosis and treatment of viral myocarditis. Mayo Clin Proc 2009;84:1001. [PMID: 19880690]

	HEART AND VESSELS
	Infective endocarditis

Organism	Specimen/Diagnostic Tests	Comments
Infective endocarditis *S. aureus* (GPC), coagulase-negative staphylococci (GPC), viridans group streptococci (GPC in chains), enterococci (GPC), *Abiotrophia* sp., nutritionally deficient streptococcus (GPC), other β-hemolytic streptococci (GPC), *Erysipelothrix rhusiopathiae* (GPR), brucella (GVCB), other gram-negative bacilli, *Coxiella burnetii*, *C. pneumoniae*, bartonella, yeast. Slow-growing fastidious GNRs: HACEK (*H. aphrophilus*, *Aggregatibacter actinomycetemcomitans*, *Cardiobacterium hominis*, *Eikenella corrodens*, *Kingella kingae*).	Blood cultures for bacteria are positive in 97%, if two to three sets are drawn from peripheral venous sites and before start of antibiotic therapy. Blood cultures are frequently positive with gram-positive organisms but can be negative (5%) with gram-negative or anaerobic organisms, fungi, HACEK, and organisms that grow slowly. Request that the laboratory hold blood cultures 10–14 days to detect slow-growing organisms. Echocardiography can identify valvular vegetations in 50% of cases. Transesophageal echocardiography (TEE) can help in diagnosis by demonstrating the presence of valvular vegetations (sensitivity >90%), prosthetic valve dysfunction, valvular regurgitation, secondary "jet" or "kissing" lesions, and paravalvular abscess. TEE has greater sensitivity than transthoracic echocardiography (TTE) (see Chapter 7).	Patients with congenital or valvular heart disease, or prosthetic valves should receive prophylaxis before dental procedures or surgery of the upper respiratory, genitourinary, or gastrointestinal tract. In left-sided endocarditis, patients should be watched carefully for development of valvular regurgitation or ring abscess. The size and mobility of valvular vegetations on TEE can help to predict the risk of arterial embolization. Streptococci account for 60–80% of cases and currently *S. aureus* and coagulase negative staphylococci account for 20–35% of infectious endocarditis cases. Fungi (2–4%) and mixed infections (1–2%) can also be etiologic agents. Almost any structural heart disease can predispose to infectious endocarditis, especially if there is increased turbulence of blood flow. Prosthetic valve endocarditis and intravascular infections due to cardiac devices (pacemakers, defibrillators) have been increasing. Ansari A et al. Infective endocarditis: an update on the role of echocardiography. Curr Cardiol Rep 2010;12:265. [PMID: 20424971] Boumis E et al; GISIG (Gruppo Italiano di Studio sulle Infezioni Gravi) Working Group on Bloodstream Infections and Endocarditis. Consensus document on controversial issues in the diagnosis and treatment of bloodstream infections and endocarditis. Int J Infect Dis 2010;14 (Suppl 4):S23. [PMID: 20843723] Brook I. Infective endocarditis caused by anaerobic bacteria. Arch Cardiovasc Dis 2008;101:665–76. [PMID: 19056073] Fitzsimmons K et al. Infective endocarditis: changing aetiology of disease. Br J Biomed Sci 2010;67:35. [PMID: 20373682] Herregods MC et al. Infective endocarditis. Acta Clin Belg 2008;63:414. [PMID: 19170360] Kern WV. Management of *Staphylococcus aureus* bacteremia and endocarditis: progresses and challenges. Curr Opin Infect Dis 2010;23:346. [PMID: 20592532] McDonald JR. Acute infective endocarditis. Infect Dis Clin North Am 2009;23:643. [PMID: 19665088] Luttenberger K et al. Subacute bacterial endocarditis: making the diagnosis. Nurse Pract 2011 Mar;36(3):31. [PMID: 21325924] McDonald JR. Acute infective endocarditis. Infect Dis Clin North Am 2009;23:643. [PMID: 19665088] Nataloni M et al. Prosthetic valve endocarditis. J Cardiovasc Med (Hagerstown) 2010;11:869. [PMID: 20154632]

HEART AND VESSELS

Infectious thrombophlebitis

Infectious thrombophlebitis

Associated with venous catheters: *S. aureus* (GPC) (65–78%), coagulase-negative staphylococci (GPC), *Candida* sp. (yeast), *Pseudomonas* sp. (GNR), Enterobacteriaceae (GNR), streptococci (GPC), enterococci (GPC), anaerobes.

Hyperalimentation with catheter: *Candida* sp., *Malassezia furfur* (yeast).

Indwelling venous catheter (eg, Broviac, Hickman): *S. aureus*, coagulase-negative staphylococci, diphtheroids (GPR), *Pseudomonas* sp., Enterobacteriaceae, *Candida* sp.

Postpartum or postabortion pelvic thrombophlebitis: Bacteroides (GNR), Enterobacteriaceae, clostridium (GPR), streptococcus (GPC).

Blood cultures for bacteria are positive in 97%, if three sets are drawn from peripheral venous sites and before start of antibiotic therapy. Catheter tip for bacterial culture to document etiology. More than 15 colonies (CFUs) suggests colonization or infection.

CT and MRI are the studies of choice in the evaluation of puerperal septic pelvic thrombophlebitis.

Thrombophlebitis is an inflammation of the vein wall. Infectious thrombophlebitis with microbial invasion of the vessel is associated with bacteremia and thrombosis.

Risk of infection from an indwelling peripheral venous catheter goes up significantly after 4 days.

Liu WC et al. Extended septic thrombophlebitis in a patient with duplicated inferior vena cava: case report and review of literature. Int Angiol 2009;28:156. [PMID: 19174747]

Nezhat C et al. Septic pelvic thrombophlebitis following laparoscopic hysterectomy. JSLS 2009;13:84. [PMID: 19366549]

Schifferdecker B et al. Endovascular treatment of septic thrombophlebitis: a case report of a rare complication and review of the literature. Vasc Med 2009;14:47. [PMID: 19144779]

	ABDOMEN	

Organism	Specimen/Diagnostic Tests	Comments
Gastritis *Helicobacter pylori*.	Serum for antibody test (76–90% sensitivity but low specificity). Stool for antigen detection test (90%) and can be used to monitor therapeutic effect. [^{13}C] and [^{14}C] urea breath test (99%) are specific, relatively noninvasive tests. Gastric mucosal biopsy for rapid urea test (90%), culture (89%), histology (92%).	Also associated with duodenal ulcer, gastric carcinoma, and gastroesophageal reflux disease. Proton pump inhibitors may cause false-negative urea breath tests and fecal antigen tests, and should be withheld for at least 7 days before testing. de Vries AC, Kuipers EJ. *Helicobacter pylori* infection and non-malignant diseases. Helicobacter 2010;15(Suppl 1):29. [PMID: 21054650] Genta RM et al. *Helicobacter pylori*-negative gastritis: seek, yet ye shall not always find. Am J Surg Pathol 2010;34:e25. [PMID: 20631607] Tan VP et al. *Helicobacter pylori* and gastritis: Untangling a complex relationship 27 years on. J Gastroenterol Hepatol 2011;26 (Suppl 1):42. [PMID: 21199513]
Infectious esophagitis *Candida* sp. (yeast), HSV, CMV,HIV (Rare causes: *M. tuberculosis* [AFB], MAC, cryptosporidium, histoplasma, VZV, Epstein-Barr).	Rule out noninfectious causes of esophagitis, especially gastroesophageal reflux. Barium esophagram reveals abnormalities in the majority of cases of candidal esophagitis. Endoscopy with biopsy and brushings for culture and cytology has the highest diagnostic yield (57%) and should be performed if clinically indicated or if empiric antifungal therapy is unsuccessful.	Thrush (25%) and odynophagia (50%) in an immunocompromised patient warrant empiric therapy for candida. Factors predisposing to infectious esophagitis include HIV infection, exposure to radiation, cytotoxic chemotherapy, recent antibiotic therapy, corticosteroid therapy, and neutropenia. Baroco AL et al. Gastrointestinal cytomegalovirus disease in the immunocompromised patient. Curr Gastroenterol Rep 2008;10:409. [PMID: 18627655] Canalejo Castrillero E et al. Herpes esophagitis in healthy adults and adolescents: report of 3 cases and review of the literature. Medicine (Baltimore) 2010;89:204. [PMID: 20616659]

ABDOMEN
Infectious colitis/dysentery

Infectious colitis/dysentery

Infant: E. coli (enteropathogenic), rotavirus. Child/adult without travel, afebrile, diarrhea with no gross blood or WBCs in stool: Rotavirus, norovirus and other caliciviruses, E. coli (GNR).

Child/adult with acute watery diarrhea, low-grade fever: E. coli (GNR) (enterotoxigenic (ETEC), enteroinvasive (EIEC), Clostridium difficile (GPR), norovirus.

Child/adult with fever and dysentery (WBC in stool): E. coli (EIEC), shigella (GNR), Campylobacter sp. (GNR)

Child/Adult with diarrhea, bloody stool or history of travel to subtropics/tropics (or Western Europe in 2011) (varies with epidemiology): E. coli (GNR), enterohemorrhagic (EHEC, 0157:H7, STEC 0104:H4), and other shiga-toxin-producing E. coli serotypes).

Other causes of acute diarrhea: salmonella (GNR), Yersinia enterocolitica (GNR), aeromonas (GNR), plesiomonas (GNR), vibrio (GNR), cryptosporidium, Entamoeba histolytica, Giardia lamblia, cyclospora, strongyloides, microsporidia (in HIV infection).

Child/adult with diarrhea and vomiting: E. coli (EPEC, enteropathogenic), norovirus.

Stool cultures routinely done for salmonella, shigella, and campylobacter.

Special stool culture techniques are needed for detection of yersinia, E. coli 0157:H7, vibrio, aeromonas, plesiomonas.

Stool cultures for salmonella, shigella, and campylobacter are not helpful for patients who have been hospitalized for >3 days.

Sensitivity of stool culture is 72%, but its specificity is 100%.

For patients who have been hospitalized for >3 days, test for toxigenic C. difficile or its toxins.

Stool ova and parasite exam or antigen EIAs (minimum 3 stool specimens over 10 days) for detection of parasites.

Modified trichrome stain for microsporidia.

Shiga toxin EIA for suspected enterohemorrhagic E. coli infection.

RT-PCR on stool for diagnosis of norovirus infection. Highly contagious.

Proctosigmoidoscopy is indicated in patients with chronic or recurrent diarrhea or in diarrhea of unknown cause for smears of aspirates and biopsy. Culture of a biopsy specimen has a slightly higher sensitivity than routine stool culture.

Obtain rectal and jejunal biopsies on HIV-infected patients, culture for bacterial pathogens and Mycobacteria (eg, MAC), and perform modified acid-fast stains for cryptosporidium, isospora, and cyclospora.

Acute dysentery is diarrhea with bloody, mucoid stools, tenesmus, and pain on defecation and implies an inflammatory invasion of the colonic mucosa. BUN and serum electrolytes may be indicated for supportive care. Severe dehydration is a medical emergency.

Necrotizing enterocolitis is a fulminant disease of premature newborns; cause is unknown, but human breast milk is protective. Air in the intestinal wall (pneumatosis intestinalis), in the portal venous system, or in the peritoneal cavity seen on plain x-ray can confirm diagnosis. 30–50% of these infants will have bacteremia or peritonitis.

Risk factors for infectious colitis include poor hygiene and immune compromise (infancy, advanced age, corticosteroid or immunosuppressive therapy, HIV infection).

The 2011 outbreak of E. coli 0104 (STEC 0104:H4) originated from Germany and caused > 800 cases of hemolytic–uremic syndrome (HUS) and > 30 deaths.

DuPont HL. Clinical practice. Bacterial diarrhea. N Engl J Med 2009;361:1560. [PMID: 19828533]

Frank C et al; HUS Investigation Team. Epidemic profile of Shiga-toxin-producing Escherichia coli 0104:H4 outbreak in Germany—preliminary report. N Engl J Med 2011;365(19):1771-80. [PMID: 21696328]

Hansen R et al. The role of infection in the aetiology of inflammatory bowel disease. J Gastroenterol 2010;45:266. [PMID: 20076977]

Holtz LR et al. Acute bloody diarrhea: a medical emergency for patients of all ages. Gastroenterology 2009;136:1887. [PMID: 19457417]

Pawlowski SW et al. Diagnosis and treatment of acute or persistent diarrhea. Gastroenterology 2009;136:1874. [PMID: 19457416]

	ABDOMEN
	Antibiotic-associated colitis

Organism	Specimen/Diagnostic Tests	Comments
Antibiotic-associated pseudomembranous colitis *Clostridium difficile* (GPR) (90%), *Clostridium perfringens* (GPR) (8%), *Candida albicans* (yeast) in elderly, hospitalized patients.	*C. difficile* produces two toxins: Toxin A is an enterotoxin and toxin B is a cytotoxin. Send stool for detection of *C. difficile* cytotoxin B by tissue culture (test takes >48 hours with sensitivity 60–80%, specificity 99%). Stool for rapid EIA to detect toxin A or toxin A and B takes only 2–4 hours (sensitivity 70–90%, specificity 99%), but these assays are no longer recommended for primary testing. New molecular assays (>90% sensitive) that detect the gene for toxin B are more sensitive and specific and can give rapid results to aid in patient contact isolation procedures. Test only one watery stool specimen and do not repeat testing unless relapse infection is suspected. Colonoscopy and visualization of characteristic 1–5 mm raised yellow plaques provides a definitive diagnosis. Antibiotic-associated diarrhea may include uncomplicated diarrhea, colitis, or pseudomembranous colitis. Only 10–20% of cases are caused by infection with *C. difficile*. Most clinically mild cases are due to functional disturbances of intestinal carbohydrate or bile acid metabolism, to allergic and toxic effects of antibiotics on intestinal mucosa, or to their pharmacologic effects on motility.	Antibiotics cause changes in normal intestinal flora, allowing overgrowth of *C. difficile* and elaboration of toxins. Other risk factors for *C. difficile*-induced colitis are GI manipulations, advanced age, female sex, inflammatory bowel disease, HIV, chemotherapy, and renal disease. Other risk factors for *C. difficile*-induced colitis are GI manipulations, advanced age, female sex, inflammatory bowel disease, HIV, chemotherapy, and renal disease. Over the past 10 years, the incidence of *C. difficile* disease has increased and the disease has become more severe. *C. difficile* nosocomial infection can be controlled by hand washing. Note that alcohol gels do not kill *C. difficile* spores on hands or in the environment. Calls for increased control of antibiotic usage, use of new molecular assays and tighter infection control practices have been put forward to prevent spread and outbreaks of *C. difficile* disease. Adams SD et al. Fulminant *Clostridium difficile* colitis. Curr Opin Crit Care 2007;13:450. [PMID: 17599017] Bartlett JG et al. Clinical recognition and diagnosis of *Clostridium difficile* infection. Clin Infect Dis 2008;46(Suppl 1):S12. [PMID: 18177217] Blondeau JM. What have we learned about antimicrobial use and the risks for *Clostridium difficile*-associated diarrhea? J Antimicrob Chemother 2009;63: 238. [PMID: 19028718] Clements AC et al. *Clostridium difficile* PCR ribotype 027: assessing the risks of further worldwide spread. Lancet Infect Dis 2010;10:395. [PMID: 20510280]

ABDOMEN
Diarrhea in HIV

Diarrhea in the HIV-infected host

Same as child-adult infectious colitis with addition of CMV, adenovirus, cryptosporidium, *Isospora belli*, microsporidia (*Enterocytozoon bieneusi* and *E. intestinalis*), *C. difficile*, *Giardia intestinalis*, *M. avium-intracellulare* complex (MAC, [AFB]), HSV, *Entamoeba histolytica*, *Balantidium coli*, *Sarcocystis* sp.

Stool for culture (especially for salmonella, shigella, yersinia, and campylobacter), *C. difficile* tissue culture or molecular assays, ova and parasite examination. Multiple samples are often needed. Proctosigmoidoscopy with fluio espiration and biopsy is indicated in patients with chronic or recurrent diarrhea or in diarrhea of unknown cause for smears of aspirates (may show organisms) and histologic examination and culture of tissue. Rectal and jejunal biopsies may be necessary, especially in patients with tenesmus or bloody stools. Need modified acid-fast stain for cryptosporidium, isospora, and cyclospora. Intranuclear inclusion bodies on histologic examination suggest CMV. Immunodiagnosis of giardia, cryptosporidium, and *E. histolytica* cysts in stool is highly sensitive and specific.

Most patients with HIV infection develop diarrhea at some point, which can be difficult to diagnose and treat. Antiretroviral therapy decreases disease incidence.

Cryptosporidium causes a chronic debilitating diarrheal infection that rarely remits spontaneously and is still without effective treatment. Diarrhea seems to be the result of malabsorption and produces a cholera-like syndrome.

Between 15% and 50% of HIV-infected patients with diarrhea have no identifiable pathogen.

Derouin F et al. Treatment of parasitic diarrhea in HIV-infected patients. Expert Rev Anti Infect Ther 2008;6:337. [PMID: 18588498]

Hwi A et al. Risk factors for gastrointestinal adverse events in HIV treated and untreated patients. AIDS Rev 2009;11:30. [PMID: 19290032]

	ABDOMEN
	Peritonitis

Organism	Specimen/Diagnostic Tests	Comments
Peritonitis Primary or spontaneous (associated with nephrosis or cirrhosis) (SBP): Enterobacteriaceae (GNR) (69%), enterococci (GPC), *S. viridans* streptococci (GPC in chains), *S. pneumoniae* (GPC), group A streptococcus (GPC), *S. aureus* (GPC), anaerobes (5%). Secondary (bowel perforation, hospital acquired, or antecedent antibiotic therapy): Enterobacteriaceae, enterococcus (GPC), *Bacteroides fragilis* group (GNR), *Pseudomonas aeruginosa* (GNR) (3–15%). Chronic ambulatory peritoneal dialysis (CAPD): Coagulase-negative staphylococci (GPC) (43%), *S. aureus* (14%), *Streptococcus* sp. (12%), Enterobacteriaceae (14%), *Pseudomonas aeruginosa*, *Corynebacterium* sp. (GPR), candida (2%), aspergillus (rare), cryptococcus (rare).	Peritoneal fluid sent for WBC (>1000/mcL in SPB, >100/mcL in CAPD) with PMN (>250/mcL in SBP and secondary peritonitis, 50% PMN in CAPD); total protein (>1 g/dL); glucose (<0 mg/dL), and LDH (<225 units/mL) in secondary; pH (<7.35 in 57% of SBP). Gram stain (sensitivity 22–77% for SBP); submit large volumes of peritoneal fluid for bacterial culture. (See Ascitic fluid profiles, Table 8–5.) Blood cultures for bacteria positive in 85% of SBP cases. Catheter-related infection is associated with a WBC >500/mcL.	In nephrotic patients, Enterobacteriaceae and *S. aureus* are most common. In cirrhotics, 69% of cases are due to Enterobacteriaceae. Cirrhotic patients (40%) with low ascitic fluid protein levels (≤1 g/dL) and high bilirubin level or low platelet count are at high risk of developing spontaneous bacterial peritonitis. "Bacterascites," a positive ascitic fluid culture without an elevated PMN count, is seen in 8% of cases of SBP and probably represents early infection. Neurocytic ascites can have a negative culture in 10–30% of cases. In secondary peritonitis, factors influencing the incidence of postoperative complications and death include age, presence of certain concomitant diseases, site of origin of peritonitis, type of admission, and the ability of the surgeon to eliminate the source of infection (appendicitis [with or without rupture], diverticulitis, perforated ulcer, perforated gallbladder). Cardenas A et al. What's new in the treatment of ascites and spontaneous bacterial peritonitis. Curr Gastroenterol Rep 2008;10:7. [PMID: 18417037] Emmi V et al. Clinical diagnosis of intra-abdominal infections. J Chemother 2009;21(Suppl 1):12. [PMID: 19622446] Mazuski JE et al. Intra-abdominal infections. Surg Clin North Am 2009;89:421. [PMID: 19281892]

ABDOMEN
Tuberculous peritonitis/enterocolitis

Tuberculous peritonitis/ enterocolitis *Mycobacterium tuberculosis* (MTb, AFB, acid-fast beaded rods).	Ascitic fluid for appearance (clear, hemorrhagic, or chylous), RBCs (can be high), WBCs (>1000/mcL, >71% lymphs) protein (>3.5 g/dL), serum/ascites albumin gradient (SAAG) (<1.1), LDH (>90 units/L), AFB culture (<50% positive). (See Ascitic fluid profiles, Table 8–5.) With coexistent chronic liver disease, protein level and SAAG are usually not helpful, but LDH >90 units/L is a useful predictor. Culture or AFB smear from other sources (especially from respiratory tract) can help confirm diagnosis. Abdominal ultrasound may demonstrate free or loculated intra-abdominal fluid, intra-abdominal abscess, ileocecal mass, and retroperitoneal lymphadenopathy. Ascites with fine, mobile septations shown by ultrasound and peritoneal and omental thickening detected by CT strongly suggest tuberculous peritonitis. Marked elevations of serum CA 125 have been noted; levels decline to normal with antituberculous therapy. Diagnosis of enterocolitis rests on biopsy of colonic lesions via endoscopy if pulmonary or other extrapulmonary infection cannot be documented. Diagnosis is best confirmed by laparoscopy with peritoneal biopsy and culture. Operative procedure may be needed to relieve obstruction or for diagnosis.	Infection of the intestines can occur anywhere along the GI tract but occurs most frequently in the ileocecal area or mesenteric lymph nodes. It often complicates pulmonary infection. Peritoneal infection usually is an extension of intestinal disease. Symptoms may be minimal even with extensive disease. In the United States, 29% of patients with abdominal tuberculosis have a normal chest x-ray. Presence of AFB in the feces does not correlate with intestinal involvement. Akpolat T. Tuberculous peritonitis. Perit Dial Int 2009;29(Suppl 2):S166. [PMID: 19270209] Emmi V et al. Clinical diagnosis of intra-abdominal infections. J Chemother 2009;21(Suppl 1):12. [PMID: 19622446] Jacob JT et al. Acute forms of tuberculosis in adults. Am J Med 2009;122:12. [PMID: 19114163] Rosselli S et al. Peritoneal tuberculosis: modern peril for an ancient disease. South Med J 2009;102:57. [PMID: 19077748]

	ABDOMEN
	Diverticulitis

Organism	Specimen/Diagnostic Tests	Comments
Diverticulitis Polymicrobial Enterobacteriaceae (GNR), *Bacteroides* sp. (GNR), Peptostreptococcus (GPC), enterococcus (GPC in chains), viridans streptococci (GPC in chains).	Identification of organism is not usually sought. Ultrasonography or flat and upright x-rays of abdomen can rule out perforation (free air under diaphragm) and localize abscess (air-fluid collections). CT is the diagnostic procedure of choice. CT-guided percutaneous drainage of abscesses can be performed.	Pain usually is localized to the left lower quadrant because the sigmoid and descending colon are the most common sites for diverticula. Fever, nausea, vomiting and changes in bowel habits may be present. It is important to rule out other abdominal disease (eg, colon carcinoma, Crohn disease, ischemic colitis, *C. difficile*-associated colitis, appendicitis), and gynecologic disorders (eg, ectopic pregnancy, ovarian cyst, or torsion). Hall J et al. New paradigms in the management of diverticular disease. Curr Probl Surg 2010;47:680. [PMID: 20684920] Hemming J et al. Features and management of colonic diverticular disease. Curr Gastroenterol Rep 2010;12:399. [PMID: 20694839] Spirt MJ. Complicated intra-abdominal infections: a focus on appendicitis and diverticulitis. Postgrad Med 2010;122:39. [PMID: 20107288]

ABDOMEN		
Liver abscess		
Liver abscess		
Usually polymicrobial: Enterobacteriaceae, especially *E. coli, Enterobacter* sp., *Proteus* sp., *Klebsiella* sp. (GNR), enterococcus (GPC in chains), *Bacteroides* sp. (GNR), actinomyces (GPR), *S. aureus* (GPC) (MRSA), viridans streptococci (GPC), *Candida* sp., *Entamoeba histolytica*.	CT scan with contrast and ultrasonography are the most accurate tests for the diagnosis of liver abscess. An antibody test against *E. histolytica* (95%) should be obtained on all patients (see Amebic serology, Chapter 3). Uncomplicated amebic liver abscesses can be treated medically without drainage. *E. histolytica* invades the intestinal wall and it can be carried to the liver by the blood where it may produce abscesses. Complete removal of abscess material obtained via surgery or percutaneous aspiration is recommended for large abscesses and for culture and direct examination to distinguish pyogenic abscess from *E. histolytica* abscess. Complications of drainage or removal of *E. histolytica* abscess are rupture of an echinococcal cyst, amebic peritonitis, and death.	Travel to and origin in an endemic area are important risk factors for amebic liver abscess. 60% of patients have a single lesion; 40% have multiple lesions. Biliary tract disease is the most common underlying disease, accounting for 40–60% of cases, followed by malignancy (biliary tract or pancreatic), colonic disease (diverticulitis), diabetes mellitus, liver disease, and alcoholism. In mid-1980s, a syndrome of monomicrobial *K. pneumonia* pyogenic liver abscess, often in diabetics, was described in Taiwan. Infections were caused by hypermucoid strains of *K. pneumonia* of capsular K1 serotype. This is now a major health problem in Asia. Fang CT et al. *Klebsiella pneumonia* genotype K1: an emerging pathogen that causes septic ocular or central nervous system complications from pyogenic liver abscess. Clin Infect Dis 2007;45:284. [PMID: 17599305] Santi-Rocca J et al. Host-microbe interactions and defense mechanisms in the development of amoebic liver abscesses. Clin Microbiol Rev 2009;22:65. [PMID: 19136434]

	ABDOMEN
	Cholangitis/cholecystitis

Organism	Specimen/Diagnostic Tests	Comments
Cholangitis/cholecystitis Enterobacteriaceae (GNR) (68%), enterococcus (GPC in chains) (14%), *Pseudomonas aeruginosa* (GNR), bacteroides (GNR) (10%), *Clostridium* sp. (GPR) (7%), fusobacterium, *M. avium-intracellulare* complex (MAC) in AIDS patients. Parasites: microsporidia (*Enterocytozoon bieneusi*) cryptosporidia, *Ascaris lumbricoides, Opisthorchis viverrini, O. felineus, Clonorchis sinensis, Fasciola hepatica, Echinococcus granulosus, E. multilocularis.* Viruses: CMV in AIDS.	Ultrasonography is the best test to quickly demonstrate gallstones or phlegmon around the gallbladder or dilation of the biliary tree. (See Abdominal Ultrasound, Chapter 6.) CT scanning is useful in cholangitis in detecting the site and cause of obstruction. (See Abdominal CT, Chapter 6.) Blood cultures for bacteria. WBC elevated (12,000–15,000 per mcL). Serum total bilirubin elevated (1–4 mg/dL). Serum aminotransferase and alkaline phosphatase may be elevated.	90% of cases of acute cholecystitis are calculous, 10% are acalculous. Risk factors for acalculous disease include prolonged illness, trauma, burns, sepsis, immunosuppression, diabetes mellitus, HIV infection, and carcinoma of the gallbladder or bile ducts. Biliary obstruction and cholangitis (inflammation or infection of common bile duct) can develop before biliary dilation is detected. Common bile duct obstruction secondary to tumor or pancreatitis seldom results in infection (0–15%). In the era of potent antiretroviral therapy, AIDS cholangiopathy is now rare. Most common pathogen in cholangitis in AIDS is cryptosporidium. De Angelis C et al. An update on AIDS-related cholangiopathy. Minerva Gastroenterol Dietol 2009;55:79. [PMID: 19212310] Julka K et al. Infectious diseases and the gallbladder. Infect Dis Clin North Am 2010;24:885. [PMID: 20937456] Lee JG. Diagnosis and management of acute cholangitis. Nat Rev Gastroenterol Hepatol 2009;6:533. [PMID: 19652653]

GENITOURINARY		
Urinary tract infection		
Urinary tract infection (UTI)/ cystitis/pyuria-dysuria syndrome Enterobacteriaceae (GNR, especially *E. coli* [80%]), *Chlamydia trachomatis*, *Staphylococcus saprophyticus* (GPC) (in young women), enterococcus (GPC), group B streptococci (GPC), *Candida* sp. (yeast), *N. gonorrhoeae* (GNCB), *Corynebacterium urealyticum* (GPR), *Ureaplasma urealyticum* (GPR), HSV, adenovirus.	Urinalysis and culture reveal the two most important signs: bacteriuria and pyuria (>10 WBCs/mcL). 30% of patients have hematuria. Cystitis (95%) is diagnosed by >10^2 CFU/mL of bacteria; other urinary infections (90%) by >10^5 CFU/mL. Culture is generally not necessary for uncomplicated cystitis in women. Combination of current symptoms (eg, dysuria, frequency, and hematuria) and prior history yields a >90% probability of UTI. However, pregnant women should be screened for asymptomatic bacteriuria and promptly treated. Both Gram stain for bacteria and dipstick analysis for nitrite and leukocyte esterase perform similarly in detecting UTI in children and are superior to microscopic analysis for pyuria. Nitrite or leukocyte esterase may be negative in 19% of patients with bacteremia due to enterococci and staphylococci. DNA amplification tests for chlamydia and gonorrhea are available.	Most men with UTIs have a functional or anatomic genitourinary abnormality. In catheter-related UTI, cure is unlikely unless the catheter is removed. In asymptomatic catheter-related UTI, antibiotics should be given only if patients are at risk for sepsis (old age, underlying disease, diabetes mellitus, pregnancy). Up to one-third of cases of acute cystitis have "silent" upper tract involvement. Bader MS et al. Management of complicated urinary tract infections in the era of antimicrobial resistance. Postgrad Med 2010;122:7. [PMID: 21084776] Chenoweth CE et al. Urinary tract infections. Infect Dis Clin North Am 2011;25:103. [PMID: 21315996] Dielubanza EJ et al. Urinary tract infections in women. Med Clin North Am 2011;95:27. [PMID: 21095409] Larcombe J. Urinary tract infection in children. Am Fam Physician 2010;82:1252. [PMID: 21121537]

	GENITOURINARY
	Prostatitis

Organism	Specimen/Diagnostic Tests	Comments
Prostatitis Acute and chronic: *E. coli* (80%) (GNR), other Enterobacteriaceae (GNR), *Pseudomonas* sp. (GNR), enterococci (GPC in chains), CMV, *Staphylococcus* sp. (GPC), chlamydiae, mycoplasma, ureaplasma. HIV: *M. tuberculosis*, *Candida* sp., coccidioides, cryptococcus, histoplasma.	Urinalysis shows pyuria, bacteriuria, and hematuria (variable). Urine culture usually identifies causative organism. Prostatic massage is useful in chronic prostatitis to retrieve organisms but is contraindicated in acute prostatitis (it may cause bacteremia). Bacteriuria is first cleared by antibiotic treatment. Then urine cultures are obtained from first-void, bladder, and postprostatic massage urine specimens. A higher organism count in the postprostatic massage specimen localizes infection to the prostate (91%) (Meares-Stamey 3-glass test).	Acute prostatitis is a severe illness characterized by fever, dysuria, and a boggy or tender prostate. Chronic prostatitis often has no symptoms of dysuria, but may present with perineal or pelvic pain and discomfort. Nonbacterial prostatitis (prostatodynia) represents 90% of prostatitis cases. Its cause is unknown, although chlamydia antigen can be found in up to 25% of patients. Anothaisintawee T et al. Management of chronic prostatitis/chronic pelvic pain syndrome: a systematic review and network meta-analysis. JAMA 2011;305:78. [PMID: 21205969] Sharp VJ et al. Prostatitis: diagnosis and treatment. Am Fam Physician 2010;82:397. [PMID: 20704171] Touma NJ et al. Prostatitis and chronic pelvic pain syndrome in men. Med Clin North Am 2011;95:75. [PMID: 21095412]

	GENITOURINARY	
	Pyelonephritis	
Organism	**Specimen/Diagnostic Tests**	**Comments**
Pyelonephritis	Urine culture is indicated when pyelonephritis is suspected. Urinalysis will usually show pyuria (>5 WBC/hpf) and may show WBC casts. Blood cultures for bacteria if sepsis is suspected. In uncomplicated pyelonephritis, ultrasonography is not necessary. In severe cases, however, ultrasound is the optimal procedure for ruling out urinary tract obstruction, pyonephrosis, and calculi. Doppler ultrasonography (88%) has a specificity of 100% for acute pyelonephritis.	Patients usually present with fever, chills, nausea, vomiting, and costovertebral angle tenderness. 20–30% of pregnant women with untreated bacteriuria develop pyelonephritis. Abreu DA et al. Retroperitoneal infections by community acquired methicillin resistant *Staphylococcus aureus.* J Urol 2008;179:172. [PMID: 18001799] Gupta K et al; Infectious Diseases Society of America; European Society for Microbiology and Infectious Diseases: International clinical practice guidelines for the treatment of acute uncomplicated cystitis and pyelonephritis in women: a 2010 update. Clin Infect Dis 2011;52:e103. [PMID: 21292654] Litza JA et al. Urinary tract infections. Prim Care 2010;37:491. [PMID: 20705195] Nicolle LE. Uncomplicated urinary tract infection in adults including uncomplicated pyelonephritis. Urol Clin North Am 2008;35:1. [PMID: 18061019]
Acute, uncomplicated (usually young women): Enterobacteriaceae (especially *E. coli*) (GNR), enterococci (GPC in chains), *Staphylococcus saprophyticus* (GPC), *S. aureus* (GPC). Complicated (older women, men; postcatheterization, obstruction, post-renal transplant): Enterobacteriaceae (especially *E. coli*), *Pseudomonas aeruginosa* (GNR), enterococcus (GPC), *S. aureus* (GPC).		

	GENITOURINARY
	Perinephric abscess

Organism	Specimen/Diagnostic Tests	Comments
Perinephric abscess Associated with staphylococcal bacteremia: *S. aureus* (GPC). Associated with pyelonephritis: Enterobacteriaceae (GNR), *Candida* sp. (yeast), coagulase-negative staphylococci (GPC).	CT scan with contrast is more sensitive than ultrasound in imaging abscess and confirming diagnosis. (See Abdominal CT, Chapter 6.) Plain films of abdomen and ultrasonography can detect stones and abscesses. Urinalysis may be normal or may show pyuria. Urine culture (positive in 60–72%). Blood cultures for bacteria (positive in 20–40%). Bacterial culture of abscess fluid via needle aspiration or drainage (percutaneous or surgical).	Uncommon complication of urinary tract infection. Predisposing factors are urinary tract calculi and diabetes mellitus. Most perinephric abscesses are the result of extension of an ascending urinary tract infection. Often they are very difficult to diagnose. Perinephric abscesses should be considered in patients who fail to respond to antibiotic therapy, in patients with anatomic abnormalities of the urinary tract, and in patients with diabetes mellitus. Baradkar VP et al. Renal and perinephric abscess due to *Staphylococcus aureus*. Indian J Pathol Microbiol 2009;52:440. [PMID: 19679989] Gardiner RA et al. Perinephric abscess. BJU Int 2011;107(Suppl 3):20. [PMID: 21492371] Malik ZA et al. Perinephric abscess caused by community-acquired methicillin resistant *Staphylococcus aureus*. Pediatr Infect Dis J 2007;26:764. [PMID: 17846900] Wani NA et al. Perinephric abscess caused by ruptured retrocecal appendix: MDCT demonstration. Urol Ann 2010;2:29. [PMID: 20842255]

GENITOURINARY		
Urethritis		
Urethritis (gonococcal and nongonococcal) Gonococcal (GC): *Neisseria gonorrhoeae* (GNDC). Nongonococcal (NGU): *Chlamydia trachomatis* (50%), *Ureaplasma urealyticum*, *Trichomonas vaginalis*, HSV, *Mycoplasma genitalium*, adenoviruses, *Gardnerella vaginalis*.	Urethral discharge collected with urethral swab usually shows >4 WBCs per oil-immersion field; Gram stain (identify gonococcal organisms as gram-negative intracellular diplococci), PMNs (in GC urethritis, >95% of WBCs are PMNs; in NGU usually <80% are PMNs). Urethral discharge for GC culture (80%). Bacterial culture. Special culture needed for *Ureaplasma urealyticum*. Molecular amplification assays for gonorrhea and chlamydia are the preferred diagnostic method (urine or urethral swab for men; vaginal swab, endocervical specimen or urine for women). Wet mount for *T. vaginalis*. RPR or VDRL should be checked in all patients because of high incidence of associated syphilis.	About 50% of patients with GC urethritis have concomitant NGU infection. Always treat sexual partners. Recurrence may be secondary to failure to treat partners. Frequently, no pathogen can be isolated. Persistent or recurrent episodes with adequate treatment of patient and partners may warrant further evaluation for other causes (eg, prostatitis). Brill JR. Diagnosis and treatment of urethritis in men. Am Fam Physician 2010;81:873. [PMID: 20353145] Hobbs MM et al. Methods for detection of *Trichomonas vaginalis* in the male partners of infected women: implications for control of trichomoniasis. J Clin Microbiol 2006;44:3994. [PMID:16971646] Holder NA. Gonococcal infections. Pediatr Rev 2008;29:228. [PMID: 18593752] Horner P. The etiology of acute nongonococcal urethritis—the enigma of idiopathic urethritis? Sex Transm Dis. 2011;38:187. [PMID: 21285913] Martin DH. Nongonococcal urethritis: new views through the prism of modern molecular microbiology. Curr Infect Dis Rep 2008;10:128-32. [PMID: 18462587] Miller KE. Diagnosis and treatment of *Chlamydia trachomatis* infection. Am Fam Physician 2006;73:1411. Erratum in: Am Fam Physician 2008;77:920. [PMID: 16669564] Taylor-Robinson D. Nongonococcal urethritis and antibiotic-resistant *Mycoplasma genitalium* infection. Clin Infect Dis 2008;47:1554. [PMID: 18990063] Wendel KA et al. Trichomoniasis: challenges to appropriate management. Clin Infect Dis 2007;44(Suppl 3):S123. [PMID: 17342665]

GENITOURINARY		
Epididymitis/orchitis		
Organism	**Specimen/Diagnostic Tests**	**Comments**
Epididymitis/orchitis Age <35 years, homosexual men: *Chlamydia trachomatis, U. urealyticum,* *E. coli* (GNR), *Enterococcus faecalis* (GPC), *P. aeruginosa* (GNR), brucella (GVCB). Age >35 years, or children: Enterobac- teriaceae (especially *E. coli*) (GNR), *Pseudomonas* sp. (GNR), salmonella (GNR), *Haemophilus influenzae* (GNCB), VZV, mumps. Immunosuppression: *H. influenzae,* *Mycobacterium tuberculosis* (AFB), *Candida* sp. (yeast), CMV.	Urinalysis may reveal pyuria. Patients aged >35 years often have midstream pyuria and scrotal pain and edema. Culture urine and expressible urethral discharge when present. Prostatic secretions for Gram stain and bacterial culture are helpful in older patients. When testicular torsion is considered, Doppler ultrasound or radionuclide scan can be useful in diagnosis.	Testicular torsion is a surgical emergency that is often confused with orchitis or epididymitis. Sexual partners should be examined for signs of sexually transmitted diseases. In non-sexually transmitted disease, evaluation for underlying urinary tract infection or structural defect is recommended. Tracy CR et al. Diagnosis and management of epididymitis. Urol Clin North Am. 2008;35:101. [PMID: 18061028] Trojian TH et al. Epididymitis and orchitis: an overview. Am Fam Physician 2009;79:583. [PMID: 19378875]

	GENITOURINARY
	Vaginitis/vaginosis

Vaginitis/vaginosis

Candida sp. (yeast), *Trichomonas vaginalis*, *Gardnerella vaginalis* (GPR), bacteroides (non-*fragilis*) (GNR), mobiluncus (GPR), peptostreptococcus (GPC), *Mycoplasma hominis*, groups A and B streptococci (GPC), HSV.

Vaginal discharge for appearance (in candidiasis, area is pruritic with thick "cheesy" discharge: in trichomoniasis, copious foamy, yellow-green, or discolored discharge), pH (about 4.5 for candida; 5.0–7.0 in trichomonas; 5.0–6.0 with bacterial), saline ("wet") preparation (motile organisms seen in trichomonas; cells covered with organisms—clue cells—in gardnerella; yeast and hyphae in candida, "fishy" odor on addition of KOH with gardnerella infection). Vaginal fluid pH as a screening test for bacterial vaginosis showed a sensitivity of 74.3%, but combined with clinical symptoms and signs its sensitivity increased to 81.3%. (See Vaginal Discharge table, Table 8–29.)

Atrophic vaginitis is seen in postmenopausal patients, often with bleeding, scant discharge, and pH 6.0–7.0.

Cultures for gardnerella are not useful and are not recommended. Culture for *T. vaginalis* has greater sensitivity than wet mount. Culture for groups A and B streptococci and rare causes of bacterial vaginosis may be indicated. Gram stain of discharge is more reliable than wet mount for diagnosis of bacterial vaginosis (93% vs. 70%, respectively).

Bacterial vaginosis results from massive overgrowth of anaerobic vaginal bacterial flora (especially gardnerella).

Serious infectious sequelae associated with bacterial vaginosis include abscesses, endometritis and pelvic inflammatory disease. There is also a danger of miscarriage, premature rupture of the membranes, and premature labor.

Donders G. Diagnosis and management of bacterial vaginosis and other types of abnormal vaginal bacterial flora: a review. Obstet Gynecol Surv 2010;65:462. [PMID: 20723268]

Quan M. Vaginitis: diagnosis and management. Postgrad Med 2010;122:117. [PMID: 21084788]

	GENITOURINARY
	Cervicitis

Organism	Specimen/Diagnostic Tests	Comments
Cervicitis, mucopurulent *Chlamydia trachomatis* (50%), *N. gonorrhoeae* (GNDC) (8%), HSV, *Mycoplasma genitalium*.	Cervical swab specimen for appearance (yellow or green purulent material), cell count (>10 WBCs per high-power oil immersion field and culture (58–80%) or nucleic acid assay (93%) for GC; urine for nucleic acid assay (93%) for GC; vaginal swab (97%), or cervical swab (97%) for detection of *C. trachomatis* by nucleic acid amplification. Culture (52%) or nonamplified assays (50–80%) are considerably less sensitive for diagnosis of *C. trachomatis*.	Because of the danger of false-positive amplified nucleic acid assays, culture is the preferred method in cases of suspected child abuse. In one study of pregnant women, a wet mount preparation of endocervical secretions with <10 PMNs per high-power field had a negative predictive value of 99% for gonococcus-induced cervicitis and of 96% for *C. trachomatis*-induced cervicitis. In family planning clinics, however, a mucopurulent discharge with >10 PMNs/hpf had a low positive predictive value of 29.2% for *C. trachomatis*-related cervicitis. Mucopurulent discharge may persist for 3 months or more even after appropriate therapy. Gaydos C et al. *Mycoplasma genitalium* as a contributor to the multiple etiologies of cervicitis in women attending sexually transmitted disease clinics. Sex Transm Dis 2009;36:598. [PMID: 19704398] Holder NA. Gonococcal infections. Pediatr Rev 2008;29:228. [PMID: 18593752] Lusk MJ et al. Cervicitis: a review. Curr Opin Infect Dis 2008;21:49. [PMID: 18192786] Lusk MJ et al. *Mycoplasma genitalium* is associated with cervicitis and HIV infection in an urban Australian STI clinic population. Sex Transm Infect 2011;87:107. [PMID: 21071566] Short VL et al. Clinical presentation of *Mycoplasma genitalium* infection versus *Neisseria gonorrhoeae* infection among women with pelvic inflammatory disease. Clin Infect Dis 2009;48:41. [PMID: 19025498] Workowski KA et al; Centers for Disease Control and Prevention (CDC). Sexually transmitted diseases treatment guidelines, 2010. MMWR Recomm Rep 2010;59:1. Erratum in: MMWR Recomm Rep 2011;60:18. [PMID: 21160459]

GENITOURINARY		
Salpingitis		**Chorioamnionitis/endometritis**

Salpingitis/pelvic inflammatory disease (PID)

Usually polymicrobial: *N. gonorrhoeae* (GNDC), *Chlamydia trachomatis*, bacteroides, peptostreptococcus, *G. vaginalis*, and other anaerobes, Enterobacteriaceae (GNR), streptococci (GPC in chains), *Mycoplasma hominis* (debatable).

Gram stain and culture or amplified nucleic acid assays of urethral or endocervical exudate.

Ultrasonographic findings include thickened fluid-filled tubes, polycystic-like ovaries, and free pelvic fluid. MRI imaging findings for PID (95%) include fluid-filled tube, pyosalpinx, tubo-ovarian abscess, or polycystic-like ovaries and free fluid. Laparoscopy supplemented by microbiologic tests and fimbrial biopsy is the diagnostic standard for PID. Transvaginal ultrasonography (81%) has a lower specificity than MRI.

Laparoscopy is the most specific test to confirm the diagnosis of PID.

RPR or VDRL should be checked in all patients because of the high incidence of associated syphilis.

PID typically progresses from cervicitis to endometritis to salpingitis. PID is a sexually transmitted disease in some cases, not in others.

All sexual partners should be examined.

All IUDs should be removed.

A strategy of identifying, testing, and treating women at increased risk for cervical chlamydial infection can lead to a reduced incidence of PID. All patients with diagnosis of acute PID should also be tested for HIV infection.

Jaiyeoba O et al. Recommendations and rationale for the treatment of pelvic inflammatory disease. Expert Rev Anti Infect Ther 2011;9:61. [PMID: 21171878]

Judlin P. Current concepts in managing pelvic inflammatory disease. Curr Opin Infect Dis 2010;23:83. [PMID: 19935421]

Paavonen J. *Chlamydia trachomatis's* infections of the female genital tract: state of the art. Ann Med 2012;44(1):18. [PMID: 21284529]

Schnee DM. Pelvic inflammatory disease. J Pediatr Adolesc Gynecol 2009;22:387. [PMID: 19885975]

Soper DE. Pelvic inflammatory disease. Obstet Gynecol 2010;116(2 Pt 1):419. [PMID: 20664404]

Chorioamnionitis/endometritis

Group B streptococcus (GPC), *E. coli* (GNR), *Listeria monocytogenes* (GPR), *Mycoplasma hominis*, *M. genitalium*, *Ureaplasma urealyticum*, *Gardnerella vaginalis*, enterococci (GPC), viridans streptococci (GPC in chains), *N. gonorrhoeae* (GNDC), bacteroides (GNR), prevotella (GNR), and other anaerobic flora, *Chlamydia trachomatis*, group A streptococcus (GPC).

Diagnosis based mostly on clinical findings. Amniotic fluid for Gram stain, glucose levels <10–20 mg/dL, and aerobic and anaerobic culture, blood for culture (10–20%). Sonographic evaluation of fetus can be helpful, but findings are nonspecific.

Risk factors include bacterial vaginosis, preterm labor, duration of labor, parity, internal fetal monitoring.

Czikk MJ et al. Chorioamnionitis: from pathogenesis to treatment. Clin Microbiol Infect 2011;17:1304. [PMID: 21672080]

Saxena S et al. Chorioamnionitis due to *Arcanobacterium haemolyticum*. J Glob Infect Dis 2011;3:92. [PMID: 21572617]

Tita AT et al. Diagnosis and management of clinical chorioamnionitis. Clin Perinatol 2010;37:339. [PMID: 20569811]

Weinstein SA et al. A review of the epidemiology, diagnosis and evidence-based management of *Mycoplasma genitalium*. Sex Health 2011;8:143. [PMID: 21592428]

BONE

Osteomyelitis

Organism	Specimen/Diagnostic Tests	Comments
Osteomyelitis *Staphylococcus aureus* (GPC) (60%). Infant: *S. aureus*, Enterobacteriaceae (GNR), groups A and B streptococci (GPC). Child (<3 years): *H. influenzae* (GNCB), *S. aureus*, streptococci. Child (>3 years) to adult: *S. aureus*, coagulase negative staphylococci, Group A streptococcus, *Pseudomonas aeruginosa*. Postoperative: *S. aureus*, Enterobacteriaceae, *Pseudomonas* sp. (GNR), *Bartonella henselae* (GNR). Joint prosthesis: Coagulase-negative staphylococci, peptostreptococcus (GPC), *Propionibacterium acnes* (GPR), viridans streptococci (GPC in chains). Immunocompromised patients (eg, elderly, HIV-infected): *M. tuberculosis*, *Candida* sp., cryptococcus, coccidioides, histoplasma.	Blood cultures for bacteria are positive in about 60%. Cultures of percutaneous needle biopsy or open bone biopsy are needed if blood cultures are negative and osteomyelitis is suspected. Imaging with bone scan or gallium plus indium scan (sensitivity 95%, specificity 60–97%) can localize areas of suspicion. Technetium methylene diphosphonate bone scan can suggest osteomyelitis days or weeks before plain bone films. Plain bone films are abnormal in acute cases after about 2 weeks of illness (33%). Indium-labeled WBC scan is useful in detecting abscesses. Ultrasound to detect subperiosteal abscesses and ultrasound-guided aspiration can assist in diagnosis and management of osteomyelitis. Ultrasound can differentiate acute osteomyelitis from vaso-occlusive crisis in patients with sickle cell disease. CT scan is useful, but MRI is more sensitive and is now the standard of care. When bone x-rays and scintigraphy are negative, MRI (98%) is useful for detecting early osteomyelitis (specificity 89%), in defining extent, and in distinguishing osteomyelitis from cellulitis.	Hematogenous or contiguous infection (eg, infected prosthetic joint, chronic cutaneous ulcer) may lead to osteomyelitis in children (metaphyses of long bones) or adults (vertebrae, metaphyses of long bones). Hematogenous osteomyelitis in drug addicts occurs in unusual locations (vertebrae, clavicle, ribs). In infants, osteomyelitis is often associated with contiguous joint involvement. Chihara S et al. Osteomyelitis. Dis Mon 2010;56:5. [PMID: 19995624] Howell WR et al. Osteomyelitis: an update for hospitalists. Hosp Pract (Minneap) 2011;39:153. [PMID: 21441771] Jorge LS et al. Osteomyelitis: a current challenge. Braz J Infect Dis 2010;14:310. [PMID: 20835519]

JOINT
Bacterial/septic arthritis

Bacterial/septic arthritis

Infant (<3 months): *S. aureus* (GPC), Group A streptococci (GPC), Enterobacteriaceae (GNR), *Kingella kingae* (GNCB), *Haemophilus influenzae* (GNCB).
Child (3 months to 6 years): *S. aureus* (35%), *H. influenzae*, group A streptococcus (GPC) (10%), Enterobacteriaceae (6%), *Borrelia burgdorferi* (Lyme), *S. pneumoniae* (GPC), *K. kingae.*
Adult, STD not likely: *S. aureus* (40%), group A streptococcus (27%), Enterobacteriaceae (23%), *Streptobacillus moniliformis* (GNR) (rat bite fever), brucella (GVCB (*Neisseria* sp.), *Mycobacterium marinum* (AFB).
Adult, STD likely: *N. gonorrhoeae* (GNDC) (disseminated gonococcal infection [DGI]).
Prosthetic joint, postoperative or following intraarticular injection: Coagulase-negative staphylococci (40%), *S. aureus* (20%), viridans streptococcus (GPC in chains), enterococci (GPC), peptostreptococcus (GPC), *Propionibacterium acnes* (GPR), Enterobacteriaceae, *Pseudomonas* sp.

Joint aspiration (synovial) fluid for WBCs (in non-gonococcal infection, mean WBC is 100,000/mcL). Gram stain (best on centrifuged concentrated specimen, positive in one-third of cases), culture (non-gonococcal infection in adults [85–95%], disseminated gonococcal infection (DGI) [25%]). (See Arthritis: Synovial fluid profiles, Table 8–4.)
Yield of culture is greatest when 10 mL of synovial fluid is inoculated onto a plate or into culture media.
Blood cultures for bacteria may be useful, especially in infants, nongonococcal infection in adults (50%), DGI (13%). *B. burgdorferi* serology for Lyme disease.
Genitourinary, throat, or rectal culture: DGI may be diagnosed by positive culture from a nonarticular source and by a compatible clinical picture.
In difficult cases, MRI can help differentiate septic arthritis from transient synovitis.

It is important to obtain synovial fluid and blood for culture before starting antimicrobial treatment.
Septic arthritis is usually hematogenously acquired. Prosthetic joint and diminished host defenses secondary to cancer, HIV, liver disease, or hypogammaglobulinemia are common predisposing factors.
Nongonococcal bacterial arthritis is usually monarticular (and typically affects one knee joint).
DGI is the most common cause of septic arthritis in urban centers and is usually polyarticular with associated tenosynovitis.
García-De La Torre I et al. Gonococcal and nongonococcal arthritis. Rheum Dis Clin North Am 2009;35:63. [PMID: 19480997]
Mathews CJ et al. Bacterial septic arthritis in adults. Lancet 2010;375:846. [PMID: 20206778]
Mathews CJ et al. Septic arthritis: current diagnostic and therapeutic algorithm. Curr Opin Rheumatol 2008;20:457. [PMID: 18525361]

	MUSCLE
	Gas gangrene

Organism	Specimen/Diagnostic Tests	Comments
Gas gangrene *Clostridium perfringens* (GPR) (80–95%), other *Clostridium* sp.: *C. ramosum, C. bifermentans, C. histolyticum, C. septicum, C. sordellii, C. tertium.*	Diagnosis should be suspected in areas of devitalized tissue when gas is discovered by palpation (subcutaneous crepitation) or x-ray. Gram stain of foul-smelling, brown, or blood-tinged watery exudate from lesion or abscess, if present, can be diagnostic with gram-positive rods (can be gram variable) and a remarkable absence of neutrophils. Anaerobic culture of discharge is confirmatory.	Gas gangrene occurs in the setting of a contaminated wound. *C. perfringens* produces potent exotoxins, including alpha toxin and theta toxin, which depress myocardial contractility, induce shock, and cause direct vascular injury at the site of infection. Infections with enterobacteriacae, other gram-negative rods, *S. aureus,* streptococci, and mixed aerobic and anaerobic infections can also cause gas formation. These agents cause cellulitis rather than myonecrosis. Crum-Cianflone NF. Bacterial, fungal, parasitic, and viral myositis. Clin Microbiol Rev 2008;21:473. [PMID: 18625683] Park H et al. Complex wounds and their management. Surg Clin North Am 2010;90:1181. [PMID: 21074035]

SKIN		
Impetigo		

Impetigo

Infant (impetigo neonatorum): *Staphylococcus* (GPC).

Nonbullous or "vesicular": *S. pyogenes* (GPC), *S. aureus* (GPC), anaerobes.

Bullous: *S. aureus*.

Gram stain, culture, and smear for HSV and VZV antigen detection by direct fluorescent antibody (DFA) of scrapings from lesions may be useful in differentiating impetigo from other vesicular or pustular lesions (HSV, VZV, contact dermatitis). DFA smear can be performed by scraping the contents, base, and roof of vesicle and applying to glass slide. After fixing, the slide is stained with DFA reagents for identification of HSV or VZV.

Impetigo neonatorum requires prompt treatment and protection of other infants (isolation).

Polymicrobial aerobic-anaerobic infections are present in some patients.

Patients with recurrent impetigo should have cultures of the anterior nares to identify and treat carriage of *S. aureus*.

Bernard P. Management of common bacterial infections of the skin. Curr Opin Infect Dis 2008;21:122. [PMID: 18317033]

Cohen PR. Community-acquired methicillin-resistant *Staphylococcus aureus* skin infections: a review of epidemiology, clinical features, management, and prevention. Int J Dermatol 2007;46:1. Erratum in: Int J Dermatol 2007;46:230. [PMID: 17214713]

Geria AN et al. Impetigo update: new challenges in the era of methicillin resistance. Cutis 2010;85:6570. [PMID: 20349679]

Odell CA. Community-associated methicillin-resistant *Staphylococcus aureus* (CA-MRSA) skin infections. Curr Opin Pediatr 2010;22:273. [PMID: 20386450]

Stanley JR et al. Pemphigus, bullous impetigo, and the staphylococcal scalded-skin syndrome. N Engl J Med 2006;355:1800. [PMID: 17065642]

	SKIN	
	Cellulitis	
Organism	**Specimen/Diagnostic Tests**	**Comments**
Cellulitis	Skin culture: In spontaneous cellulitis, isolation of the causative organism is difficult. In traumatic and postoperative wounds, Gram stain may allow rapid diagnosis of staphylococcal or clostridial infection. Culture of wound or abscess material after disinfection of the skin site almost always yields the diagnosis. MRI can aid in diagnosis of secondary abscess formation, necrotizing fasciitis, or pyomyositis. Frozen section of biopsy specimen may be useful.	Cellulitis has long been considered to be the result of an antecedent bacterial invasion with subsequent bacterial proliferation. However, the difficulty in isolating putative pathogens from cellulitic skin has cast doubt on this theory. Predisposing factors for cellulitis include diabetes mellitus, edema, peripheral vascular disease, venous insufficiency, leg ulcer or wound, tinea pedis, dry skin, obesity, and history of cellulitis. Consider updating anti-tetanus prophylaxis for all wounds. In the diabetic patient, and in postoperative and traumatic wounds, consider prompt surgical debridement for necrotizing fasciitis. With abscess formation, surgical drainage is the mainstay of therapy and may be sufficient. Hemolytic streptococcal gangrene may follow minor trauma and involves specific strains of streptococcus. Kilburn SA et al. Interventions for cellulitis and erysipelas. Cochrane Database Syst Rev 2010;(6):CD004299. [PMID: 20556757] Morgan MS. Diagnosis and management of necrotising fasciitis: a multiparametric approach. J Hosp Infect 2010;75:249. [PMID: 20542593] Shimizu T et al. Necrotizing fasciitis. Intern Med 2010;49:1051. [PMID: 20558917] Stevens DL et al. Cellulitis and soft-tissue infections. Ann Intern Med 2009;150:ITC11. [PMID: 19124814]
Spontaneous, traumatic wound: Polymicrobial: *S. aureus* (GPC), groups A, C, and G streptococci (GPC), enterococci (GPC), Enterobacteriaceae (GNR), *Clostridium perfringens* (GPR), *Clostridium tetani*, *Pseudomonas* sp. (GNR) (if water exposure).		
Postoperative wound (not GI or GU): *S. aureus*, group A streptococcus, Enterobacteriaceae, *Pseudomonas* sp.		
Postoperative wound (GI or GU): Must add *Bacteroides* sp., anaerobes, enterococcus (GPC), groups B or C streptococci.		
Diabetes mellitus: Polymicrobial: *S. pyogenes*, enterococcus, *S. aureus*, Enterobacteriaceae, anaerobes.		
Bullous lesions, sea water contaminated abrasion, after raw seafood consumption: *Vibrio vulnificus* (GNR).		
Vein graft donor site: Beta-hemolytic streptococci.		
Decubitus ulcers: Polymicrobial: *S. aureus*, anaerobic streptococci, Enterobacteriaceae, *Pseudomonas* sp., *Bacteroides* sp. other anaerobes.		
Necrotizing fasciitis, type 1: streptococcus, anaerobes, Enterobacteriaceae; type 2: Group A streptococcus (hemolytic streptococcal gangrene).		

BLOOD

Bacteremia of unknown source

Bacteremia of unknown source		
Neonate (<4 days): Group B streptococcus (GPC), E. coli (GNR), klebsiella (GNR), enterobacter (GNR), S. aureus (GPC), coagulase-negative staphylococci (GPC), Candida sp. **Neonate (>5 days):** Add H. influenzae (GNCB). **Child (nonimmunocompromised):** S. pneumoniae (GPDC), N. meningitidis (GNDC), S. aureus (GPC), enterococci (GPC). **Adult (IV drug use):** S. aureus or viridans streptococci (GPC in chains), enterococci (GPC). **Adult (catheter-related, "line" sepsis):** coagulase-negative staphylococci (30%), S. aureus (12%), Candida sp. (11%), enterococci (9%), other streptococci (9%), Klebsiella pneumoniae (9%), Enterobacter sp. (4%), Serratia sp. (4%), Pseudomonas sp. (4%), Acinetobacter baumanii (1–4%), Corynebacterium jeikeium (1%), other yeast (1%). **Adult (splenectomized):** S. pneumoniae, H. influenzae, N. meningitidis. **Neutropenia (<500 PMN/mcL):** Enterobacteriaceae, Pseudomonas sp., S. aureus, coagulase-negative staphylococci, viridans streptococci (GPC in chains). **Immunocompromised:** Bartonella sp. (GNR), Mycobacterium avium/intracellulare (AFB).	Blood cultures are mandatory for all patients with fever and no obvious source of infection. Often they are negative, especially in neonates. Cultures (2–3 sets) should be drawn from different sites before start of antibiotic therapy. Culture should not be drawn from an IV line or from a femoral site if possible. Culture and Gram stain of urine, wounds, and other potentially infected sites may provide a more rapid diagnosis than blood cultures. Blood cultures are incubated for 5 days. New methods are being introduced that rapidly (within 3–5 hours) identify bacteria or yeast genus and species from a positive blood culture bottle (eg, peptide nucleic acid fluorescence in situ hybridization [FNA-FISH], bacteriophage methods).	Occult bacteremia affects approximately 5% of febrile children ages 2–36 months. In infants, the findings of an elevated total WBC count (>15,000 mcL) and absolute neutrophil count (ANC >10,000/mcL) are equally sensitive in predicting bacteremia, but the ANC is more specific. Predisposing factors in adults include IV drug use, neutropenia, urinary tract infection, cancer, diabetes mellitus, venous catheterization, hemodialysis, and plasmapheresis. Catheter-related infection in patients with long-term venous access (Broviac, Hickman, etc) may be treated successfully without removal of the line, but recurrence of bacteremia is frequent. Riedel S et al. Blood cultures: key elements for best practices and future directions. J Infect Chemother 2010;16:301. [PMID: 20490596] Rodríguez-Baño J et al. Current management of bloodstream infections. Expert Rev Anti Infect Ther 2010;8:815. [PMID: 20586566] Thwaites GE et al; UK Clinical Infection Research Group. Clinical management of Staphylococcus aureus bacteraemia. Lancet Infect Dis 2011;11:208. [PMID:21371655]

PART II. EMERGING (NEW) AND RE-EMERGING PATHOGENS/INFECTIOUS AGENTS.[1]

Organism	Specimen/Diagnostic Tests	Comments
Avian influenza A/H5N1 and Novel H1N1 influenza A Influenza A virus subtype, H5N1, has greater virulence, easier (more efficient) human-to-human transmission, and resistance to antiviral drugs. Novel H1N1 influenza A virus caused a pandemic in 2009.	Sputum for viral culture (H5N1 virus should not be cultured in routine laboratory—send to CDC or reference laboratory). Molecular methods for strain typing. Blood and sputum for RT-PCR for influenza A identification and strain typing; RT-PCR testing is limited to local and state public health laboratories. Molecular assays for influenza A and B with identification of H1N1 strain are now commercially available for clinical laboratories. Healthcare workers who have close contact with patients with influenza-like symptoms should follow CDC guidelines for personal protective equipment (masks, etc) to prevent infection.	The first documented case of bird-to-human transmission of avian influenza A (H5N1) occured in 1997 in Hong Kong. The H5N1 virus is carried by birds that shed the virus in saliva, nasal secretions, and feces. Other birds/fowls are infected by fecal-oral transmission through contact with contaminated surface, feed, water, grout, etc. By 2006, almost every country in the world had reported at least one case of H5N1 influenza. Clinical symptoms and signs: mild-to-severe respiratory symptoms and fever. High mortality in humans. There are fears of a future pandemic with H5N1 influenza A. Novel H1N1 influenza A caused mostly mild illness except for severe illness in young children, pregnant women, and obese patients. Caliendo AM. Multiplex PCR and emerging technologies for the detection of respiratory pathogens. Clin Infect Dis 2011;52(Suppl 4):S326. [PMID: 21460291] Ison MG et al. Influenza 2010–2011: lessons from the 2009 pandemic. Cleve Clin J Med 2010;77:812. [PMID: 21048054] Landry ML. Diagnostic tests for influenza infection. Curr Opin Pediatr 2011;23:91. [PMID: 21150446] Loeffelholz MJ. Avian influenza A H5N1 virus. Clin Lab Med 2010;30:1. [PMID: 20513539] Swerdlow DL et al. 2009 H1N1 influenza pandemic: field and epidemiologic investigations in the United States at the start of the first pandemic of the 21st century. Clin Infect Dis 2011;52(Suppl 1):S1. [PMID: 21342879] Tang JW et al. Emerging, novel, and known influenza virus infections in humans. Infect Dis Clin North Am 2010;24:603. [PMID: 20674794]

[1]Nearly 70% of emerging infectious disease outbreaks during the last 10 years have been zoonotic diseases transmitted from animals to humans. Controlling the diseases caused by new/re-emerging infectious agents is difficult owing to the diversity of geographic sources, the potential for rapid global dissemination from the source, and ecologic and social/economic influences.

Human metapneumovirus (huMPV)

HuMPV is the causative agent of infant bronchiolitis in 5–15% of cases.

There have been documented cases of co-infection with huMPV and RSV.

From the family of Paramyxoviridae, the organism is a new metapneumovirus related to the turkey tracheitis virus. The first documented case of huMPV occurred in 2001 in the US.

Respiratory specimens for viral culture, and RT-PCR. DFA reagents also available for antigen detection in some laboratories.

huMPV is a respiratory pathogen that causes infections ranging from colds to severe bronchiolitis and pneumonia.

Clinical symptoms and signs: 70–80% of infected individuals are asymptomatic, 20% have mild flu-like symptoms, 6% have symptoms indistinguishable from RSV, bronchiolitis, croup, asthma, or pneumonia.

Broor S et al. Human metapneumovirus: a new respiratory pathogen. J Biosci 2008;33:483. [PMID: 19208974]

Hermos CR et al. Human metapneumovirus. Clin Lab Med 2010;30:131. [PMID: 20513544]

Papenburg J et al. The distinguishing features of human metapneumovirus and respiratory syncytial virus. Rev Med Virol 2010;20:245. [PMID: 20586081]

Organism	Specimen/Diagnostic Tests	Comments
Human monkeypox Monkeypox is in the family of Orthopoxvirus, which is in the same genus as the smallpox (variola) virus. First documented case occurred in US in June 2003. The infected humans had contact with prairie dogs that had been housed with infected Gambian giant rats from Ghana. This outbreak of 72 cases, as reported to the CDC, involved patients in six states.	Respiratory samples and skin lesion specimens submitted for viral culture. Blood and/or CSF samples for monkeypox virus DNA by PCR and for IGM antibodies by ELISA. Tissue samples for immunohistochemical testing or by demonstrating virus morphologically consistent with orthopoxvirus by electron microscopy.	History: Exposure to wild mammalian pet or exotic animal. Clinical symptoms and signs: Fever, chills or sweats, headaches, backache, sore throat, cough, shortness of breath, lymphadenopathy, rash (macular, papular, vesicular or pustular, generalized or localized, discrete or confluent), encephalitis. Mortality rate in Africa: approximately 10%, higher in immunocompromised patients. Centers for Disease Control Monkeypox Homepage http://www.cdc.gov/ncidod/monkeypox Nalca A et al. Reemergence of monkeypox: prevalence, diagnostics, and countermeasures. Clin Infect Dis 2005;41:1765. [PMID: 16288402] Weaver JR et al. Monkeypox virus and insights into its immunomodulatory proteins. Immunol Rev 2008;225:96. [PMID: 18837778]

Severe acute respiratory syndrome—coronavirus A (SARS-CoA)

First reported in Southern China in 2002; by mid-2003 over 8500 cases had been reported with nearly 800 deaths.

Identified in 2003 as a Coronavirus; infection originates from wildlife (eg, civets and other mammals).

Highly infectious, spread by close person-to-person contact.

Obtain CBC, activated PTT, serum liver tests, creatine phosphokinase (CPK), lactate dehydrogenase (LDH), chest radiograph, blood cultures, pleural fluid culture, sputum for bacterial culture and respiratory virus panel (rule out influenzae A and B, and RSV).

Viral culture of respiratory specimens is not recommended. Respiratory sample, stool, plasma/serum may be sent to CDC for SAR-CoA RT-PCR assay.

Blood or serum for SAR-CoA antibody EIA assay performed by State Public Health laboratories.

Laboratory abnormalities: normal or low WBC with decreased lymphocytes, prolonged activated PTT, increased transaminases, increased CPK, increased LDH.

Clinical symptoms and signs: Early symptoms include fever, chills, rigors, myalgia, and headaches. Respiratory symptoms appear 2–7 days after onset, with shortness of breath and/or dry cough; pneumonia in 60–100%.

Healthcare workers who have close contact with patients with symptoms consistent with a respiratory viral illness should follow CDC guidelines for use of personal protective equipment (masks, etc) to prevent infection. CDC SARS http://www.cdc.gov/sars/index.html

Cheng VC et al. Severe acute respiratory syndrome coronavirus as an agent of emerging and reemerging infection. Clin Microbiol Rev 2007;20:660. [PMID: 17934078]

Cleri DJ et al. Severe acute respiratory syndrome (SARS). Infect Dis Clin North Am 2010;24:175. [PMID: 20171552]

Hui DS et al. Severe acute respiratory syndrome and coronavirus. Infect Dis Clin North Am 2010;24:619. [PMID: 20674795]

Hui DS et al. Clinical features, pathogenesis and immunobiology of severe acute respiratory syndrome. Curr Opin Pulm Med 2008;14:241. [PMID: 18427248]

Organism	Specimen/Diagnostic Tests	Comments
West Nile virus (WNV) Although it first appeared in the US in 1999, within 5 years WNV had established itself as endemic in the US. Responsible agent is a single-strand RNA virus of the family Flavivirus. Its enzootic cycle involves several species of mosquitoes and birds before infecting humans; however, it is transmitted to humans from the bite of *Culex* species of mosquitoes. Incubation period of 2–14 days.	Serum, CSF, or tissue collected within 8 days of illness for IgM antibody ELISA; test performed by state public health laboratories or reference laboratories.	Clinical symptoms and signs: 80% of those infected are asymptomatic, 20% have mild flulike symptoms: fever, headache, myalgias, skin rash, and lymphadenopathy. In immunocompetent patients, illness is self-limited, lasting 3–6 days. Central nervous system infection (encephalitis or meningitis or flaccid paralysis) develops in 1%, with change in mental status, movement disorders, and focal neurologic deficits (more common with increased age). Gastrointestinal symptoms also occur. Centers for Disease Control and Prevention: West Nile Virus http://www.cdc.gov/ncidod/dvbid/westnile/index.htm National Institute of Allergy and Infectious Diseases: West Nile Virus http://www.niaid.nih.gov/topics/westnile/Pages/default.aspx
Mumps A virus from the family Paramyxovirus. Disease is spread by respiratory droplets; infectivity precedes the symptom by 1 day and may last a week. Incubation period is 14–21 days, average 18 days.	Buccal/oral swab for viral culture (gold standard) or mumps viral RNA by RT-PCR. Blood for serologic tests for acute mumps infection (IgM) and test of immunity (IgG) antibodies using EIA assay. Blood for serologic tests for mumps include detection of virus-specific IgM in a single sample or a fourfold or greater increase in IgG antibodies between acute- and convalescent-phase specimens using indirect EIA assay. In previously vaccinated persons, serologic tests have limited use. In a recent outbreak, mumps virus IgM antibodies were detected in <15% of infected persons who were previously vaccinated; 95% had mumps virus IgG antibodies. Virus detection can also vary owing to low viral loads in immunized persons.	Clinical symptoms and signs: Acute onset of unilateral or bilateral, tender, self-limited swelling of the parotids (75%) or other salivary glands, lasting 2 or more days, without other apparent causes; fever, malaise, stiff neck, headaches. Complications include meningitis (30%), orchitis, pancreatitis, oophoritis, thyroiditis, neuritis, hepatitis, myocarditis, thrombocytopenia, arthralgias and nephritis. Centers for Disease Control and Prevention: Mumps http://www.cdc.gov/vaccines/vpd-vac/mumps/default.htm Hviid A et al. Mumps. Lancet 2008;371:932. [PMID: 18342688] MacDonald N et al. Mumps is back: why is mumps eradication not working? Adv Exp Med Biol 2011;697:197. [PMID: 21120728] Senanayake SN. Mumps: a resurgent disease with protean manifestations. Med J Aust 2008;189:456. [PMID: 18928441]

Transmissible spongiform encephalopathy (TSE)

TSE is a progressive, fatal, incurable, neurodegenerative prion disease occurring in both animals and humans. TSEs include bovine spongiform encephalopathy (BSE) in cattle; scrapie in sheep; chronic wasting disease in deer and elk; kuru in humans; Creutzfeldt–Jakob disease (CJD) in humans; and certain genetically determined or familial disorders (eg, fatal familial insomnia and Gerstmann–Straussler-Scheinker syndrome).

There is the potential for bovine spongiform encephalopathy (BSE) transmission to humans from eating infected meat or meat products. Another public health issue involves the potential transmission through blood transfusions or via corneal, dura mater, and other transplants.

Tissue from brain, spinal cord, eyes, tonsils, lymphoid tissue, spleen, pancreas, and nerves for immunohistochemical (IHC) analysis; and for conformation-dependent immunoassay (CDI), which is faster and uses specific antibodies that bind to all disease-causing prions in the brain. Use great caution when handling tissue from brain or spinal cord of a potential TSE patient.

Clinical symptoms and signs: rapidly progressive dementia, myoclonic fasciculations, ataxia, tremor, psychiatric symptoms.
Brown K et al. The prion diseases. J Geriatr Psychiatry Neurol 2010;23:277–8. [PMID: 20938044]
Venneti S. Prion diseases. Clin Lab Med 2010;30:293–309. [PMID: 20513552]

Organism	Specimen/Diagnostic Tests	Comments
Lyme disease Causative agent is *Borrelia burgdorferi*. Found primarily in the Northeast, mid-Atlantic coastal areas, and north-central US. *Borrelia burgdorferi* is transmitted primarily by the deer tick (*Ixodes* species) after it has been attached to a host for more than 24 hours.	Serum for IgM and IgG antibodies by ELISA, need confirmation by Western immunoblot (CDC recommendation).	Clinical symptoms and signs: *Acute stage*: erythema migrans (expanding rash with area of central clearing) at the site of tick bite within 10 days, low-grade fever, headache, myalgia, arthralgia, and regional lymphadenopathy for 3–4 weeks. *Musculoskeletal symptoms*: asymmetric arthritis; may require 3–4 years to resolve (regardless of treatment). *Early neurologic involvement*: cranial neuritis, meningitis, and encephalitis. *Chronic neurologic disease*: subacute encephalopathy, axonal polyneuropathy, and leukoencephalopathy. Marques AR. Lyme disease: a review. Curr Allergy Asthma Rep 2010;10:13. [PMID: 20425509] Murray TS et al. Lyme disease. Clin Lab Med 2010;30:311. [PMID: 20513553] National Institute of Allergy and Infectious Diseases: Lyme Disease http://www.niaid.nih.gov/topics/lymedisease/Pages/lymedisease.aspx O'Connell S. Lyme borreliosis: current issues in diagnosis and management. Curr Opin Infect Dis 2010;23:231. [PMID: 20407371]

Human monocytic ehrlichiosis (HME)

Causative agent is *Ehrlichia chaffeensis*.
Transmitted to humans and animals by various ticks: *Dermacentor*, *Ixodes* and *Amblyomma* species.
Note: Human granulocytic ehrlichiosis, where morulae are found in WBC granulocytes (neutrophils), has been renamed. This disease, which is clinically indistinguishable from HME, is now called human granulocytic anaplasmosis (HGA), since the intracellular bacteria, *Anaplasma phagocytophilum*, has been identified as the infecting organism. The vectors for HGA are *Ixodes* ticks.

Blood/serum: for IgM or IgG antibodies by IFA or ELISA.
Blood/serum/bone marrow for ehrlichial DNA by PCR.
CBC, liver tests. Blood abnormalities may include leukopenia, thrombocytopenia, and morulas (clusters of *Ehrlichia* bacteria in the cytoplasma of white blood cell monocytes). Increased transaminases.

Clinical symptoms and signs: Illness is mild to fatal; most patients recover completely without treatment. Disease can resemble Rocky Mountain spotted fever, lasting 1–2 weeks with rash (20%), fever, headache, chills, nausea, vomiting, anorexia, myalgias, cough, diarrhea, lymphadenopathy.
Severe complications (rare) include meningoencephalitis and toxic shock with multiorgan failure; these complications are more common in immunocompromised patients.
E. chaffeensis is found primarily in North Atlantic and South Central states of the US.
A phagocytophilum is found primarily in the Northeast and upper Midwestern areas of US.

Centers for Disease Control & Prevention: Human Ehrlichiosis http://www.cdc.gov/ehrlichiosis/
Ismail N et al. Human ehrlichiosis and anaplasmosis. Clin Lab Med 2010;30:261. [PMID: 20513551]
National Institute of Allergy and Infectious Diseases: Ehrlichiosis and Anaplasmosis http://www.niaid.nih.gov/topics/ehrlichiosisanaplasmosis/pages/default.aspx
Rikihisa Y. Mechanisms of obligatory intracellular infection with *Anaplasma phagocytophilum*. Clin Micro Rev 2011;24:469. [PMID: 21734244]
Standart S et al. Primary isolation of *Ehrlichia chaffeensis* from patients with febrile illnesses: clinical and molecular characteristics. J Infect Dis 2000;181:1082. [PMID: 10720534]

Organism	Specimen/Diagnostic Tests	Comments
Acinetobacter *Acinetobacter* species are gram-negative rods, and nosocomial pathogens.	Stool, respiratory, or blood culture. Most common in debilitated ICU patients. Organism can survive for a long period of time in the environment and on the hands of healthcare workers.	Healthcare-associated infection caused by *Acinetobacter* has increased in the last decade during which this strain has developed multidrug resistance. In 2006, *Acinetobacter* was 92% susceptible to tigecycline in the US. Multidrug-resistant strains are universally susceptible to the polymyxins (colistin, polymyxin B); however, these drugs have significant side effects. Garnacho-Montero J et al. Multiresistant *Acinetobacter baumannii* infections: epidemiology and management. Curr Opin Infect Dis 2010;23:332. [PMID: 20581674] Guerrero DM et al. *Acinetobacter baumannii*-associated skin and soft tissue infections: recognizing a broadening spectrum of disease. Surg Infect (Larchmt) 2010;11:49. [PMID: 19788383] Neonakis IK et al. Confronting multidrug-resistant *Acinetobacter baumannii*: a review. Int J Antimicrob Agents 2011;37:102. [PMID: 21130607]

Clostridium difficile

Clostridium difficile is a gram-positive anaerobic rod. *C. difficile* produces 2 toxins: toxin A, which is an enterotoxin, and toxin B, which is a cytotoxin.

C. difficile has been found in stool in 15–25% of patients with antibiotic-associated diarrhea, 10% of patients treated with antibiotics who do not have diarrhea, and in 95% of patients with diarrhea associated with pseudomembranous colitis.

Stool for culture is a sensitive test (99–100%), but 25% of isolates recovered are nonpathogenic and test takes 72 hours. A toxin assay on the isolated organism must still be completed.

Stool for cytotoxicity assay (toxin B) using tissue cultures has been considered a good test, but recent reports suggest a lower sensitivity of 60–80% for toxin detection and the test takes 48 hours.

Toxigenic culture of stool (demonstrates production of toxin from a *C. difficile* isolate) has become the new "gold standard" assay, but this assay also takes several days.

Stool for EIA testing for toxin A and B has a 70–80% sensitivity and rapid tests are available. However, the EIA assays are no longer recommended for routine testing for the toxins.

A rapid lateral flow assay that detects both toxins A and B and an enzyme, glutamate dehydrogenase (GDH), by EIA is available and useful for screening for presence of toxigenic *C. difficile* in stool.

Molecular assays that detect the toxin B gene are very sensitive (95%) and specific. These assays are becoming the standard of care in many laboratories.

Flexible sigmoidoscopy or colonoscopy may be performed in patients with severe symptomatology to detect plaques of pseudomembranous colitis when a rapid diagnosis is needed; sensitivity is 51%.

Clinical symptoms and signs: watery diarrhea, fever, anorexia, and abdominal pain and tenderness. Diarrhea can be mild to severe. Severe diarrhea can lead to ulceration and bleeding from the colon (colitis) and to perforation of the intestine (peritonitis).

A new emerging type of *C. difficile* is ribotype O27, also known as NAP-1, which produces 16–23 times more toxin A and B and is resistant to fluoroquinolones. This emerging *C. difficile* strain causes more severe disease, increased need for surgical procedures, and death.

Bartlett JG. *Clostridium difficile*: progress and challenges. Ann N Y Acad Sci 2010;1213:62. [PMID: 21175676]

Bartlett JG. Detection of *Clostridium difficile* infection. Infect Control Hosp Epidemiol 2010;31(Suppl 10):S35. [PMID: 20920365]

Curry S. *Clostridium difficile*. Clin Lab Med 2010;30:3292. [PMID: 20513554]

Gerding DN et al. *Clostridium difficile* infection in 2010: advances in pathogenesis, diagnosis and management of CDI. Nat Rev Gastroenterol Hepatol 2011;8:67. [PMID: 21293502]

Hessen MT. *Clostridium difficile* infection. Ann Intern Med 2010;153:ITC41-15. [PMID: 20921540]

Organism	Specimen/Diagnostic Tests	Comments
Diarrheagenic *Escherichia coli* *Escherichia coli* is a member of genus Escherichia within the family Enterobacteriaceae. *E. coli* can be characterized by shared lipopolysaccharide (O) and flagellar (H) antigens that define serogroups (O antigen only) or serotypes (O and H antigens). More than 175 O antigens and 53 H antigens have been recognized, but only a few serotype combinations are associated with diarrheal diseases.	Stool culture, with special tests (see entries below). *E. coli* has at least 6 different mechanisms by which to cause diarrhea, and each is associated with a different pathotype and different virulence determinants. The 6 pathotypes are Enteropathogenic *E. coli* (**EPEC**), Enterohemorrhagic *E. coli* (**EHEC**) (also known as Shiga toxin (Stx)-producing *E. coli* (**STEC**), Enterotoxigenic *E. coli* (**ETEC**), Enteroaggregative *E. coli* (**EAEC**), Enteroinvasive *E. coli* (**EIEC**), and diffusely adherent *E. coli* (**DAEC**). Over 200 types of *E. coli* are known to produce shiga toxins. Approximately 1% of stool samples tested in clinical laboratories contain (STEC) shiga toxins. EIAs are available for detection of shiga toxins.	The principal reservoir of EHEC/STEC is the intestinal tract of cattle and herbivorous animals (eg, sheep, deer, goats, birds). EHEC/STEC strains are most frequently identified as diarrheagenic *E. coli* serotypes. Over 60 STEC serotypes are associated with human diseases. *E. coli* O157:H7 is the most common STEC serotype, but there was an outbreak of several thousand cases of *E. coli* O104:H4 in Western Europe in 2011. The source was thought to be contaminated raw sprouts originating from a farm in Germany. It was associated with > 800 cases of hemolytic-uremic syndrome and >30 deaths. Several US cases and 1 HUS death were documented. Bavaro MF. *Escherichia coli* O157: what every internist and gastroenterologist should know. Curr Gastroenterol Rep 2009;11:301. [PMID: 19615306] Bitzan M. Treatment options for HUS secondary to *Escherichia coli* O157:H7. Kidney Int Suppl 2009;112:S62. [PMID: 19180140] Centers for Disease Control & Prevention: Investigation Update: Outbreak of Shiga toxin-producing *E. coli* O104 (STEC O104:H4) Infections Associated with Travel to Germany, June 23, 2011. [http://www.cdc.gov/ecoli/2011/ecoliO104/] Frank C et al; the HUS Investigation Team. Epidemic profile of Shiga-toxin-producing *Escherichia coli* O104:H4 outbreak in Germany—preliminary report. N Engl J Med 2011;365:1771. [PMID: 21696328]
Enteroinvasive *E. coli* (EIEC) Organism invades colonic epithelial cells, lyses the phagosome, multiplies intracellularly, and moves through the cell, exits and re-enters the basolateral plasma membrane. It is closely related to *Shigella* species genetically, biochemically and pathogenetically.	Stool for PCR or DNA probes for *inv* genes; test performed by state public health laboratories or research laboratories.	Clinical symptoms and signs: watery diarrhea with a mechanism similar to shigella-related diarrhea and also related to induced apoptosis in infected macrophages; fever, abdominal cramps. Clinical symptoms and signs: mild to severe diarrhea Johnson TJ et al: Pathogenomics of the virulence plasmids of *Escherichia coli*. Microbiol Mol Biol Rev 2009;73:750. Erratum in: Microbiol Mol Biol Rev 2010;74:477. [PMID: 19946140]

Diffusely adherent *E. coli* (DAEC) Organism elicits a characteristic diffuse aggregative pattern of adherence to HEP-2 cells.	Stool for tissue culture assay for diffuse adherence; test performed by state public health laboratories.	Centers for Disease Control & Prevention: Diarrheagenic *Escherichia coli* http://www.cdc.gov/nczved/divisions/dfbmd/diseases/diarrheagenic_ecoli/technical.htm
Enterotoxigenic *E. coli* (ETEC) Organism adheres to small bowel enterocytes and the enterotoxin causes mild to severe watery diarrhea. Produces two types of toxin: heat-labile (LT) or heat-stable (ST) toxins.	Stool for detection of toxin-producing *E. coli*; test performed by state public health laboratories. Stool does not contain WBCs, mucus, or RBCs.	Clinical symptoms and signs: watery diarrhea, usually lasting for 3–7 days, which can be prolonged or can relapse for months; abdominal cramps; occasional nausea; fever usually absent. Frequent cause of traveler's diarrhea. Navaneethan U et al. Mechanisms of infectious diarrhea. Nat Clin Pract Gastroenterol Hepatol 2008;5:637. [PMID: 18813221]
Enteroaggregative *E. coli* (EAEC) Organism adheres to small and large bowel epithelial cells and expresses secretory enterotoxins and cytotoxins.	Stool for tissue culture adhesion assay; test performed by state public health laboratories. DNA and PCR tests lack sufficient sensitivity and specificity.	Clinical symptoms and signs: intestinal colic, bloody stool, and mucus. Persistant diarrhea in children. Chronic diarrhea in HIV-infected patients/immunocompromised patients. Correlated with interleukin-8 production. Navarro-Garcia F. Enteroaggregative *Escherichia coli* plasmid-encoded toxin. Future Microbiol 2010;5:1005. [PMID: 20632801]
Enteropathogenic *E. coli* (EPEC) Organism adheres to small bowel enterocytes and destroys the normal microvillar structure.	Stool for EPEC PCR or DNA probes may be offered in Public Health Laboratories or research laboratories.	Leading cause of pediatric diarrhea in developing countries. Clinical symptoms and signs: severe diarrhea, low-grade fever, vomiting. Prolonged diarrhea resulting in weight loss, malnutrition, and death. Infantile diarrhea, dehydration. Ochoa TJ et al. New insights into the epidemiology of enteropathogenic *Escherichia coli* infection. Trans R Soc Trop Med Hyg 2008;102:852. [PMID: 18455741] Trabulsi LR et al. Typical and atypical enteropahtogenic *Escherichia coli*. Emerg Infect Dis 2002;8:509. [PMID: 11996687]

Organism	Specimen/Diagnostic Tests	Comments
Enterohemorrhagic E. coli / Shiga-toxin-producing E. coli (EHEC/STEC) Organism colonizes enterocytes of the large bowel and causes a characteristic attaching and effacing pathology. It produces Shiga toxin (Stx) 1 or 2, which inhibit protein synthesis.	Stool for bacterial culture, special media for testing 0157:H7 and 0104:H4. Stool for Shiga toxin by EIA.	Clinical symptoms and signs: frequently bloody diarrhea (although diarrhea without blood can occur), abdominal pain, vomiting, fever usually absent. Hemolytic uremic syndrome (HUS) develops in up to 10%. E. coli 0157:H7 and 0104:H4. EHEC/STEC cause >80% of cases of HUS. Among those with HUS, up to 30–50% have long-term kidney damage; and up to 5–10% die.
Methicillin-resistant Staphylococcus aureus (MRSA) MRSA infections are divided into 2 categories by source: (1) health care-associated (HA-MRSA) secondary to hospitalization, surgery, long-term care, dialysis, invasive device, etc; and (2) community-associated (CA-MRSA). Methicillin resistance is associated with the acquisition of the mecA gene, which encodes the mutant penicillin-binding protein, PBP 2a.	Cultures of skin, soft tissue, blood with isolation of S. aureus and susceptibility testing for methicillin resistance. Swab of anterior nares to screen for MRSA using molecular assays, chromogenic plates (MRSA colonies are pink or blue on chromogenic media), or standard bacterial culture and susceptibility testing.	Clinical symptoms and signs: cellulitis, erysipelas, bacteremia, endocarditis, pneumonia, death. Increasing prevalence of community-associated MRSA, which can cause severe disease in immunocompetent persons, has led to recommendations to screen for MRSA colonization in vulnerable patient populations. This includes patients in ICUs, dialysis centers, or long-term-care facilities, patients admitted for elective surgery, or patients with history of recent hospitalization. Barnes BE ET AL. A literature review on community-acquired methicillin-resistant *Staphylococcus aureus* in the United States: clinical information for primary care nurse practitioners. J Am Acad Nurse Pract 2011;23:23. [PMID: 21208311] Boucher H et al. Serious infections caused by methicillin-resistant *Staphylococcus aureus*. Clin Infect Dis 2010;51(Suppl 2):S183. [PMID: 20731576] Chua K et al. Antimicrobial resistance: not community-associated methicillin-resistant *Staphylococcus aureus* (CA-MRSA)! A clinician's guide to community MRSA—its evolving antimicrobial resistance and implications for therapy. Clin Infect Dis 2011;52:99. [PMID: 21148528] Deleo FR et al. Community-associated methicillin-resistant *Staphylococcus aureus*. Lancet 2010;375:1557. [PMID: 20206987] Kurlenda J et al. Current diagnostic tools for methicillin-resistant *Staphylococcus aureus* infections. Mol Diagn Ther 2010;14:73. [PMID: 20359250]

Streptococcus pneumoniae, resistant

Streptococcus pneumoniae is a gram-positive diplococcus that was generally susceptible to all classes of antimicrobial agents in the 1970s. With increased usage of antibiotics in patients with viral infections, *S. pneumoniae* has acquired genetic material that encodes resistance to many commonly used antibiotics.

It has developed resistance to β-lactamases (45%) at altered penicillin-binding protein sites, to macrolides (40%) at macrolide efflux pump (*mef* genes) and erythromycin-ribosomal methylases (*erm* genes) sites, to lincosamines (14%), to tetracycline, to folate-inhibitors (14–21%), and to fluoroquinolones (1–2%) with mutations in genes that code for DNA gyrase and to topoisomerase IV sites. Emergence of the multidrug-resistant *S. pneumoniae* serotype 19A is due in part to routine use of protein-conjugated pneumococcal vaccine in the US, since this serotype is not included in the vaccine.

Vancomycin-resistant *Enterococcus* (VRE)

Emergence of VRE seen in both *E. faecalis* and *E. faecium* (most common) and at least 7 phenotypes (van A through van G). VRE, especially *E. faecium*, usually demonstrates intrinsic resistance to cephalosporins, aminoglycosides, and β-lactam antibiotics. Enterococci that acquire the van A gene are highly resistant to vancomycin and to teicoplanin. The location of this gene on a plasmid means that it can be spread between strains, and therefore identification of VRE may require contact isolation in the hospital by infection control. Enterococci can also pass the van A gene cluster to *S. aureus* resulting in vancomycin-resistant *S. aureus*.

Cultures of sputum, blood, cerebrospinal fluid.

Cultures of stool, blood, wound, abscesses, CSF.

Jacobs MR. Antimicrobial-resistant *Streptococcus pneumoniae*: trends and management. Expert Rev Anti Infect Ther 2008;6:619. [PMID: 18847402]

Jones RN et al. Evolving trends in *Streptococcus pneumoniae* resistance: implications for therapy of community-acquired bacterial pneumonia. Int J Antimicrob Agents 2010;36:197. [PMID: 20558045]

Linares J et al. Changes in antimicrobial resistance, serotypes and genotypes in *Streptococcus pneumoniae* over a 30-year period. Clin Microbiol Infect 2010;16:402. [PMID: 20132251]

Lynch JP 3rd et al. *Streptococcus pneumoniae*: epidemiology and risk factors, evolution of antimicrobial resistance, and impact of vaccines. Curr Opin Pulm Med 2010;16:217. [PMID: 20375783]

Reinert RR. The antimicrobial resistance profile of *Streptococcus pneumoniae*. Clin Microbiol Infect 2009;15(Suppl 3):7. [PMID: 19366363]

Heintz BH et al. Vancomycin-resistant enterococcal urinary tract infections. Pharmacotherapy 2010;30:1136. [PMID: 20973687]

Lin MY et al. Methicillin-resistant *Staphylococcus aureus* and vancomycin-resistant enterococcus: recognition and prevention in intensive care units. Crit Care Med 2010;38 (Suppl 8):S335. [PMID: 20647791]

6

Diagnostic Imaging: Test Selection and Interpretation

Benjamin M. Yeh, MD

HOW TO USE THIS SECTION

Information in this chapter is arranged anatomically from superior to inferior. It would not be feasible to include all available imaging tests in one chapter in a book of this size, but we have attempted to summarize the essential features of those examinations that are most frequently ordered in modern clinical practice or those that may be associated with difficulty or risk. Indications, advantages and disadvantages, contraindications, and patient preparation are presented. Costs of the studies are approximate and represent averages reported from several large medical centers.

$$\begin{aligned} \$ &= <\$250 \\ \$\$ &= \$250–\$750 \\ \$\$\$ &= \$750–\$1000 \\ \$\$\$\$ &= >\$1000 \end{aligned}$$

RISKS OF CT AND ANGIOGRAPHIC INTRAVENOUS CONTRAST AGENTS

Although intravenous contrast is an important tool in radiology, it is not without substantial risks. Minor reactions (nausea, vomiting, hives) occur with an overall incidence between 1% and 12%. Major reactions (laryngeal edema, bronchospasm, cardiac arrest) occur in 0.16–1 cases per 1000 patients. Deaths have been reported in 1:40,000 to 1:170,000 cases. Patients with an allergic history (asthma, hay fever, allergy to foods or drugs) have a slightly increased risk. A history of allergic-type reaction to contrast material is associated with an increased risk of a subsequent severe reaction.

Prophylactic measures that may be required in such cases include corticosteroids and H_1 and H_2 blockers.

In addition, there is a risk of contrast-induced renal failure, which is usually mild and reversible. Persons at increased risk for potentially *irreversible* renal damage include patients with preexisting renal disease (particularly diabetics with borderline renal function), multiple myeloma, and severe hyperuricemia.

MRI INTRAVENOUS CONTRAST AGENTS

Contrast agents used in MRI are different from those used in most other radiology studies. Most MRI contrast agents are teratogenic and relatively contraindicated in pregnancy. Rarely, patients with severe renal dysfunction, particularly if on dialysis, or those with acute renal failure may develop irreversible nephrogenic systemic fibrosis after receiving gadolinium-based intravenous contrast. Immediate contrast reactions are rare (minor reactions in approximately 0.07% and major reactions in 0.001%). Contrast-induced renal failure is not associated with MRI intravenous contrast.

In summary, intravenous contrast should be viewed in the same manner as other medications—that is, risks and benefits must be balanced before an examination using this pharmaceutical is ordered.

	Test	Indications	Advantages	Disadvantages/Contraindications	Preparation
HEAD					
CT					
HEAD **Computed tomography** (CT) $$$		Evaluation of acute craniofacial trauma, acute neurologic dysfunction (<72 hours) from suspected intracranial or subarachnoid hemorrhage. Further characterization of intracranial masses identified by MRI (presence or absence of calcium or involvement of the bony calvarium). Evaluation of sinus disease and temporal bone disease.	Rapid acquisition makes it the modality of choice for trauma. Superb spatial resolution. Superior to MRI in detection of hemorrhage within the first 24–48 hours.	Artifacts from bone may interfere with detection of disease at the skull base and in the posterior fossa. Generally limited to transaxial views. Direct coronal images of paranasal sinuses and temporal bones are routinely obtained if patient can lie prone. **Contraindications and risks:** Caution in pregnancy because of the potential harm of ionizing radiation to the fetus. See Risks of CT and Angiographic Intravenous Contrast Agents, p. 375.	Normal hydration. Sedation of agitated patients. Recent serum creatinine determination if intravenous contrast is to be used.

			BRAIN	
			CTA	MRI
Test	**Indications**	**Advantages**	**Disadvantages/Contraindications**	**Preparation**
BRAIN **CT angiography** (CTA) $$$	Evaluation of cerebral arteriovenous malformations, intracranial aneurysm.	Rapid acquisition makes it an excellent choice for evaluation of blood vessels in stroke. Can cover a large territory, including down to the heart. Superb spatial resolution.	Artifacts from bone may interfere with detection of disease at the skull base and in the posterior fossa. Generally limited to transaxial views. Direct coronal images of paranasal sinuses and temporal bones are routinely obtained if patient can lie prone. **Contraindications and risks:** Caution in pregnancy because of the potential harm of ionizing radiation to the fetus. See Risks of CT and Angiographic Intravenous Contrast Agents, p. 375.	Normal hydration. Sedation of agitated patients. Recent serum creatinine determination if intravenous contrast is to be used.
HEAD **Magnetic resonance imaging** (MRI) $$$$	Evaluation of essentially all intracranial disease except those listed above for CT.	Provides excellent tissue contrast resolution, multiplanar capability. Can detect flowing blood and cryptic vascular malformations. Can detect demyelinating and dysmyelinating disease. No ionizing radiation.	Subject to motion artifacts. Inferior to CT in the setting of acute trauma because it is insensitive to acute hemorrhage, incompatible with traction devices, inferior in detection of bony injury and foreign bodies, and requires longer image acquisition time. Special instrumentation required for patients on life support. **Contraindications and risks:** Contraindicated in patients with cardiac pacemakers, intraocular metallic foreign bodies, intracranial aneurysm clips, cochlear implants, and some artificial heart valves.	Sedation of agitated patients. Screening CT or plain radiograph images of orbits if history suggests possible metallic foreign body in the eye.

BRAIN		
	MRA/MRV	**Brain scan**
BRAIN **Magnetic resonance angiography/ venography** (MRA/MRV) $$$$	Evaluation of cerebral arterio-venous malformations, intracranial aneurysm, and blood supply of vascular tumors as aid to operative planning (MRA). Evaluation of dural sinus thrombosis (MRV).	No ionizing radiation. No iodinated contrast needed.	Subject to motion artifacts. Special instrumentation required for patients on life support. **Contraindications and risks:** Contraindicated in patients with cardiac pacemakers, intraocular metallic foreign bodies, intracranial aneurysm clips, cochlear implants, and some artificial heart valves.	Sedation of agitated patients. Screening CT or plain radiograph images of orbits if history suggests possible metallic foreign body in the eye.
BRAIN **Brain scan** (radionuclide) $$	Confirmation of brain death.	Confirmation of brain death not impeded by hypothermia or barbiturate coma. Can be portable.	Limited resolution. Delayed imaging required with some agents. Cannot be used alone to establish diagnosis of brain death. Must be used in combination with clinical examination or cerebral angiography to establish diagnosis. **Contraindications and risks:** Caution in pregnancy because of the potential harm of ionizing radiation to the fetus.	Premedicate with potassium perchlorate when using TcO_4 to block choroid plexus uptake.

		BRAIN	
		Brain PET/SPECT	**Cisternography**

Test	Indications	Advantages	Disadvantages/Contraindications	Preparation
BRAIN **Positron emission tomography (PET)/Single Photon Emission Computed Tomography (SPECT)** brain scan $$$	Evaluation of suspected dementia. Evaluation of medically refractory seizures.	Provides functional information. Can localize seizure focus prior to surgical excision. Up to 82% positive predictive value for Alzheimer's dementia in appropriate clinical settings. Provides cross-sectional images and therefore improved lesion localization compared with planar imaging techniques.	Limited resolution compared with MRI and CT. Limited application in work-up of dementia due to low specificity of images and fact that test results do not alter clinical management. **Contraindications and risks:** Caution in pregnancy because of potential harm of ionizing radiation to the fetus.	Sedation of agitated patients.
BRAIN **Cisternography** (radionuclide) $$	Evaluation of hydrocephalus (particularly normal pressure), CSF rhinorrhea or otorrhea, and ventricular shunt patency.	Provides functional information. Can help distinguish normal pressure hydrocephalus from senile atrophy. Can detect CSF leaks.	Requires multiple delayed imaging sessions up to 48–72 hours after injection. **Contraindications and risks:** Caution in pregnancy because of the potential harm of ionizing radiation to the fetus.	Sedation of agitated patients. For suspected CSF leak, pack the patient's nose or ears with cotton pledgets before administration of dose. Must follow strict sterile precautions for intrathecal injection.

NECK			
MRI			**MRA**
NECK **Magnetic resonance imaging** (MRI) $$$$	Evaluation of upper aerodigestive tract. Staging of neck masses. Differentiation of lymphadenopathy from blood vessels. Evaluation of head and neck malignancy, thyroid nodules, parathyroid adenoma, lymphadenopathy, retropharyngeal abscess, brachial plexopathy.	Provides excellent tissue contrast resolution. Tissue differentiation of malignancy or abscess from benign tumor often possible. Sagittal and coronal planar imaging possible. Multiplanar capability especially advantageous regarding brachial plexus. No iodinated contrast needed to distinguish lymphadenopathy from blood vessels.	Subject to motion artifacts, particularly those of carotid pulsation and swallowing. Special instrumentation required for patients on life support. **Contraindications and risks:** Contraindicated in patients with cardiac pacemakers, intraocular metallic foreign bodies, intracranial aneurysm clips, cochlear implants, and some artificial heart valves.	Sedation of agitated patients. Screening CT or plain radiograph images of orbits if history suggests possible metallic foreign body in the eye.
NECK **Magnetic resonance angiography** (MRA) $$$$	Evaluation of carotid bifurcation atherosclerosis, cervicocranial arterial dissection.	No ionizing radiation. No iodinated contrast needed. MRA of the carotid arteries can be a sufficient preoperative evaluation regarding critical stenosis when local expertise exists.	Subject to motion artifacts, particularly from carotid pulsation and swallowing. Special instrumentation required for patients on life support. **Contraindications and risks:** Contraindicated in patients with cardiac pacemakers, intraocular metallic foreign bodies, intracranial aneurysm clips, cochlear implants, and some artificial heart valves.	Sedation of agitated patients. Screening CT or plain radiograph images of orbits if history suggests possible metallic foreign body in the eye.

Test	Indications	Advantages	Disadvantages/Contraindications	Preparation
			NECK	
		CT		Ultrasound
NECK **Computed tomography** (CT) $$$	Evaluation of the upper aerodigestive tract. Staging of neck masses for patients who are not candidates for MRI. Evaluation of suspected abscess.	Rapid. Superb spatial resolution. Can guide percutaneous fine-needle aspiration of possible tumor or abscess.	Adequate intravenous contrast enhancement of vascular structures is mandatory for accurate interpretation. **Contraindications and risks:** See Risks of CT and Angiographic Intravenous Contrast Agents, p. 375.	Normal hydration. Sedation of agitated patients. Recent serum creatinine determination.
NECK **Ultrasound** (US) $$	Patency and morphology of arteries and veins. Evaluation of thyroid and parathyroid. Guidance for percutaneous fine-needle aspiration biopsy of neck lesions.	Can detect and monitor for atherosclerotic stenosis of carotid arteries noninvasively and without iodinated contrast.	Technically demanding, operator-dependent. Patient must lie supine and still for 1 hour.	None.

THYROID

Modality	Indications	Advantages / Function	Comments — Contraindications and risks	Patient preparation
THYROID **Ultrasound** (US) $$	Determination whether a palpable nodule is a cyst or solid mass and whether multiple nodules are present. Assessment of response to suppressive therapy. Screening patients with a history of radiation to the head and neck. Guidance for biopsy.	Noninvasive. No ionizing radiation. Can be portable. Can image in all planes.	Cannot distinguish between benign and malignant lesions unless local invasion is demonstrated. Technique very operator-dependent. **Contraindications and risks:** None.	None.
THYROID **Thyroid uptake and scan** (radionuclide) $$	Uptake indicated for evaluation of clinical hypothyroidism, hyperthyroidism, thyroiditis, effects of thyroid-stimulating and thyroid-suppressing medications, and for calculation of therapeutic radiation dosage. Scanning indicated for above as well as evaluation of palpable nodules, mediastinal mass, and screening of patients with history of head and neck irradiation for thyroid cancer. Total body scanning used for postoperative evaluation of thyroid cancer metastases.	Demonstrates both morphology and function. Can identify ectopic thyroid tissue and "cold" nodules that have a greater risk of malignancy. Imaging of whole body with one dose (^{131}I).	Substances interfering with test include iodides in vitamins and medicines, antithyroid drugs, corticosteroids, and intravascular contrast agents. Delayed imaging is required with iodides (^{123}I, 6 hours and 24 hours; ^{131}I total body, 72 hours). Test may not visualize thyroid gland in subacute thyroiditis. **Contraindications and risks:** Not advised in pregnancy because of the risk of ionizing radiation to the fetus (iodides cross placenta and concentrate in fetal thyroid). Significant radiation exposure occurs in total body scanning with ^{131}I; patients should be instructed about precautionary measures by nuclear medicine personnel.	Administration of dose after a 4- to 6-hour fast aids absorption. Discontinue all interfering substances prior to test, especially thyroid-suppressing medications: T_3 (1 week), T_4 (4–6 weeks), propylthiouracil (2 weeks).

	THYROID
	Radionuclide therapy

Test	Indications	Advantages	Disadvantages/Contraindications	Preparation
THYROID **Thyroid therapy** (radionuclide) $$$	Hyperthyroidism and some thyroid carcinomas (papillary and follicular types are amenable to treatment, whereas medullary and anaplastic types are not).	Noninvasive alternative to surgery.	Rarely, radiation thyroiditis may occur 1–3 days after therapy. Hypothyroidism occurs commonly as a long-term complication. Higher doses that are required to treat thyroid carcinoma may result in pulmonary fibrosis. **Contraindications and risks:** Contraindicated in pregnancy and lactation. Contraindicated in patients with metastatic thyroid cancer to the brain, because treatment may result in brain edema and subsequent herniation, and in those <20 years of age with hyperthyroidism because of possible increased risk of thyroid cancer later in life. After treatment, a patient's activities are restricted to limit total exposure of any member of the general public until radiation level is ≤ 0.5 rem.	After treatment, patients must isolate all bodily secretions from household members. High doses for treatment of thyroid carcinoma may necessitate hospitalization.

PARATHYROID	Evaluation of suspected parathyroid adenoma.	Identifies hyperfunctioning tissue, which is useful when planning surgery.	Small adenomas (<500 mg) may not be detected. **Contraindications and risks:** Caution in pregnancy is advised because of the risk of ionizing radiation to the fetus.	Requires strict patient immobility during scanning.
Parathyroid scan (radionuclide) $$				

PARATHYROID

Radionuclide scan

Test	Indications	Advantages	Disadvantages/Contraindications	Preparation	
CHEST **Chest radiograph** $	Evaluation of pleural and parenchymal pulmonary disease, mediastinal disease, cardiogenic and noncardiogenic pulmonary edema, congenital and acquired cardiac disease. Screening for traumatic aortic rupture (though CT is playing an increasing role). Evaluation of possible pneumothorax (expiratory upright film) or pleural effusion.	Inexpensive. Widely available.	Difficult to distinguish between causes of hilar and mediastinal enlargement (ie, vasculature versus adenopathy). Not sensitive for small pulmonary nodules. **Contraindications and risks:** Caution in pregnancy because of the potential harm of ionizing radiation to the fetus.	None.	CHEST Chest radiograph
CHEST **Computed tomography** (CT) $$$	Evaluation of thoracic trauma. Evaluation of mediastinal and hilar tumor. Evaluation and staging of primary and metastatic lung neoplasm. Characterization of pulmonary nodules. Differentiation of parenchymal versus pleural process (ie, lung abscess versus empyema). Evaluation of interstitial lung disease (1-mm thin sections), aortic dissection, and aneurysm. Screening for lung cancer in high-risk populations.	Rapid. Superb spatial resolution. Can guide percutaneous fine-needle aspiration of possible tumor or abscess.	Patient cooperation required for appropriate breath-holding. **Contraindications and risks:** Caution in pregnancy because of the potential harm of ionizing radiation to the fetus. See Risks of CT and Angiographic Intravenous Contrast Agents, p. 375.	Preferably NPO for 2 hours before study. Normal hydration. Sedation of agitated patients. Recent serum creatinine determination.	CHEST CT

CHEST		
	MRI	**PET/CT**
CHEST **Magnetic resonance imaging** (MRI) $$$$	Evaluation of mediastinal masses. Discrimination between hilar vessels and enlarged lymph nodes. Tumor staging (especially when invasion of vessels or pericardium is suspected). Evaluation of aortic dissection, aortic aneurysm, congenital and acquired cardiac disease.	Provides excellent tissue contrast resolution and multiplanar capability. No ionizing radiation.	Subject to motion artifacts. **Contraindications and risks:** Contraindicated in patients with cardiac pacemakers, intraocular metallic foreign bodies, intracranial aneurysm clips, cochlear implants, and some artificial heart valves.	Sedation of agitated patients. Screening CT of the orbits if history suggests possible metallic foreign body in the eye.
CHEST **Positron emission tomography/ Computed tomography** (PET/CT) $$$$	Evaluation for mediastinal masses and metastases. Discrimination between benign and malignant lymph nodes. Tumor staging and treatment monitoring.	Combines metabolic and anatomic information. Large area of coverage (can image whole body).	Patient cooperation required for appropriate breath-holding. **Contraindications and risks:** Contraindicated in pregnancy because of the potential harm of ionizing radiation to the fetus. See Risks of CT and Angiographic Intravenous Contrast Agents, p. 375.	Preferably NPO for 2 hours before study. Normal hydration. Sedation of agitated patients. Recent serum creatinine determination.

		LUNG	
		Ventilation-perfusion scan	CT
Test	**Indications**	**Advantages**	**Disadvantages/Contraindications**	**Preparation**

Test	Indications	Advantages	Disadvantages/Contraindications	Preparation
LUNG **Ventilation-perfusion scan** (radionuclide) $\dot{V}$ = \$\$ $\dot{Q}$ = \$\$ $\dot{V}+\dot{Q}$ = \$\$\$ – \$\$\$\$	Evaluation of pulmonary embolism or burn inhalation injury. Preoperative evaluation of patients with chronic obstructive pulmonary disease and of those who are candidates for pneumonectomy.	Noninvasive. Provides functional information in preoperative assessment. Permits determination of differential and regional lung function in preoperative assessment. Documented pulmonary embolism is extremely rare with normal perfusion scan.	Patients must be able to cooperate for ventilation portion of the examination. There is a high proportion of intermediate probability studies in patients with underlying lung disease. The likelihood of pulmonary embolism ranges from 20%–80% in these cases. A patient who has a low probability scan still has a chance ranging from nil to 19% of having a pulmonary embolus. **Contraindications and risks:** Patients with severe pulmonary artery hypertension or significant right-to-left shunts should have fewer particles injected. Caution advised in pregnancy because of risk of ionizing radiation to the fetus.	Current chest radiograph is mandatory for interpretation.
LUNG **Computed tomography** (CT) \$\$\$	Evaluation of clinically suspected pulmonary embolism.	Rapid. High sensitivity and specificity for clinically relevant pulmonary emboli. Allows determination of causes other than pulmonary embolism for dyspnea. Evaluation of pulmonary vein anatomy before electrophysiology ablation.	Respiratory motion artifacts can be a problem in dyspneic patients and older CT scanners. High-quality study requires breath-holding of approximately 10–20 seconds. Specific imaging protocol utilized which limits diagnostic information for other abnormalities. **Contraindications and risks:** Caution in pregnancy because of potential harm of ionizing radiation to fetus. See Risks of CT and Angiographic Intravenous Contrast Agents, p. 375.	Large-gauge intravenous access (minimum 20-gauge) required. Prebreathing oxygen may help dyspneic patients perform adequate breath hold. Normal hydration. Preferably NPO for 2 hours before study. Recent serum creatinine determination.

BREAST			
Mammogram			
BREAST			
Mammogram $	Screening for breast cancer in asymptomatic women: (1) every 1–2 years between ages 40 and 49; (2) every year after age 50. If history of breast cancer, mammogram should be performed yearly at any age. Indicated at any age for symptoms (palpable mass, bloody discharge) or before breast surgery.	Newer digital and film screen techniques generate lower radiation doses (0.1–0.2 cGy per film, mean glandular dose). A 23% lower mortality rate has been demonstrated in patients screened with combined mammogram and physical examination compared with physical examination alone. In a screening population, more than 40% of cancers are detected by mammography alone and cannot be palpated on physical examination.	Detection of breast masses is more difficult in patients with radiographically dense breasts. Breast compression may cause patient discomfort. In a screening population, 9% of cancers are detected by physical examination alone and are not detectable by mammography. **Contraindications and risks:** Radiation from repeated mammograms can theoretically cause breast cancer; however, the benefits of screening mammograms greatly outweigh the risks.	None.

Test	Indications	Advantages	Disadvantages/Contraindications	Preparation
BREAST				
Breast MRI				
BREAST **MRI** $$$$	Screening for breast cancer in very high-risk women. May be used to guide breast biopsy of MRI-detected abnormalities.	Improved cancer detection, compared with mammograms, particularly for women with radiographically dense breasts. No ionizing radiation.	Higher rate of false positives than mammography. Utilizes intravenous contrast material. **Contraindications and risks:** Contraindicated in patients with cardiac pacemakers, intraocular metallic foreign bodies, intracranial aneurysm clips, cochlear implants, and some artificial heart valves.	Screening CT of the orbits if history suggests possible metallic foreign body in the eye.

HEART			
Myocardial perfusion scan			
HEART **Myocardial perfusion scan** (thallium scan, technetium-99m methoxy-isobutyl isonitrile (sestamibi) scan, others) $-$$-$$$ (broad range)	Evaluation of atypical chest pain. Detection of presence, location, and extent of myocardial ischemia.	Highly sensitive for detecting physiologically significant coronary stenosis. Noninvasive. Able to stratify patients according to risk for myocardial infarction. Normal examination associated with average risk of cardiac death or nonfatal myocardial infarction of <1% per year.	The patient must be carefully monitored during treadmill or pharmacologic stress—optimally, under the supervision of a cardiologist. False-positive results may be caused by exercise-induced spasm, aortic stenosis, or left bundle branch block; false-negative results may be caused by inadequate exercise, mild or distal disease, or balanced diffuse ischemia. **Contraindications and risks:** Aminophylline (inhibitor of dipyridamole) is a contraindication to the use of dipyridamole. Treadmill or pharmacologic stress carries a risk of arrhythmia, ischemia, infarct, and, rarely, death. Caution in pregnancy because of the risk of ionizing radiation to the fetus.	In case of severe peripheral vascular disease, severe pulmonary disease, or musculoskeletal disorder, pharmacologic stress with dipyridamole or other agents may be used. Tests should be performed in the fasting state. Patient should not exercise between stress and redistribution scans.

		HEART	
		CT Coronary artery calcium scoring/angiography	Ventriculography

Test	Indications	Advantages	Disadvantages/Contraindications	Preparation
HEART **Computed tomography coronary artery calcium scoring/ angiography** $$-$$$	Screening evaluation for coronary artery calcification. Evaluation for coronary artery stenoses and congenital anomalies.	Noninvasive. Higher coronary artery calcium score correlates with increased risk for significant coronary artery stenosis.	Gated data acquisition may be difficult in patients with severe arrhythmias or rapid heart rate. If high calcium score or coronary artery stenosis is found, patient may need additional treatment (to reduce risk of myocardial infarction). **Contraindications and risks:** Caution in pregnancy because of potential harm of ionizing radiation to fetus. See Risks of CT and Angiographic Intravenous Contrast Agents, p. 375.	May require medication with β-blocker to decrease heart rate.
HEART **Radionuclide ventriculography** (multigated acquisition [MUGA]) $$-$$$-$$$$	Evaluation of patients with ischemic heart disease and other cardiomyopathies. Evaluation of response to pharmacologic therapy and effects of cardiotoxic drugs.	Noninvasive. Ejection fraction is a reproducible index that can be used to follow course of disease and response to therapy.	Gated data acquisition may be difficult in patients with severe arrhythmias. **Contraindications and risks:** Recent infarct is a contraindication to exercise ventriculography (arrhythmia, ischemia, infarct, and rarely death may occur with exercise). Caution is advised in pregnancy because of the risk of ionizing radiation to the fetus.	Requires harvesting, labeling, and reinjecting the patient's red blood cells. Sterile technique required in handling of red cells.

ABDOMEN		
	KUB	**Ultrasound**
		None.
ABDOMEN	Assessment of bowel gas patterns (eg, to distinguish ileus from obstruction). To rule out pneumoperitoneum, order an upright abdomen and chest radiograph (acute abdominal series).	NPO for 6 hours.
Abdominal plain radiograph (KUB [kidneys, ureters, bladder] x-ray) $	Inexpensive. Widely available.	Supine film alone is inadequate to rule out pneumoperitoneum (see Indications). Obstipation may obscure lesions. **Contraindications and risks:** Contraindicated in pregnancy because of the risk of ionizing radiation to the fetus.
ABDOMEN **Ultrasound** (US) $$	Differentiation of cystic versus solid lesions of the liver and kidneys. Detection of intra- and extrahepatic biliary ductal dilation, cholelithiasis, gallbladder wall thickness, pericholecystic fluid, peripancreatic fluid and pseudocyst, hydronephrosis, abdominal aortic aneurysm, appendicitis, ascites, primary and metastatic liver carcinoma.	Noninvasive. No ionizing radiation. Can be portable. Imaging in all planes. Can guide percutaneous fine-needle aspiration of tumor or abscess. Technique very operator-dependent. Organs (particularly pancreas and distal aorta) may be obscured by bowel gas. **Contraindications and risks:** None.

	ABDOMEN			
	CT			
Test	Indications	Advantages	Disadvantages/Contraindications	Preparation
ABDOMEN **Computed tomography** (CT) $$$–$$$$	Morphologic evaluation of all abdominal and pelvic organs. Evaluation of abscess, trauma, mesenteric and retroperitoneal lymphadenopathy, bowel obstruction, obstructive biliary disease, pancreatitis, appendicitis, peritonitis, visceral infarction, and retroperitoneal hemorrhage. Staging and monitoring of malignancy in the liver, pancreas, kidneys, and other abdominopelvic organs and spaces. Determination of tumor resectability. Excellent screening tool for evaluation of suspected renal and ureteral stones or other cause of upper urinary tract bleeding. CT angiography evaluates the aorta and its branches. Can provide preoperative assessment of abdominal aortic aneurysm and dissection size, proximal and distal extent, relationship to renal arteries, and presence of anatomic anomalies. CT colonography useful in patients with failed colonoscopy or those unable to undergo colonoscopy. Differentiation of benign from malignant adrenal adenoma.	Rapid. Complete coverage of abdomen and pelvis. Superb spatial resolution. Not limited by overlying bowel gas, as with ultrasound. Can guide fine-needle aspiration and percutaneous drainage. Noncontrast is the standard of reference for determining the extent and locations of urinary tract stone disease.	Barium or Hypaque, surgical clips, and metallic prostheses can cause artifacts and degrade image quality. **Contraindications and risks:** Contraindicated in pregnancy because of the potential harm of ionizing radiation to the fetus. See Risks of CT and Angiographic Intravenous Contrast Studies, p. 375.	Preferably NPO for 4–6 hours. Normal hydration. Distention of gastrointestinal tract with water or oral contrast material. Sedation of agitated patients. Recent serum creatinine determination if intravenous contrast material is to be given.

	ABDOMEN	
	MRI	**PET/CT**

ABDOMEN **Magnetic resonance imaging** (MRI) $$$$	Assessment and preoperative staging of intraabdominal cancers. Differentiation of benign from malignant adrenal masses. Complementary to CT in evaluation of liver lesions (especially metastatic disease and possible tumor invasion of hepatic or portal veins). Differentiation of benign from malignant liver tumors. Differentiation of retroperitoneal lymphadenopathy from blood vessels or the diaphragmatic crus.	Provides excellent tissue contrast resolution, multiplanar capability. No ionizing radiation.	Subject to motion artifacts. Gastrointestinal opacification not yet readily available. Special instrumentation required for patients on life support. **Contraindications and risks:** Contraindicated in patients with cardiac pacemakers, intraocular metallic foreign bodies, intracranial aneurysm clips, cochlear implants, and some artificial heart valves.	NPO for 4–6 hours. Intramuscular glucagon to inhibit peristalsis. Sedation of agitated patients. Screening CT or plain radiograph images of orbits if history suggests possible metallic foreign body in the eye.
ABDOMEN/ PELVIS **Positron emission tomography/ computed tomography** (PET/CT) $$$$	Evaluation for abdominopelvic malignancy and metastases. Discrimination between benign and malignant lymph nodes. Tumor staging and treatment monitoring.	Combines metabolic and anatomic information. Large area of coverage (can image whole body).	Patient cooperation required for appropriate breath-holding. **Contraindications and risks:** Contraindicated in pregnancy because of the potential harm of ionizing radiation to the fetus. See Risks of CT and Angiographic Intravenous Contrast Agents, p. 375.	Preferably NPO for 2 hours before study. Normal hydration. Sedation of agitated patients. Recent serum creatinine determination.

	ABDOMEN			
	Mesenteric angiography			
Test	Indications	Advantages	Disadvantages/Contraindications	Preparation
ABDOMEN **Mesenteric angiography** $$$$	Gastrointestinal hemorrhage that does not resolve with conservative therapy and cannot be treated endoscopically. Localization of gastrointestinal bleeding site. Acute mesenteric ischemia, intestinal angina, splenic or other splanchnic artery aneurysm. Evaluation of possible vasculitis, such as polyarteritis nodosa. Detection of islet cell tumors not identified by other studies. Abdominal trauma.	Therapeutic embolization of gastrointestinal vessels during hemorrhage is often possible.	Invasive. Patient may need to remain supine with leg extended for 6 hours after the procedure to protect the common femoral artery at the catheter entry site. **Contraindications and risks:** Allergy to iodinated contrast material may require corticosteroid and H_1 blocker or H_2 blocker premedication. Contraindicated in pregnancy because of the potential harm of ionizing radiation to the fetus. Contrast nephrotoxicity may occur, especially with preexisting impaired renal function due to diabetes mellitus or multiple myeloma; however, any creatinine elevation following the procedure is usually reversible (see Risks of CT and Angiographic Contrast Agents, p. 375).	NPO for 4–6 hours. Good hydration to limit possible renal insult due to iodinated contrast material. Recent serum creatinine determination, assessment of clotting parameters, reversal of anticoagulation. Performed with conscious sedation. Requires cardiac, respiratory, blood pressure, and pulse oximetry monitoring.

GASTROINTESTINAL				

GI **Upper GI study** (UGI) $$	Double-contrast barium technique demonstrates esophageal, gastric, and duodenal mucosa for evaluation of inflammatory disease and other subtle mucosal abnormalities. Single-contrast technique assesses bowel motility, peristalsis, possible outlet obstruction, gastroesophageal reflux and hiatal hernia, esophageal cancer, and varices. Water-soluble contrast (Gastrografin) is suitable for evaluation of anastomotic leak or gastrointestinal perforation.	Good evaluation of mucosa with double-contrast examination. No sedation required. Less expensive than endoscopy.	Aspiration of water-soluble contrast material may occur, resulting in severe pulmonary edema. Leakage of barium from a perforation may cause granulomatous inflammatory reaction. Identification of a lesion does not prove it to be the site of blood loss in patients with gastrointestinal bleeding. Barium precludes endoscopy and body CT examination. Retained gastric secretions prevent mucosal coating with barium. **Contraindications and risks:** Caution in pregnancy because of the potential harm of ionizing radiation to the fetus.	NPO for 8 hours.
GI **Enteroclysis** $$	Barium fluoroscopic study for location of site of intermittent partial small bowel obstruction. Evaluation of extent of Crohn disease or small bowel disease in patient with persistent gastrointestinal bleeding and normal UGI and colonic evaluations. Evaluation of metastatic disease to the small bowel.	Clarifies lesions noted on more traditional barium examination of the small bowel. Best means of establishing small bowel as normal.	Requires nasogastric or orogastric tube placement and manipulation to beyond the ligament of Treitz. **Contraindications and risks:** Radiation exposure is substantial, because lengthy fluoroscopic examination is required. Therefore, the test is contraindicated in pregnant women and should be used sparingly in children and women of child-bearing age.	Clear liquid diet for 24 hours. Colonic cleansing.

		GASTROINTESTINAL	
Test		CT Enterography	Small bowel follow-through
GI **CT enterography** $$$	Indications	Assessment for small bowel strictures before capsule endoscopy. Assess for extent of inflammatory bowel disease, postoperative adhesions, and small bowel tumors.	Barium fluoroscopic study for location of site of intermittent partial small bowel obstruction. Evaluation of extent of Crohn disease or small bowel disease in patient with normal endoscopy and colonic evaluations. Evaluation of metastatic disease to the small bowel.
	Advantages	Noninvasive. Complete visualization of the small bowel. Evaluates extraluminal disease, including extent of intraabdominal abscesses and fistulas.	Less invasive and better tolerated than enteroclysis. May be combined with UGI.
	Disadvantages/Contraindications	Requires drinking large amounts of water or oral contrast material. Improved images obtained if antiperistaltic agent given at time of examination. **Contraindications and risks:** Caution in pregnancy because of the potential harm of ionizing radiation to the fetus. Caution in repeated examinations of young patients because of cumulative radiation dose.	Less diagnostic power than enteroclysis for mucosal detail. Requires nasogastric or orogastric tube placement and manipulation to beyond the ligament of Treitz. **Contraindications and risks:** Radiation exposure is substantial, because lengthy fluoroscopic examination is required. Therefore, the test is contraindicated in pregnant women and should be used sparingly in children and women of child-bearing age.
	Preparation	NPO for 4–6 hours. Consume 1–2 liters of water orally or contrast material 45 minutes before scan.	Clear liquid diet for 24 hours. Colonic cleansing.
GI **Small bowel follow-through** $$			

GASTROINTESTINAL				
Barium enema				
CT colonography				

GI — Barium enema (BE) — $$

Double-contrast technique for evaluation of colonic mucosa for suspected inflammatory bowel disease or neoplasm. Single-contrast technique for investigation of possible fistulous tracts, anastomotic leak, bowel obstruction, and for examination of debilitated patients.

Good mucosal evaluation. No sedation required.

Retained fecal material limits evaluation of mucosa. Requires patient cooperation. Marked diverticulosis precludes evaluation for possible neoplasm in involved area. Evaluation of right colon occasionally incomplete or limited by reflux of barium across ileocecal valve and overlapping opacified small bowel. Use of barium delays subsequent colonoscopy and body CT. **Contraindications and risks:** Contraindicated in patients with toxic megacolon and immediately after full-thickness colonoscopic biopsy.

Colon cleansing with enemas, cathartic, and clear liquid diet (1 day in young patients, 2 days in older patients). Intravenous glucagon (which inhibits peristalsis) sometimes given to distinguish colonic spasm from a mass lesion.

GI — CT colonography — $$

Thin section CT for evaluation of possible colonic polyps and masses.

Has ability to evaluate extracolonic intraabdominal disease (AAA, renal cell carcinoma, kidney stones). No IV contrast. Better tolerated than colonoscopy.

Retained fecal material may limit study. Requires patient cooperation. If polyps or masses are found, patient will still need to undergo colonoscopy or sigmoidoscopy for tissue diagnosis.

Requires colonic preparation that varies from institution to institution.

		GASTROINTESTINAL	
		Hypaque enema	**Esophageal reflux study**
Test		GI **Hypaque enema** $$	GI **Esophageal reflux study** (radionuclide) $$
Indications		Water-soluble contrast for fluoroscopic evaluation of colonic anatomy, anastomotic leak, or other perforation. Differentiation of colonic versus small bowel obstruction. Therapy for obstipation.	Evaluation of heartburn, regurgitation, recurrent aspiration pneumonia.
Advantages		Water-soluble contrast medium is evacuated much faster than barium because it does not adhere to the mucosa. Therefore, Hypaque enema can be followed immediately by oral ingestion of barium for evaluation of possible distal small bowel obstruction.	Noninvasive and well tolerated. More sensitive for reflux than fluoroscopy, endoscopy, and manometry; sensitivity similar to that of acid reflux test. Permits quantitation of reflux. Can identify aspiration into the lung.
Disadvantages/Contraindications		Demonstrates only colonic morphologic features and not mucosal changes. Incidental findings can be noted. **Contraindications and risks:** Caution in repeated examinations because of cumulative radiation dose. Contraindicated in patients with toxic megacolon. Hypertonic solution may lead to fluid imbalance in debilitated patients and children.	Incomplete emptying of esophagus may mimic reflux. Abdominal binder—used to increase pressure in the lower esophagus—may not be tolerated in patients who have undergone recent abdominal surgery. **Contraindications and risks:** Contraindicated in pregnancy because of the potential harm of ionizing radiation to the fetus.
Preparation		Colonic cleansing is desirable but not always necessary.	NPO for 4–6 hours. During test, patient must be able to consume 300 mL of liquid.

GASTROINTESTINAL	
Gastric emptying study	GI bleeding scan

| GI

Gastric emptying study (radionuclide)

$$ | Evaluation of dumping syndrome, vagotomy, gastric outlet obstruction due to inflammatory or neoplastic disease, effects of drugs, and other causes of gastroparesis (eg, diabetes mellitus). | Gives functional information not available by other means. | Reporting of meaningful data requires adherence to standard protocol and establishment of normal values.
Contraindications and risks: Contraindicated in pregnancy because of the potential harm of ionizing radiation to the fetus. | NPO for 4–6 hours. During test, patient must be able to eat a 300 g meal consisting of both liquids and solids. |
| GI

GI bleeding scan (labeled red cell scan, radionuclide)

$$–$$$ | Evaluation of upper or lower gastrointestinal blood loss. Distinguishing hemangioma of the liver from other mass lesions of the liver. | Noninvasive compared with angiography. Longer period of imaging possible, which aids in detection of intermittent bleeding. Labeled red cells and sulfur colloid can detect a bleeding rates as low as 0.05–0.10 mL/min (angiography can detect a bleeding rate of about 0.5 mL/min). 90% sensitivity for blood loss >500 mL/24 h. | Bleeding must be active during time of imaging.
Presence of free TcO₄ (poor labeling efficiency) can lead to gastric, kidney, and bladder activity that can be misinterpreted as sites of bleeding. Uptake in hepatic hemangioma, varices, arteriovenous malformation, abdominal aortic aneurysm, and bowel wall inflammation can also lead to false-positive examination.
Contraindications and risks: Contraindicated in pregnancy because of the potential harm of ionizing radiation to the fetus. | Sterile technique required during in vitro labeling of red cells. |

| | BLOOD |
| | Indium scan |

Test	Indications	Advantages	Disadvantages/Contraindications	Preparation
BLOOD **Leukocyte scan** (indium scan, labeled white blood cell [WBC] scan, technetium-99m hexamethyl-propylene amine oxime [Tc99m-HMPAO]-labeled WBC scan, radionuclide) $$–$$$	Evaluation of fever of unknown origin, suspected abscess, pyelonephritis, osteomyelitis, inflammatory bowel disease. Examination of choice for evaluation of suspected vascular graft infection.	Highly specific (98%) for infection (in contrast to gallium). Highly sensitive in detecting abdominal source of infection. In patients with fever of unknown origin, total body imaging is advantageous compared with CT scan or ultrasound. Preliminary imaging as early as 4 hours is possible with indium but less sensitive (30–50% of abscesses are detected at 24 hours).	24 hour delayed imaging may limit the utility of indium scan in critically ill patients. False-negative scans occur with antibiotic administration or in chronic infection. Perihepatic or splenic infection can be missed because of normal leukocyte accumulation in these organs; liver and spleen scan is necessary adjunct in this situation. False-positive scans occur with swallowed leukocytes, bleeding, indwelling tubes and catheters, surgical skin wound uptake, and bowel activity due to inflammatory processes. Pulmonary uptake is nonspecific and has low predictive value for infection. Patients must be able to hold still during relatively long acquisition times (5–10 minutes). Tc99m-HMPAO WBC may be suboptimal for detecting infection involving the genitourinary and gastrointestinal tracts because of normal distribution of the agent to these organs. **Contraindications and risks:** Contraindicated in pregnancy because of the hazard of ionizing radiation to the fetus. High radiation dose to spleen.	Leukocytes from the patient are harvested, labeled in vitro, and then reinjected; process requires 12 hours. Scanning takes place 24 hours after injection of indium-labeled WBC and 1–2 hours after injection of Tc99m-HMPAO WBC. Homologous donor leukocytes should be used in neutropenic patients.

GALLBLADDER	Indications	Advantages	Disadvantages	Preparation/Comments
GALLBLADDER **Ultrasound** (US) $	Demonstrates cholelithiasis (95% sensitive), sonographic Murphy sign, gallbladder wall thickening, pericholecystic fluid, intra- and extrahepatic biliary dilation.	Noninvasive. No ionizing radiation. Can be portable. Imaging in all planes. Can guide fine-needle aspiration, percutaneous transhepatic cholangiography, and biliary drainage procedures.	Technique very operator-dependent. Presence of barium obscures sound waves. Difficult in obese patients. Administration of excessive pain medication before examination limits accuracy of diagnosing acute cholecystitis. **Contraindications and risks:** None.	**Ultrasound** Preferably NPO for 6 hours to enhance visualization of gallbladder.
GALLBLADDER **Hepatic iminodiacetic acid scan** (HIDA) $$	Evaluation of suspected acute cholecystitis or common bile duct obstruction. Evaluation of bile leaks, biliary atresia, and biliary enteric bypass patency.	95% sensitive and 99% specific for diagnosis of acute cholecystitis. Hepatobiliary function assessed. Defines pathophysiology underlying acute cholecystitis. Rapid. Can be performed in patients with elevated serum bilirubin. No intravenous contrast used.	Does not demonstrate the cause of obstruction (eg, tumor or gallstone). Not able to evaluate biliary excretion if hepatocellular function is severely impaired. Sensitivity may be lower in acalculous cholecystitis. False-positive results can occur with hyperalimentation, prolonged fasting, and acute pancreatitis. **Contraindications and risks:** Contraindicated in pregnancy because of the potential harm of ionizing radiation to the fetus.	**HIDA scan** NPO for at least 4 hours but preferably less than 24 hours. Premedication with cholecystokinin can prevent false-positive examination in patients who are receiving hyperalimentation or who have been fasting longer than 24 hours. Avoid administration of morphine prior to examination if possible.

Test	Indications	Advantages	Disadvantages/Contraindications	Preparation
PANCREAS/BILIARY TREE				
			PANCREAS/BILIARY TREE	
			ERCP	
Endoscopic retrograde cholangiopancreatography (ERCP) $$$$	Demonstrates cause, location, and extent of extrahepatic biliary obstruction (eg, choledocholithiasis). Can diagnose chronic pancreatitis. Primary sclerosing cholangitis, AIDS-associated cholangitis, and cholangiocarcinomas.	Avoids surgery. Less invasive than percutaneous transhepatic cholangiography. Offers therapeutic potential (sphincterotomy and extraction of common bile duct stone, balloon dilation of strictures, placement of stents). Finds gallstones in up to 14% of patients with symptoms but negative ultrasound.	Requires endoscopy. May cause pancreatitis (1%), cholangitis (<1%), peritonitis, hemorrhage (if sphincterotomy performed), and death (rare). **Contraindications and risks:** Relatively contraindicated in patients with concurrent or recent (<6 weeks) acute pancreatitis or suspected pancreatic pseudocyst. Contraindicated in pregnancy because of the potential harm of ionizing radiation to the fetus.	NPO for 6 hours. Sedation required. Vital signs should be monitored by the nursing staff. Not possible in patient who has undergone Roux-en-Y hepaticojejunostomy.
PANCREAS/BILIARY TREE **Magnetic resonance cholangiopancreatography (MRCP)** $$$$	Evaluation of intra- and extrahepatic biliary and pancreatic duct dilatation, and the cause of obstruction.	Noninvasive. No ionizing radiation. Imaging in all planes. Can image ducts beyond the point of obstruction. Evaluates extraluminal disease.	Special instrumentation required for patients on life support. **Contraindications and risks:** Contraindicated in patients with cardiac pacemakers, intraocular metallic foreign bodies, intracranial aneurysm clips, cochlear implants, and some artificial heart valves.	Preferably NPO for 6 hours.

LIVER		
	Ultrasound	**CT**
LIVER **Ultrasound** (US) $	Differentiation of cystic versus solid intrahepatic lesions. Evaluation of intra- and extrahepatic biliary dilation, primary and metastatic liver tumors, and ascites. Evaluation of patency and flow velocity of portal vein, hepatic arteries, and hepatic veins.	
	Noninvasive. No radiation. Can be portable. Imaging in all planes. Can guide fine-needle aspiration, percutaneous transhepatic cholangiography, and biliary drainage procedures.	
	Technique very operator-dependent. May miss solid liver lesions, including hepatocellular carcinoma. More difficult in obese patients. The presence of fatty liver or cirrhosis can limit the sensitivity of ultrasound for focal mass lesions. **Contraindications and risks:** None.	
	Preferably NPO for 6 hours.	
LIVER **Computed tomography** (CT) $$$–$$$$	Suspected metastatic or primary tumor, gallbladder carcinoma, biliary obstruction, abscess.	
	Excellent spatial resolution. Can direct percutaneous fine-needle aspiration biopsy. Excellent evaluation of hepatic vasculature.	
	Requires iodinated contrast material administered intravenously. **Contraindications and risks:** Contraindicated in pregnancy because of the potential harm of ionizing radiation to the fetus. See Risks of CT and Angiographic Intravenous Contrast Agents, p. 375.	
	NPO for 4–6 hours. Recent creatinine determination. Administration of oral contrast material for opacification of stomach and small bowel. Specific hepatic protocol with arterial, portal venous, and delayed images used for evaluation of neoplasm.	

	LIVER
	MRI

Test	Indications	Advantages	Disadvantages/Contraindications	Preparation
LIVER **Magnetic resonance imaging** (MRI) $$$$	Characterization of hepatic lesions, including suspected cyst, hepatocellular carcinoma, focal nodular hyperplasia, and metastasis. Suspected metastatic or primary tumor. Differentiation of benign cavernous hemangioma from malignant tumor. Evaluation of hemochromatosis, hemosiderosis, fatty liver, and suspected focal fatty infiltration.	Requires no iodinated contrast material. Provides excellent tissue contrast resolution, multiplanar capability.	Subject to motion artifacts, particularly those of respiration. Special instrumentation required for patients on life support. **Contraindications and risks:** Contraindicated in patients with cardiac pacemakers, intraocular metallic foreign bodies, intracranial aneurysm clips, cochlear implants, some artificial heart valves.	Screening CT or plain radiograph images of orbits if history suggests possible metallic foreign body in the eye. Intramuscular glucagon is used to inhibit intestinal peristalsis.

LIVER/BILIARY TREE			
	PTC		
LIVER/BILIARY TREE **Percutaneous transhepatic cholangio-gram** (PTC) $$$	Evaluation of biliary obstruction in patients in whom ERCP has failed or patients with Roux-en-Y hepaticojejunostomy.	Can characterize tae nature of diffuse intrahepatic biliary disease such as primary sclerosing cholangitis. Provides guidance and access for percutane-ous transhepatic biliary drainage and possible stent placement to treat obstruction. Best examination to assess site and morphology of obstruction close to the hilum (as opposed to ERCP, which is better for distal obstruction).	Invasive; requires special training. Performed with conscious sedation. **Contraindications and risks:** Ascites may present a contraindication.	NPO for 4–6 hours. Sterile technique, assessment of clotting parameters, correction of coagulopathy. Performed with conscious sedation.

	LIVER			
	Hepatic angiography			
Test	Indications	Advantages	Disadvantages/Contraindications	Preparation
LIVER **Hepatic angiography** $$$$	Preoperative evaluation for liver transplantation, vascular malformations, trauma, Budd-Chiari syndrome, portal vein patency (when ultrasound equivocal) prior to transjugular intrahepatic portosystemic shunt (TIPS) procedure. In some cases, evaluation of hepatic neoplasm or transcatheter embolotherapy of hepatic malignancy.	Gold standard assessment of hepatic arterial anatomy, which is highly variable. More accurate than ultrasound with respect to portal vein patency when the latter suggests occlusion.	Invasive. Patient must remain supine with leg extended for 6 hours following the procedure to protect the common femoral artery at the catheter entry site. **Contraindications and risks:** Allergy to iodinated contrast material may require corticosteroid and H$_1$ blocker or H$_2$ blocker premedication. Contraindicated in pregnancy because of the potential harm of ionizing radiation to the fetus. Contrast nephrotoxicity may occur, especially with preexisting impaired renal function due to diabetes mellitus or multiple myeloma; however, any creatinine elevation after the procedure is usually reversible.	NPO for 4–6 hours. Good hydration to limit possible renal insult due to iodinated contrast material. Recent serum creatinine determination, assessment of clotting parameters, reversal of anticoagulation. Performed with conscious sedation. Requires cardiac, respiratory, blood pressure, and pulse oximetry monitoring.

LIVER/SPLEEN			
Liver, spleen scan			

LIVER-SPLEEN			
Liver, spleen scan (radionuclide) $$	Identification of functioning splenic tissue to localize an accessory spleen or evaluate suspected functional asplenia. Assessment of size, shape, and position of liver and spleen. Characterization of a focal liver mass with regard to inherent functioning reticuloendothelial cell activity (in particular focal nodular hyperplasia). Confirmation of patency and distribution of hepatic arterial perfusion catheters.	May detect isodense lesions missed by CT. Useful to detect location of active GI bleed (see GI bleeding scan, above).	Diminished sensitivity for small lesions (less than 1.5–2.0 cm) and deep lesions. SPECT increases sensitivity (can detect lesions of 1.0–1.5 cm). Nonspecific; unable to distinguish solid versus cystic or inflammatory versus neoplastic tissue. Lower sensitivity for diffuse hepatic tumors. **Contraindications and risks:** Caution in pregnancy advised because of the risk of ionizing radiation to the fetus.	None.

	PANCREAS	
	CT	Ultrasound
Test	**Indications**	**Advantages**	**Disadvantages/Contraindications**	**Preparation**
PANCREAS **Computed tomography** (CT) $$$–$$$$	Evaluation of pancreatic and biliary obstruction and possible adenocarcinoma. Staging of pancreatic carcinoma. Evaluation of complications and causes of acute pancreatitis.	Can guide fine-needle biopsy or placement of a drainage catheter. Can identify early necrosis in pancreatitis.	Optimal imaging requires special protocol, including precontrast plus arterial and venous phase contrast-enhanced images. **Contraindications and risks:** Contraindicated in pregnancy because of the potential harm of ionizing radiation to the fetus. See Risks of CT and Angiographic Intravenous Contrast Agents, p. 375.	Preferably NPO for 4–6 hours. Normal hydration. Opacification of gastrointestinal tract with oral Gastrografin. Sedation of agitated patients. Recent serum creatinine determination.
PANCREAS **Ultrasound** (US) $	Identification of peripancreatic fluid collections, pseudocysts, and pancreatic ductal dilation.	Noninvasive. No radiation. Can be portable. Imaging in all planes. Can guide fine-needle aspiration or placement of drainage catheter.	Pancreas may be obscured by overlying bowel gas. Technique very operator-dependent. Presence of barium obscures sound waves. Less sensitive than CT. **Contraindications and risks:** None.	Preferably NPO for 6 hours.

ADRENAL			
MIBG scan			
ADRENAL **MIBG (meta- iodobenzyl- guanidine)** (radionuclide) $$$	Suspected pheochromocytoma when CT is negative or equivocal. Also useful in evaluation of neuroblastoma, carcinoid, and medullary carcinoma of thyroid.	Test is useful for localization of pheochromocytomas (particularly extra-adrenal). 80–90% sensitive for detection of pheochromocytoma.	High radiation dose to adrenal gland. High cost and limited availability of MIBG. Delayed imaging (at 1, 2, and 3 days) necessitates return of patient. **Contraindications and risks:** Contraindicated in pregnancy because of the risk of ionizing radiation to the fetus. Because of the relatively high dose of 131I, patients should be instructed about precautionary measures by nuclear medicine personnel.	Administration of Lugol's iodine solution (to block thyroid uptake) before and after administration of MIBG.

	GENITOURINARY		
	CT	Ultrasound	MRI
Test	GENITOURI-NARY **Computed tomography** (CT) $$$	GENITOURI-NARY **Ultrasound** (US) $$	GENITOURI-NARY **Magnetic resonance imaging** (MRI) $$$$
Indications	Evaluation for possible kidney or ureteral stones. Evaluation of staging of renal parenchymal tumors, hydronephrosis, pyelonephritis, and perinephric abscess.	Evaluation of renal morphology, hydronephrosis, size of prostate, and residual urine volume. Differentiation of cystic versus solid renal lesions.	Staging of cancers of the uterus, cervix, and prostate. Can provide information additional to what is obtained by CT in some cases of renal cell and bladder carcinoma.
Advantages	Rapid. Outstanding sensitivity for nephroureterolithiasis. Can guide percutaneous procedures. Excellent spatial resolution.	Noninvasive. No radiation. Can be portable. Imaging in all planes. Can guide fine-needle aspiration or placement of drainage catheter.	Provides excellent tissue contrast resolution, multiplanar capability. No ionizing radiation.
Disadvantages/Contraindications	Generally limited to transaxial views. **Contraindications and risks:** Caution in pregnancy because of the risk of ionizing radiation to the fetus. See Risks of CT and Angiographic Intravenous Contrast Agents, p. 375.	Technique very operator-dependent. More difficult in obese patients. **Contraindications and risks:** None.	Subject to motion artifacts. Gastrointestinal opacification not yet readily available. Special instrumentation required for patients on life support. **Contraindications and risks:** Contraindicated in patients with cardiac pacemakers, intraocular metallic foreign bodies, intracranial aneurysm clips, cochlear implants, and some artificial heart valves.
Preparation	Sedation of agitated patients.	Preferably NPO for 6 hours. Full urinary bladder required for pelvic studies.	Sedation of agitated patients. Screening CT or plain radiograph images of orbits if history suggests possible metallic foreign body in the eye.

	GENITOURINARY	
	IVP	Radionuclide scan
GENITOURINARY **Intravenous pyelogram** (IVP) $$$	Fluoroscopic evaluation of uroepithelial neoplasm, calculus, papillary necrosis, and medullary sponge kidney. Screening for urinary system injury after trauma.	Permits evaluation of collecting system in less invasive manner than retrograde pyelogram. Can assess both renal morphology and function.
	Suboptimal evaluation of the renal parenchyma. Does not adequately evaluate cause of ureteral deviation. **Contraindications and risks:** Caution in pregnancy is advised because of the risk of ionizing radiation to the fetus. See Risks of CT and Angiographic Intravenous Contrast Agents, p. 375.	Adequate hydration. Colonic cleansing is preferred but not essential. Recent serum creatinine determination.
GENITOURINARY **Renal scan** (radionuclide) $$	Determination of relative renal function. Evaluation of suspected renal vascular hypertension. Differentiation of a dilated but non-obstructed system from one that has a urodynamically significant obstruction. Evaluation of renal blood flow and function in acute or chronic renal failure. Evaluation of both medical and surgical complications of renal transplant. Estimation of glomerular filtration rate and effective renal plasma flow.	Provides functional information without risk of iodinated contrast used in IVP. Provides quantitative information not available by other means.
	Finding of poor renal blood flow does not pinpoint an etiologic diagnosis. Limited utility when renal function is extremely poor. Estimation of glomerular filtration rate and renal plasma flow often is inaccurate. **Contraindications and risks:** Caution in pregnancy because of the risk of ionizing radiation to the fetus.	Normal hydration needed for evaluation of suspected obstructive uropathy because dehydration may result in false-positive examination. Blood pressure should be monitored and an intravenous line started when an angiotensin-converting enzyme (ACE) inhibitor is used to evaluate renal vascular hypertension. Patient should discontinue ACE inhibitor medication for at least 48 hours before examination if possible.

Test	Indications	Advantages	Disadvantages/Contraindications	Preparation
PELVIS				
PELVIS **Ultrasound** (US) $$	Evaluation of ovarian mass, enlarged uterus, vaginal bleeding, pelvic pain, possible ectopic pregnancy, and infertility. Monitoring of follicular development. Localization of intrauterine device.	Use of a vaginal probe enables very early detection of intrauterine pregnancy and ectopic pregnancy and does not require a full bladder.	Transabdominal scan has limited sensitivity for uterine or ovarian pathology. Vaginal probe has limited field of view and therefore may miss large masses outside the pelvis. **Contraindications and risks:** None.	Distended bladder required (only in transabdominal examination).
PELVIS **Magnetic resonance imaging** (MRI) $$$$	Evaluation of gynecologic malignancies, particularly endometrial, cervical, and vaginal carcinoma. Evaluation of prostate, bladder, and rectal carcinoma. Evaluation of congenital anomalies of the genitourinary tract. Useful in distinguishing lymphadenopathy from vasculature.	Provides excellent tissue contrast resolution, multiplanar capability. No ionizing radiation. Best imaging evaluation of uterine, cervical, prostate, and bladder carcinoma. May provide metabolic and functional information on prostate cancer.	Subject to motion artifacts. Special instrumentation required for patients on life support. **Contraindications and risks:** Contraindicated in patients with cardiac pacemakers, intraocular metallic foreign bodies, intracranial aneurysm clips, cochlear implants, and some artificial heart valves.	Intramuscular glucagon is used to inhibit intestinal peristalsis. Sedation of agitated patients. Screening CT or plain radiograph images of orbits if history suggests possible metallic foreign body in the eye. An endorectal device (radiofrequency coil) is used for prostate MRI.

BONE			
Bone scan			
BONE	Evaluation of primary or metastatic neoplasm, osteomyelitis, arthritis, metabolic disorders, trauma, avascular necrosis, joint prosthesis, and reflex sympathetic dystrophy. Evaluation of clinically suspected but radiographically occult fractures. Identification of stress fractures.	Can examine entire osseous skeleton or specific area of interest. Highly sensitive compared with plain film radiography for detection of bone neoplasm. In osteomyelitis, bone scan may be positive much earlier (24 hours) than plain film (10–14 days).	Nonspecific. Correlation with plain film radiographs often necessary. Limited utility in patients with poor renal function. Poor resolution in distal extremities, head, and spine; in these instances, SPECT is often useful. Sometimes difficult to distinguish osteomyelitis from cellulitis or septic joint; dual imaging with gallium or with indium-labeled leukocytes can be helpful. False-negative results for osteomyelitis can occur following antibiotic therapy and within the first 24 hours after trauma. In avascular necrosis, bone scan may be "hot," "cold," or normal, depending on the stage. **Contraindications and risks:** Caution in pregnancy because of the risk of ionizing radiation to the fetus.	Patient should be well hydrated and void frequently after the procedure.
Bone scan, whole body (radionuclide) **$$-$$$**			

Test	Indications	Advantages	Disadvantages/Contraindications	Preparation
			SPINE	
			CT	MRI
SPINE **Computed tomography** (CT) $$$	Evaluation of structures that are not well visualized on MRI, including ossification of the posterior longitudinal ligament, tumoral calcification, osteophytic spurring, retropulsed bone fragments after trauma. Also used for patients in whom MRI is contraindicated.	Rapid. Superb spatial resolution. Can guide percutaneous fine-needle aspiration of possible tumor or abscess.	Generally limited to transaxial views. Coronal and sagittal reformation images can be generated. MRI unequivocally superior in evaluation of the spine nerve roots and cord, except for conditions mentioned here in indications. Artifacts from metal prostheses degrade images. **Contraindications and risks:** Contraindicated in pregnancy because of the potential harm of ionizing radiation to the fetus. See Risks of CT and Angiographic Intravenous Contrast Agents, p. 375.	Normal hydration. Sedation of agitated patients.
SPINE **Magnetic resonance imaging** (MRI) $$$$	Diseases involving the spine and cord except where CT is superior (ossification of the posterior longitudinal ligament, tumoral calcification, osteophytic spurring, retropulsed bone fragments after trauma).	Provides excellent tissue contrast resolution, multiplanar capability. No ionizing radiation.	Less useful in detection of calcification, small spinal vascular malformations, acute spinal trauma (because of longer acquisition time, incompatibility with life support devices, and inferior detection of bony injury). Subject to motion artifacts. Special instrumentation required for patients on life support. **Contraindications and risks:** Contraindicated in patients with cardiac pacemakers, intraocular metallic foreign bodies, intracranial aneurysm clips, cochlear implants, and some artificial heart valves.	Sedation of agitated patients. Screening CT or plain radiograph images of orbits if history suggests possible metallic foreign body in the eye.

MUSCULOSKELETAL			
MRI			
MUSCULO-SKELETAL SYSTEM **Magnetic resonance imaging** (MRI) $$$$	Evaluation of joints except where a prosthesis is in place. Extent of primary or malignant tumor (bone and soft tissue). Evaluation of aseptic necrosis, bone and soft tissue infections, marrow space disease, and traumatic derangements.	Provides excellent tissue contrast resolution, multiplanar capability. No ionizing radiation.	Subject to motion artifacts. Less able than CT to detect calcification, ossification, and periosteal reaction. Special instrumentation required for patients on life support. **Contraindications and risks:** Contraindicated in patients with cardiac pacemakers, intravascular metallic foreign bodies, intracranial aneurysm clips, cochlear implants, and some artificial heart valves.	Sedation of agitated patients. Screening CT or plain radiograph images of orbits if history suggests possible metallic foreign body in the eye.

Test	Indications	Advantages	Disadvantages/Contraindications	Preparation
VASCULATURE				
Ultrasound				
VASCULATURE **Ultrasound** (US) $$	Evaluation of deep venous thrombosis, extremity grafts, patency of inferior vena cava, portal vein, and hepatic veins. Carotid Doppler indicated for symptomatic carotid bruit, atypical transient ischemic attack, monitoring after endarterectomy, and baseline prior to major vascular surgery. Surveillance of TIPS patency and flow.	Noninvasive. No radiation. Can be portable. Imaging in all planes.	Technique operator-dependent. Ultrasound not sensitive to detection of ulcerated plaque. May be difficult to diagnose tight stenosis versus occlusion (catheter angiography may be necessary). May be difficult to distinguish acute from chronic deep venous thrombosis. **Contraindications and risks:** None	None.

AORTA		
Angiography		
AORTA AND ITS BRANCHES **Angiography** $$$	Peripheral vascular disease, abdominal aortic aneurysm, renal artery stenosis (atherosclerotic and fibromuscular disease), visceral ischemia, thoracic aortic dissection, vasculitis, abdominal tumors, gastrointestinal hemorrhage, arteriovenous malformations, abdominopelvic trauma. Preoperative evaluation for aortofemoral bypass reconstructive surgery. Postoperative assessment of possible graft stenosis, especially femoral to popliteal or femoral to distal (foot or ankle).	Can localize athero-sclerotic stenosis and assess the severity by morphology, flow, and pressure gradient. Provides assessment of stenotic lesions and access for percutaneous transluminal balloon dilation as well as stent treatment of iliac stenoses. Provides access for thrombolytic therapy of acute or subacute occlusion of native artery or bypass graft.	Invasive. Patient must remain supine with leg extended for 6 hours following the procedure to protect the common femoral artery at the catheter entry site. **Contraindications and risks:** Allergy to iodinated contrast material may require corticosteroid and H₁ blocker or H₂ blocker premedication. Contraindicated in pregnancy because of the potential harm of ionizing radiation to the fetus. Contrast nephrotoxicity may occur, especially with preexisting impaired renal function due to diabetes mellitus or multiple myeloma; however, any creatinine elevation that occurs after the procedure is usually reversible.	NPO for 4–6 hours. Good hydration to limit possible renal insult due to iodinated contrast material. Recent serum creatinine determination, assessment of clotting parameters, reversal of anticoagulation. Performed with conscious sedation. Requires cardiac, respiratory, blood pressure, and pulse oximetry monitoring as well as non-invasive studies of peripheral vascular disease to verify indication for angiography and to guide the examination.

Test	Indications	Advantages	Disadvantages/Contraindications	Preparation
AORTA				
CTA				
AORTA AND ITS BRANCHES **Computed tomography angiography** (CTA) $$$	Preoperative assessment of aortic or branch artery aneurysms and dissections. Evaluation of thoracoabdominal trauma. Evaluation of possible aortic injury. Evaluation of mesenteric ischemia.	Rapid. Excellent spatial resolution and large territory coverage. Evaluates calcified vascular plaques.	Limited functional and hemodynamic evaluation. **Contraindications and risks:** Contraindicated in pregnancy because of potential harm of ionizing radiation to the fetus. See Risks of CT and Angiographic Intravenous Contrast Agents, p. 375.	Sedation of agitated patients. Hydration.
MRA				
AORTA AND ITS BRANCHES **Magnetic resonance angiography** (MRA) $$$$	Can provide preoperative assessment of thoracoabdominal aortic aneurysms and dissections to determine diseased arterial size, proximal and distal extent, relationship to major branch arteries, and presence of anatomic anomalies. Permits evaluation of the hemodynamic and functional significance of renal artery stenosis.	No ionizing radiation. No iodinated contrast needed.	Subject to motion artifacts. Special instrumentation required for patients on life support. **Contraindications and risks:** Contraindicated in patients with cardiac pacemakers, intraocular metallic foreign bodies, intracranial aneurysm clips, cochlear implants, and some artificial heart valves.	Sedation of agitated patients. Screening CT or plain radiograph images of orbits if history suggests possible metallic foreign body in the eye.

7

Basic Electrocardiography* and Echocardiography

Fred M. Kusumoto, MD

I. BASIC ELECTROCARDIOGRAPHY

HOW TO USE THIS SECTION

This chapter includes criteria for the diagnosis of basic electrocardiographic waveforms and cardiac arrhythmias. It is intended for use as a reference and assumes a basic understanding of the electrocardiogram (ECG).

Electrocardiographic interpretation is a "stepwise" procedure, and the first steps are to study and characterize the cardiac rhythm.

Step One (Rhythm)

Categorize what you see in the 12-lead ECG or rhythm strip, using the three major parameters that allow for systematic analysis and subsequent diagnosis of the rhythm:

1. Mean rate of the QRS complexes (slow, normal, or fast).
2. Width of the QRS complexes (wide or narrow).
3. Rhythmicity of the QRS complexes (characterization of spaces between QRS complexes) (regular or irregular).

Step Two (Morphology)

Step 2 consists of examining and characterizing the morphology of the cardiac waveforms.

1. Examine for atrial abnormalities and bundle branch blocks (BBBs) (pp. 441–444).

---

*Adapted, with permission, from Evans GT Jr.: *ECG Interpretation Cribsheets,* 4th ed. Ring Mountain Press, 1999.

2. Assess the QRS axis and the causes of axis deviations (pp. 444–446).
3. Examine for signs of left ventricular hypertrophy (pp. 447–448).
4. Examine for signs of right ventricular hypertrophy (pp. 448–449).
5. Examine for signs of myocardial infarction, if present (pp. 450–451).
6. Bear in mind conditions that may alter the ability of the ECG to diagnose a myocardial infarction (pp. 459–460).
7. Examine for abnormalities of the ST segment or T wave (pp. 462–465).
8. Assess the QT interval (pp. 466–467).
9. Examine for miscellaneous conditions (pp. 467–470).

STEP ONE: DIAGNOSIS OF THE CARDIAC RHYTHM

A. APPROACH TO DIAGNOSIS OF THE CARDIAC RHYTHM

Most electrocardiograph machines display 10 seconds of data in a standard tracing. A rhythm is defined as three or more successive P waves or QRS complexes.

Categorize the patterns seen in the tracing according to a systematic method. This method proceeds in three steps that lead to a diagnosis based on the most likely rhythm producing a particular pattern:

1. What is the mean rate of the QRS complexes?

Slow (<60 bpm): The easiest way to determine this is to count the total number of QRS complexes in a 10-second period. If there are no more than 9, the rate is slow.

Another method for determining the rate is to count the number of large boxes (0.20 s) between QRS complexes and use the following formula:

$$\text{Rate} = 300 \div (\text{number of large boxes between QRS complexes})$$

A slow heart rate (<60 bpm) has more than five large boxes between QRS complexes.

Normal (60–100 bpm): If there are 10–16 complexes in a 10-second period, the rate is normal.

In normal heart rates, the QRS complexes are separated by three–five large boxes.

Fast (>100 bpm): If there are ≥ 17 complexes in a 10-second period, the rate is fast.

Fast heart rates have fewer than three large boxes between QRS complexes.

TABLE 7–1. SUSTAINED REGULAR RHYTHMS.

Rate	Fast	Normal	Slow
Narrow QRS duration	Sinus tachycardia Atrial tachycardia Atrial flutter (2:1 AV conduction) Junctional tachycardia Orthodromic AVRT	Sinus rhythm Ectopic atrial rhythm Atrial flutter (4:1 conduction) Accelerated junctional rhythm	Sinus bradycardia Ectopic atrial bradycardia Junctional rhythm
Wide QRS duration	All rhythms listed above under narrow QRS duration, but with BBB or IVCD patterns		
	Ventricular tachycardia Antidromic AVRT	Accelerated ventricular rhythm	Ventricular escape rhythm

AV = atrioventricular; **BBB** = bundle branch blocks; **IVCD** = intraventricular conduction delay.

2. Is the duration of the dominant QRS morphology narrow (<0.12 s) or wide (≥0.12 s)? (Refer to the section on the QRS duration.)
3. What is the "rhythmicity" of the QRS complexes (defined as the spacing between QRS complexes)? Regular or irregular? (Any change in the spacing of the R-R intervals defines an irregular rhythm.)

Using the categorization above, refer to Tables 7–1 and 7–2 to select a specific diagnosis for the cardiac rhythm.

TABLE 7–2. SUSTAINED IRREGULAR RHYTHMS.

Rate	Fast	Normal	Slow
Narrow QRS duration	Atrial fibrillation Atrial flutter (variable AV conduction) Multifocal atrial tachycardia Atrial tachycardia with AV block (rare)	Atrial fibrillation Atrial flutter (variable AV conduction) Multiform atrial rhythm Atrial tachycardia with AV block (rare)	Atrial fibrillation Atrial flutter (variable AV conduction) Multiform atrial rhythm Sinus rhythm with 2° AV block
Wide QRS duration	All rhythms listed above under narrow QRS duration, but with BBB or IVCD patterns		
	Torsade de pointes Rarely, anterograde conduction of atrial fibrillation over an accessory pathway in patients with WPW syndrome		

AV = atrioventricular; **BBB** = bundle branch blocks; **IVCD** = intraventricular conduction delay; **WPW** = Wolff-Parkinson-White syndrome.

B. NORMAL HEART RATE

Sinus Rhythm

The sinus node is the primary pacemaker for the heart. Because the sinus node is located at the junction of the superior vena cava and the right atrium, in **sinus rhythm** the atria are activated from "right to left" and "high to low." The P wave in sinus rhythm is upright in lead II and inverted in lead aVR. In lead V_1, the P wave is usually biphasic with a small initial positive deflection due to right atrial activation and a terminal negative deflection due to left atrial activation.

The normal sinus rate is usually between 60 and 100 bpm but can vary significantly. During sleep, when parasympathetic tone is high, **sinus bradycardia** (sinus rates <60 bpm) is a normal finding, and during conditions associated with increased sympathetic tone (exercise, stress), **sinus tachycardia** (sinus rates >100 bpm) is common. In children and young adults, **sinus arrhythmia** (sinus rates that vary by more than 10% during 10 seconds) due to respiration is frequently observed.

Ectopic Atrial Rhythm

In some situations, the atria are activated by an ectopic atrial focus rather than the sinus node. In this case, the P wave will have an abnormal shape depending on where the ectopic focus is located. For example, if the focus arises from the left atrium, the P wave is inverted in leads I and aVL. If the depolarization rate of the ectopic focus is between 60 and 100 bpm, the patient has an **ectopic atrial rhythm.** If the rate is <60 bpm, the rhythm is defined as an ectopic atrial bradycardia.

Atrial Flutter With 4:1 Atrioventricular Conduction

In **atrial flutter**, the atria are activated rapidly (usually 300 bpm) owing to a stable reentrant circuit. Most commonly, the reentrant circuit rotates counterclockwise around the tricuspid valve. Because the left atrium and interatrial septum are activated low-to-high, "sawtooth" flutter waves that are inverted in the inferior leads (II, III, and aVF) are usually observed. If every fourth atrial beat is conducted to the ventricles (owing to slow conduction in the atrioventricular [AV] node), a relatively normal ventricular rate of 75 bpm is observed.

Accelerated Junctional Rhythm (p. 439)

Premature QRS Activity

It is common to have isolated premature QRS activity that leads to mild irregularity of the heart rhythm. A premature narrow QRS complex is most often due to a normally conducted **premature atrial complex (PAC)** or more rarely a **premature junctional complex (PJC)**. A premature wide QRS complex is usually due to a **premature ventricular complex (PVC)** or to a premature supraventricular complex (PAC or PJC) that conducts to the ventricle with aberrant conduction due to block in one of the bundle branches (p. 442). Premature supraventricular complexes (with or without aberrant conduction) are commonly observed phenomena that are not associated with cardiac disease. Although PVCs are observed in normal individuals, they are usually associated with higher risk in patients with cardiac disease.

C. TACHYCARDIA

Tachycardias are normally classified by whether the QRS complex is narrow or wide and whether the rhythm is regular or irregular. A narrow QRS tachycardia indicates normal activation of the ventricular tissue regardless of the tachycardia mechanism. Narrow QRS tachycardias are frequently grouped together as supraventricular tachycardia (SVT) and can be due to a number of mechanisms described in the following text. This grouping also has clinical usefulness because SVTs are not usually life-threatening. In addition to QRS width, it is useful to consider the anatomic site from which the tachycardia arises: atrium, atrioventricular junction, ventricle, or utilization of an accessory pathway (Figure 7–1).

Narrow QRS Tachycardia with a Regular Rhythm: Regular SVT (Figure 7–2)

A. **Sinus Tachycardia:** Under many physiologic conditions, the sinus node discharges at a rate >100 bpm. In **sinus tachycardia**, an upright P wave can be observed in II and aVF and an inverted P wave is observed in aVR. The PR interval is usually relatively normal, because conditions associated with sinus tachycardia (most commonly sympathetic activation) also cause more rapid AV conduction.

B. **Atrial Tachycardia:** Rarely, a single atrial site other than the sinus node fires rapidly. This leads to an abnormally shaped P wave. The specific shape of the P wave depends on the specific site of **atrial tachycardia.** The PR interval depends on how quickly atrioventricular conduction occurs. As the atrial tachycardia rate increases, the AV node conduction slows (decremental conduction) and the PR interval increases; decremental conduction properties of the AV node prevent rapid ventricular rates in the presence of rapid atrial rates.

C. **Atrial Flutter:** The mechanism for **atrial flutter** is described above. Most commonly atrioventricular conduction occurs with

Atrial tachycardias

   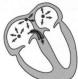

Atrial flutter   Atrial fibrillation   Atrial tachycardia   Atrial tachycardia (MAT)

Junctional tachycardias

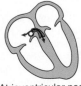 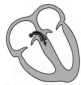

Atrioventricular node reentrant tachycardia   Atrioventricular node automatic tachycardia

Ventricular tachycardias

 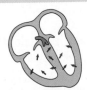

Ventricular tachycardia   Ventricular fibrillation

Accessory pathway-mediated tachycardias

Orthodromic atrioventricular reentrant tachycardia   Antidromic atrioventricular reentrant tachycardia   Atrial fibrillation with activation of the ventricles via an accessory pathway and the AV node

Figure 7–1. Anatomic classification of tachycardias. (*Adapted from Kusumoto FM: Arrhythmias. In: Cardiovascular Pathophysiology, FM Kusumoto [editor], Hayes Barton Press, 2004.*)

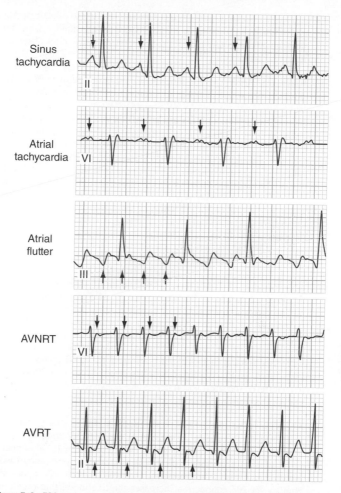

Figure 7–2. ECG appearance of different forms of regular SVTs. Arrows show the first four atrial deflections in each SVT. In *sinus tachycardia,* the P wave has a normal morphology, and the PR interval is normal. In *atrial tachycardia,* the P wave is abnormal (positive in V_1, and the PR interval is prolonged because of decremental conduction in the AV node). In *atrial flutter,* inverted "saw-tooth" waves are observed in lead III. In *AVNRT,* a pseudo-R wave due to retrograde atrial activation is observed in lead V_1. In *AVRT,* a retrograde P wave is observed in the ST segment because the atria and ventricles are activated sequentially. The P wave is usually located relatively close to the preceding QRS complex because the accessory pathway conducts rapidly.

every other flutter wave (2:1 conduction), leading to a heart rate of approximately 150 bpm. In some situations, very rapid ventricular rates can be observed due to 1:1 conduction, or slower rates observed due to 3:1 conduction.

D. Junctional Tachycardia: The most common type of tachycardia to arise from tissue near the atrioventricular junction is **AV nodal reentrant tachycardia (AVNRT)**. In AVNRT, two separate parallel pathways of conduction are present within junctional and perijunctional tissue. Usually, one of the pathways has relatively rapid conduction properties but a long refractory period ("fast pathway"), and the other has slow conduction and a short refractory period ("slow pathway"). In some cases, a premature atrial contraction can block one of the pathways (usually the fast pathway), conduct down the slow pathway, and activate the fast pathway retrogradely, initiating a reentrant circuit. In rare circumstances, a site within the AV node fires rapidly as a result of increased automaticity.

Regardless of the mechanism, because the tachycardia originates within the AV junction, the atria and ventricles are activated simultaneously. Most commonly (in approximately 50% of cases), the P wave is buried in the QRS complex and is not seen. In approximately 40% of cases, the retrograde P wave is observed in the terminal portion of the QRS complex. The easiest place to see the retrograde P wave is in lead V_1, where a low-amplitude terminal positive deflection (pseudo-R' wave) is seen (Figure 7–2). In addition, a terminal negative deflection (pseudo-S wave) is seen in the inferior leads (II, III, and aVF). Finally, in about 10% of cases, the P wave is observed in the initial portion of the QRS complex. The location of the P wave depends on the relative speeds of retrograde activation of the atria and anterograde activation of the ventricles via the His-Purkinje system.

E. Accessory Pathway–Mediated Tachycardia: Usually, the AV node and His bundle provide the only path for AV conduction. In approximately 1 in 1000 individuals, an additional AV connection called an **accessory pathway** is present. The presence of two parallel pathways (the accessory pathway and the AV node-His bundle) for AV conduction increases the likelihood that reentrant tachycardia will occur. The most common tachycardia is a reentrant narrow QRS tachycardia in which the ventricles are activated via the His-Purkinje system and the atria are activated via retrograde activation from the accessory pathway (Figure 7–3). This type of tachycardia is frequently called **orthodromic atrioventricular reentrant tachycardia (AVRT)** because conduction through the AV node and His-Purkinje fibers occurs normally (*ortho* is Greek

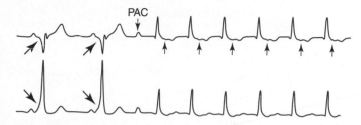

Figure 7–3. Initiation of SVT in a patient with an accessory pathway. During sinus rhythm, the ventricles are activated via the accessory pathway and the AV node-His bundle. Because the accessory pathway conducts rapidly and inserts into regular ventricular myocardium, the PR interval is short and a delta wave is observed (*large arrows*). A premature atrial complex (PAC) blocks in the accessory pathway and travels only down the AV node-His bundle, leading to a narrow QRS complex. The atria are activated retrogradely by the accessory pathway (*small arrows*), and orthodromic AVRT is initiated. (*Adapted from Kusumoto FM: Cardiovascular disorders: Heart disease. In:* Pathophysiology of Disease: An Introduction to Clinical Medicine, *6th ed. McPhee SJ, Hammer G [editors], McGraw-Hill, 2010.*)

for straight or normal). Orthodromic AVRT is one cause of SVT; the QRS complexes are narrow and normal-appearing because the ventricles are activated via the AV node and His-Purkinje system, ventricular tissue, an accessory pathway, and atrial tissue. Because the ventricles and atria are activated sequentially, the P wave is most often observed within the ST segment (Figure 7–2). As discussed later, accessory pathways can also be associated with regular and irregular wide complex tachycardias.

Narrow QRS Tachycardias with an Irregular Rhythm: Irregular SVT (Figure 7–4)

A. **Atrial Fibrillation:** Atrial fibrillation is the most common abnormal fast heart rhythm observed. Atrial fibrillation is most commonly due to multiple chaotic wandering wavelets of reentry that cause irregular activation of the atria. Because the AV node is also activated irregularly, AV conduction is variable and an irregular ventricular rhythm is observed. In atrial fibrillation, the rhythm is often called "irregularly irregular" because there is no organized atrial activity. On the ECG, continuous fibrillatory low-amplitude waves with varying morphology are observed with no easily identifiable isoelectric period. The fibrillatory waves are usually best seen in leads V_1, V_2, II, III, and aVF.

B. **Multifocal Atrial Tachycardia:** In **multifocal atrial tachycardia** (often called **MAT**), several atrial sites beat due to abnormal automa-

Atrial fibrillation

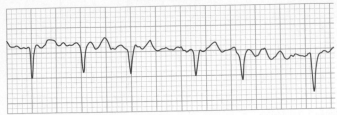

Multifocal atrial tachycardia

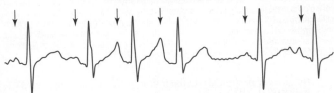

Figure 7–4. ECG appearance of atrial fibrillation and multifocal atrial tachycardia (MAT). In atrial fibrillation, continuous chaotic activation of the atria results in continuous low-amplitude fibrillatory waves. In MAT, discrete P waves (*arrows*) and an isoelectric T–P segment are observed.

ticity. This leads to P waves of three or more different morphologies. The rhythm is usually irregular; the different sites fire at different rates. MAT can be distinguished from atrial fibrillation by discrete P waves and isoelectric periods between the T wave and the P wave. The most common cause of MAT is chronic obstructive pulmonary disease (approximately 60% of cases).

C. **Atrial Flutter With Variable Block:** Atrial flutter can sometimes present as an irregular rhythm because of variable AV block. In this case, although the ventricular rhythm is irregular, there are often relatively constant intervals between the QRS complexes. For example, if the atrial flutter rate is 300 bpm, the possible ventricular rates will be 300 bpm, 150 bpm, 100 bpm, or 75 bpm for 1:1, 2:1, 3:1, and 4:1 AV conduction, respectively.

Wide QRS Complex Tachycardia With a Regular Rhythm

The most common cause of **wide QRS complex tachycardia with a regular rhythm (WCT-RR)** is sinus tachycardia with either right bundle branch block (RBBB) or left bundle branch block (LBBB). However, if a patient with structural heart disease presents with WCT-RR, one assumes a worst-case scenario and the presumptive diagnosis becomes **ventricular tachycardia (VT).** Most commonly, VT originates from a rapid reentrant circuit located at the border of infarcted and normal myocardium. Because the ventricles are not activated via the bundle branches or the Purkinje system, an abnormally wide QRS complex is observed. Any atrial or junctional tachycardias associated with aberrant conduction can also cause a WCT-RR. Finally, in very rare circumstances, patients with accessory pathways present with **antidromic AVRT** in which the ventricles are activated via the accessory pathway (leading to a wide and bizarre QRS complex) and the atria are activated retrogradely via the His bundle-AV node (*anti* is Greek for against).

The ECG differentiation between regular SVTs with aberrant conduction (sinus tachycardia, atrial tachycardia, atrial flutter, junctional tachycardia, orthodromic AVRT) and VT can sometimes be difficult. Accurate diagnosis of VT is critical because this rhythm is frequently life-threatening. The two principal techniques for identifying VT are the presence of AV dissociation and abnormal QRS morphology.

A. **Atrioventricular Dissociation:** In **AV dissociation,** the atria and ventricles are not related in one-to-one fashion. AV dissociation can be due to several conditions:

1. Atrioventricular conduction block (p. 439).
2. Slowing of the primary pacemaker, most commonly due to sinus bradycardia or sinus pauses with junctional escape rhythm (p. 439).
3. Acceleration of a subsidiary pacemaker, most commonly due to VT or much less commonly due to junctional tachycardia.

The most important reason to identify AV dissociation is in wide complex tachycardia for the differentiation of SVT with aberrancy from VT. In VT, the rapid ventricular rate is often associated with retrograde block within the His-Purkinje system (ventriculoatrial block). This leads to P waves (from sinus node depolarization) that are not associated in 1:1 fashion with the QRS complexes (Figure 7–5). The presence of AV dissociation makes VT the most likely diagnosis in a patient with a regular wide complex tachycardia. In some circumstances, AV dissociation can be identified by the presence of **capture beats** or **fusion beats**. Occasionally, a properly timed P wave conducts to the ventricles and a portion (fusion beat) or all (capture beat) of ventricular tissue is activated by the His-Purkinje tissue for one QRS complex. It is always easier to identify AV dissociation rather than AV association; T waves can often be confused with P waves. Always examine the entire ECG for unexpected deflections in the QRS complex, ST segment, and T waves that are dissociated P waves. The P waves are usually most obvious in the inferior leads (II, III, and aVF) or V_1.

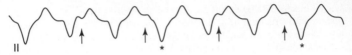

Figure 7–5. Lead II from a wide complex tachycardia. The arrows mark P waves that are not associated with every QRS complex (AV dissociation). The QRS complexes marked with an * are slightly narrower owing to partial activation from the preceding P wave (fusion complex).

MORPHOLOGY ALGORITHMS FOR IDENTIFYING VT

1. METHOD ONE: QUICK METHOD FOR DIAGNOSIS OF VT (REQUIRES LEADS I, V₁, AND V₂)

This method derives from an analysis of typical waveforms of RBBB or LBBB as seen in leads I, V_1, and V_2. If the waveforms do not conform to either the common or uncommon typical morphologic patterns, the diagnosis defaults to VT.

Step One

Determine the morphologic classification of the wide QRS complexes (RB type or LB type), using the criteria below.

  A. **Determination of the Morphologic Type of Wide QRS Complexes:** Use lead V_1 only to determine the type of bundle branch block morphology of abnormally wide QRS complexes.

  1. **RBBB- and RBB-type QRS complexes as seen in lead V_1:** A wide QRS complex with a net positive area under the QRS curve is called the right bundle branch "type" of QRS. This does not mean that the QRS conforms exactly to the morphologic criteria for RBBB. Typical morphologies seen in RBBB are shown in the box at left below. Atypical morphologies at the right are most commonly seen in PVCs or during VT.

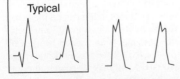

  2. **LBBB- and LBB-type QRS complexes as seen in lead V_1:** A wide QRS complex with a net negative area under the QRS curve is called a left bundle branch "type" of QRS. This does not mean

that the QRS conforms exactly to the morphologic criteria for LBBB. Typical morphologies of LBBB are shown in the box at left below. Atypical morphologies at the right are most commonly seen in PVCs or during VT.

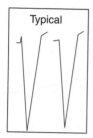
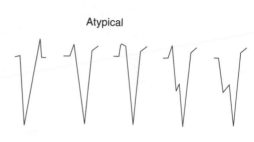

Step Two

Apply criteria for common and uncommon normal forms of either RBBB or LBBB, as described below. The waveforms may not be identical, but the morphologic descriptions must match. If the QRS complexes do not match, the rhythm is probably VT.

A. **RBBB: Lead I must have a terminal broad S wave, but the R/S ratio may be <1.**

In lead V_1, the QRS complex is usually triphasic but sometimes is notched and monophasic. The latter must have notching on the ascending limb of the R wave, usually at the lower left.

B. **LBBB: Lead I must have a monophasic, usually notched R wave and may not have Q waves or S waves.**

Both lead V_1 and lead V_2 must have a dominant S wave, usually with a small, narrow R wave. S descent must be rapid and smooth, without notching.

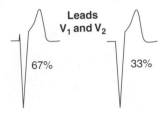

2. METHOD TWO: THE BRUGADA ALGORITHM FOR DIAGNOSIS OF VT

(Requires all six precordial leads.)

Brugada and coworkers reported on a total of 554 patients with WCTRR whose mechanism was diagnosed in the electrophysiology laboratory. Patients included 384 (69%) with VT and 170 (31%) with SVT with aberrant ventricular conduction.

1. **Is there absence of an RS complex in ALL precordial leads?**

   If Yes ($n = 83$), VT is established diagnosis (sensitivity 21%, specificity 100%). **Note:** Only QR, Qr, qR, QS, QRS, monophasic R, or rSR′ are present. qRs complexes were not mentioned in the Brugada study.

   If No ($n = 471$), proceed to next step.

2. **Is the RS interval >100 ms in ANY ONE precordial lead?**

   If Yes ($n = 175$), VT is established diagnosis (sensitivity 66%, specificity 98%). **Note:** The onset of R to the nadir of S is >100 ms (>2.5 small boxes) in a lead with an RS complex.

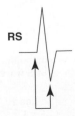

   If No ($n = 296$), proceed to next step.

3. Is there AV dissociation?

If Yes ($n = 59$), VT is established diagnosis (sensitivity 82%, specificity 98%). *Note:* AV block also implies the same diagnosis.

If No ($n = 237$), proceed to next step. *Note:* Antiarrhythmic drugs were withheld from patients in this study. Clinically, drugs that prolong the QRS duration may give a false-positive sign of VT using this criterion.

4. Are morphologic criteria for VT present?

If Yes ($n = 59$), VT is established diagnosis (sensitivity 99%, specificity 97%). *Note:* RBBB type QRS in V_1 versus LBBB type QRS in V_1 should be assessed as shown in the boxes below.

If No ($n = 169$)—and if there are no matches for VT in the boxes below—the diagnosis is SVT with aberration (sensitivity 97%, specificity 99%).

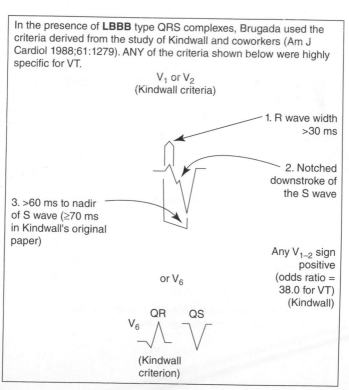

In the presence of **LBBB** type QRS complexes, Brugada used the criteria derived from the study of Kindwall and coworkers (Am J Cardiol 1988;61:1279). ANY of the criteria shown below were highly specific for VT.

V_1 or V_2
(Kindwall criteria)

1. R wave width >30 ms

2. Notched downstroke of the S wave

3. >60 ms to nadir of S wave (≥70 ms in Kindwall's original paper)

Any V_{1-2} sign positive (odds ratio = 38.0 for VT) (Kindwall)

or V_6

V_6 QR   QS

(Kindwall criterion)

In the presence of **RBBB** type QRS complexes (dominant positive in V_1), a diagnosis of VT can be made by examination of both V_1 and V_6.

V_1 only	V_6
Monophasic R wave	QS or QR
QR or RS	R/S < 1 (seen with LAD)

3. METHOD THREE: THE GRIFFITH METHOD FOR DIAGNOSIS OF VT (REQUIRES LEADS V_1 AND V_6)

This method derives from an analysis of typical waveforms of RBBB or LBBB as seen in both leads V_1 and V_6. If the waveforms do not conform to the typical morphologic patterns, the diagnosis defaults to VT.

Step One

Determine the morphologic classification of the wide QRS complexes (RB type or LB type), using the criteria above.

Step Two

Apply criteria for normal forms of either RBBB or LBBB, as described below. A negative answer to any of the three questions is inconsistent with either RBBB or LBBB, and the diagnosis defaults to VT.

    A. For QRS Complexes With RBBB Categorization:
       1. Is there an rSR′ morphology in lead V_1?

2. Is there an RS complex in V_6 (may have a small septal Q wave)?

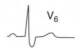

3. Is the R/S ratio in lead $V_6 > 1$?

B. For QRS Complexes With LBBB Categorization:
1. Is there an rS or QS complex in leads V_1 and V_2?

V_1 and V_2
either morphology
is acceptable

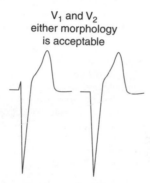

2. Is the onset of the QRS to the nadir of the S wave in lead V_1 <70 ms?
3. Is there an R wave in lead V_6, without a Q wave?

Wide QRS Tachycardia with an Irregular Rhythm

A. Polymorphic Ventricular Tachycardia and Ventricular Fibrillation In **polymorphic ventricular tachycardia** and **ventricular fibrillation,** the ventricles are often activated continuously in chaotic fashion by disorganized wavelets of activation that produce irregular QRS complexes with no isoelectric periods. Both ventricular fibrillation and polymorphic ventricular tachycardia are life-threatening conditions that require prompt defibrillation. The distinction between ventricular fibrillation and polymorphic ventricular tachycardia is simply based on the amplitude of the QRS complexes and has very little clinical utility. The most common cause of polymorphic ventricular tachycardia and ventricular fibrillation is myocardial ischemia due to coronary artery occlusion.

B. **Torsade de Pointes** Torsade de pointes ("twisting of the points") is a specific form of polymorphic VT that is often pause dependent, has a characteristic shifting morphology of the QRS complex, and occurs in the setting of a prolonged QT interval. Torsade de pointes is associated with drug-induced states, congenital long QT syndrome, and hypokalemia (p. 446).

C. **Atrial Fibrillation with Anterograde Accessory Pathway Activation** If a patient with an accessory pathway develops atrial fibrillation, the ventricles are activated by both the normal AV node-His bundle axis and the accessory pathway. Because the accessory pathway does not have decremental conduction properties, it allows very rapid activation of the ventricles. The combination of an irregular wide complex rhythm with very rapid rates (250–300 bpm) should arouse suspicion of this scenario, particularly in a young, otherwise healthy patient.

D. **Bradycardia** Slow heart rates can be due to failure of impulse formation (sinus node dysfunction) or blocked AV conduction.

Sinus Node Dysfunction

Sinus node dysfunction is manifested in a number of ECG findings. Most commonly, there is a sinus pause with a junctional escape beat. Alternatively, sinus bradycardia can be associated with sinus node dysfunction.

A. **Sinus Bradycardia:** The normal range of sinus rates changes with age. In infants less than 12 months old, the mean heart rate is 140 bpm with a range of 100–190 bpm. In contrast, the normal range for adults is probably 50–90 bpm. Sinus rates less than 60 bpm are classified as **sinus bradycardia,** but it must be remembered that sinus rates of less than 60 bpm are commonly observed (sleep, athletes). Treatment of sinus bradycardia (usually with a pacemaker) is indicated only when it is associated with symptoms, not because of a specific heart rate.

B. Sinus Pauses: In some individuals, the sinus node abruptly stops firing, leading to **sinus pauses.** Usually an escape rhythm from an ectopic atrial focus or the junction prevents asystole. Sinus pauses up to 2 seconds are seen in normal adults. Patients with sinus pauses >3 seconds should be evaluated for the presence of sinus node dysfunction.

C. Junctional Rhythm: If the sinus node rate is very low, **sustained junctional rhythm** can sometimes be observed. In junctional rhythm, the QRS is not preceded by a P wave. A retrograde P wave can sometimes be seen in the initial portion or terminal portion of the QRS complex, but most commonly it is "buried" in the QRS complex. Normally, junctional rhythms are <60 bpm. Transient junctional rhythm can be observed in normal individuals during sleep, but sinus node dysfunction should be suspected if junctional rhythm is observed when a patient is awake.

In rare circumstances, **accelerated junctional rhythms** between 60 and 100 bpm are observed due to more rapid depolarization of AV nodal cells. If the junctional rate is faster than the sinus rate, the sinus node will be suppressed by retrograde atrial activation because of repetitive depolarization from the junction. Accelerated junctional rhythms can be present in digitalis toxicity, rheumatic fever, and after cardiac surgery.

AV Block

Because AV conduction normally occurs along a single axis, the AV node and His bundle, **atrioventricular (AV) block** most commonly is due to block at one of these two sites. Block within the His bundle is associated with a worse prognosis and should be suspected in any form of AV block associated with a wide QRS complex. Electrocardiographically, AV block is usually described as first-degree, second-degree, or third-degree AV block. In **first-degree (1°) AV block,** every P wave is conducted to the ventricles, but there is an abnormal delay between atrial activation and ventricular activation (PR interval >0.2 second). In 1° AV block, the ventricular rate is not slow unless sinus bradycardia is also present.

In **second-degree (2°) AV block,** some but not all P waves are conducted to the ventricles. This leads to an irregular ventricular rhythm. Second-degree AV block is usually subclassified as **Mobitz type I block, Wenckebach block** or **Mobitz type II block.** In type I 2° AV block, progressive prolongation of the PR interval is observed; in type II 2° AV block, the PR interval remains relatively constant before the blocked P wave. The importance of this distinction is this: type I 2° AV block usually indicates that conduction is blocked within the AV node, whereas type II AV block suggests that conduction is blocked within the His bundle (regardless of the width of the QRS complex). The simplest way to differentiate between type I and type II 2° AV block is to compare the PR intervals before and after the block P wave. In type I 2° AV block, the PR interval after the blocked P wave is shorter than the PR interval before the blocked P wave; in type II 2° AV block, the PR intervals are the same.

In **third-degree (3°) or complete AV block,** no P waves are conducted to the ventricles. The P-to-P and QRS-to-QRS intervals are constant and unrelated (AV dissociation). The QRS rate and morphology depend on the site of the subsidiary intrinsic pacemaker. If the block is within the AV node, a lower AV nodal pacemaker often takes over and the rate is 40–50 bpm with a normal-appearing QRS complex (junctional rhythm). If the block is within the His bundle, a ventricular pacemaker with a rate of 20–40 bpm and a wide QRS will be noted (**ventricular escape rhythm**).

STEP TWO: MORPHOLOGIC DIAGNOSIS OF THE CARDIAC WAVEFORMS

A. THE NORMAL ECG: TWO BASIC QRST PATTERNS

The most common pattern is illustrated below and is usually seen in leads I or II and V_6. There is a small "septal" Q wave <30 ms in duration. The T wave is upright. The normal ST segment, which is never normally iso-electric except sometimes at slow rates (<60 bpm), slopes upward into an upright T wave, whose proximal angle is more obtuse than the distal angle. The normal T wave is never symmetric.

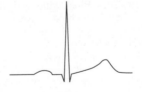

The pattern seen in the right precordial leads, usually V_{1-3}, is shown on the next page (p. 441). There is a dominant S wave. The J point—the junction between the end of the QRS complex and the ST segment—is usually slightly elevated, and the T wave is upright. The T wave in V_1 may occasionally be inverted as a normal finding in up to 50% of young women and 25% of young men, but this finding is usually abnormal in adult males. V_2 usually has the largest absolute QRS and T-wave magnitude of any of the 12 electrocardiographic leads.

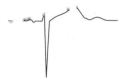

B. ATRIAL ABNORMALITIES

Right Atrial Enlargement (RAE)

Diagnostic criteria include a positive component of the P wave in lead V_1 or $V_2 \geq 1.5$ mm. Another criterion is a P-wave amplitude in lead II >2.5 mm.

Note: A tall, peaked P in lead II may represent RAE but is more commonly due to either chronic obstructive pulmonary disease (COPD) or increased sympathetic tone.

Clinical correlation: RAE is seen with right ventricular hypertrophy (RVH).

Left Atrial Enlargement (LAE)

The most sensitive lead for the diagnosis of LAE is lead V_1, but the criteria for lead II are more specific. Criteria include a terminal negative wave ≥ 1 mm deep and ≥ 40 ms wide (one small box by one small box in area) for lead V_1 and >40 ms between the first (right) and second (left) atrial components of the P wave in lead II, or a P-wave duration >110 ms in lead II.

Clinical correlations: left ventricular hypertrophy (LVH), coronary artery disease, mitral valve disease, or cardiomyopathy.

C. BUNDLE BRANCH BLOCK

The normal QRS duration in adults ranges from 67–114 ms (Glasgow cohort). If the QRS duration is ≥ 120 ms (three small boxes or more on the electrocardiographic paper), there is usually an abnormality of conduction of the ventricular impulse. The most common causes are either RBBB or LBBB (see p. 442). However, other conditions may also prolong the QRS duration.

RBBB is defined by delayed terminal QRS forces that are directed to the right and anteriorly, producing broad terminal positive waves in leads V_1 and aVR and a broad terminal negative wave in lead I.

LBBB is defined by delayed terminal QRS forces that are directed to the left and posteriorly, producing wide R waves in leads that face the left ventricular free wall and wide S waves in the right precordial leads.

RIGHT BUNDLE BRANCH BLOCK

Diagnostic Criteria

The diagnosis of uncomplicated complete RBBB is made when the following criteria are met:

1. Prolongation of the QRS duration to 120 ms or more.
2. An rsr′, rsR′, or rSR′ pattern in lead V_1 or V_2. The R′ is usually greater than the initial R wave. In a minority of cases, a wide and notched R pattern may be seen.
3. Leads V_6 and I show a QRS complex with a wide S wave (S duration is longer than the R duration or >40 ms in adults).

(See common and uncommon waveforms for RBBB under Step Two, p. 433.)

ST–T changes in RBBB

In uncomplicated RBBB, the ST–T segment is depressed and the T wave inverted in the right precordial leads with an R′ (usually only in lead V_1 but occasionally in V_2). The T wave is upright in leads I, V_5, and V_6.

LEFT BUNDLE BRANCH BLOCK

Diagnostic Criteria

The diagnosis of uncomplicated complete LBBB is made when the following criteria are met:

1. Prolongation of the QRS duration to 120 ms or more.
2. There are broad and notched or slurred R waves in left-sided precordial leads V_5 and V_6, as well as in leads I and aVL. Occasionally, an RS pattern may occur in leads V_5 and V_6 in uncomplicated LBBB associated with posterior displacement of the left ventricle.
3. With the possible exception of lead aVL, Q waves are absent in the left-sided leads, specifically in leads V_5, V_6, and I.
4. The R peak time is prolonged to >60 ms in lead V_5 or V_6 but is normal in leads V_1 and V_2 when it can be determined.
5. In the right precordial leads V_1 and V_3, there are small initial r waves in the majority of cases, followed by wide and deep S waves. The transition zone in the precordial leads is displaced to the left. Wide QS complexes may be present in leads V_1 and V_2 and rarely in lead V_3.

(See common and uncommon waveforms for LBBB under Step Two, pp. 433–434.)

ST–T Changes in LBBB

In uncomplicated LBBB, the ST segments are usually depressed and the T waves inverted in left precordial leads V_5 and V_6 as well as in leads I and aVL. Conversely, ST-segment elevations and positive T waves are recorded in leads V_1 and V_2. Only rarely is the T wave upright in the left precordial leads. As a general rule, ST–T changes in LBBB are usually in the direction opposite the direction of the QRS complex (inverted T waves and ST-segment depression if the QRS is upright).

D. INCOMPLETE BUNDLE BRANCH BLOCKS

Incomplete LBBB

The waveforms are similar to those in complete LBBB, but the QRS duration is <120 ms. Septal Q waves are absent in I and V_6. Incomplete LBBB is synonymous with LVH and commonly mimics a delta wave in leads V_5 and V_6.

Incomplete RBBB

The waveforms are similar to those in complete RBBB, but the QRS duration is <120 ms. This diagnosis suggests RVH. Occasionally, in a normal variant pattern, there is an rSr′ waveform in lead V_1. In this case, the r′ is usually smaller than the initial r wave; this pattern is not indicative of incomplete RBBB.

Intraventricular Conduction Delay or Defect

If the QRS duration is ≥120 ms but typical waveforms of either RBBB or LBBB are not present, there is an intraventricular conduction delay or defect (IVCD). This pattern is common in dilated cardiomyopathy. An IVCD with a QRS duration of ≥170 ms is highly predictive of dilated cardiomyopathy.

E. FASCICULAR BLOCKS (HEMIBLOCKS)

1. LEFT ANTERIOR FASCICULAR BLOCK (LAFB)

Diagnostic Criteria

1. Mean QRS axis from –45 degrees to –90 degrees (possibly –31 to –44 degrees).

2. A qR pattern in lead aVL, with the R peak time, that is, the onset of the Q wave to the peak of the R wave ≥45 ms (slightly more than one small box wide), as shown below.

Clinical correlations: hypertensive heart disease, coronary artery disease, or idiopathic conducting system disease.

2. LEFT POSTERIOR FASCICULAR BLOCK (LPFB)

Diagnostic Criteria

1. Mean QRS axis from +90 degrees to +180 degrees.
2. A qR complex in leads III and aVF, an rS complex in leads aVL and I, with a Q wave ≥40 ms in the inferior leads.

Clinical correlations: LPFB is a diagnosis of exclusion. It may be seen in the acute phase of inferior myocardial injury or infarction or may result from idiopathic conducting system disease.

F. DETERMINATION OF THE MEAN QRS AXIS

The mean electrical axis is the average direction of the activation or repolarization process during the cardiac cycle. Instantaneous and mean electrical axes may be determined for any deflection (P, QRS, ST–T) in the three planes (frontal, transverse, and sagittal). The determination of the electrical axis of a QRS complex is useful for the diagnosis of certain pathologic cardiac conditions.

The Mean QRS Axis in the Frontal Plane (Limb Leads)

Arzbaecher developed the **hexaxial reference system** that allowed for the display of the relationships among the six frontal plane (limb) leads. A diagram of this system is shown on the next page.

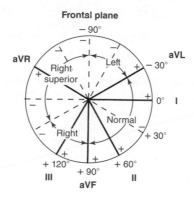

Frontal plane

The normal range of the QRS axis in adults is −30 degrees to +90 degrees.

It is rarely important to precisely determine the degrees of the mean QRS. However, the recognition of abnormal axis deviations is critical because it leads to a presumption of disease. The mean QRS axis is derived from the net area under the QRS curves. The most efficient method of determining the mean QRS axis uses the method of Grant, which requires only leads I and II (see below). If the net area under the QRS curves in these leads is positive, the axis falls between −30 degrees and +90 degrees, which is the normal range of axis in adults. (The only exception to this rule is in RBBB, in which the first 60 ms of the QRS is used. Alternatively, one may use the maximal amplitude of the R and S waves in leads I and II to assess the axis in RBBB.) Abnormal axes are shown below.

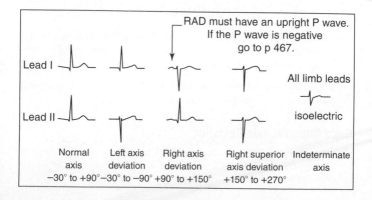

Left Axis Deviation (LAD)

The four main causes of left axis deviation are as follows:

A. **Left Anterior Fascicular Block (LAFB):** See criteria above.

B. **Inferior Myocardial Infarction:** There is a pathologic Q wave ≥30 ms either in lead aVF or lead II in the absence of ventricular preexcitation.

C. **Ventricular Preexcitation (WPW Pattern):** LAD is seen with inferior paraseptal accessory pathway locations. This can mimic inferoposterior myocardial infarction. The classic definition of the Wolff-Parkinson-White (WPW) pattern includes a short PR interval (<120 ms); an initial slurring of the QRS complex, called a delta wave; and prolongation of the QRS complex to >120 ms. However, because this pattern may not always be present despite the presence of ventricular preexcitation, a more practical definition is an absent PR segment and an initial slurring of the QRS complex in any lead. The diagnosis of the WPW pattern usually requires sinus rhythm.

D. **COPD:** LAD is seen in 10% of patients with COPD.

Right Axis Deviation (RAD)

The four main causes of right axis deviation (RAD) are as follows:

A. **Right Ventricular Hypertrophy:** This is the most common cause (refer to diagnostic criteria, p. 448). However, one must first exclude acute occlusion of the posterior descending coronary artery, causing LPFB, and exclude also items B and C below.

B. **Extensive Lateral and Apical Myocardial Infarction:** Criteria include QS or Qr patterns in leads I and aVL and in leads V_{4-6}.

C. **Ventricular Preexcitation (WPW Pattern):** RAD seen with left lateral accessory pathway locations. This can mimic lateral myocardial infarction.

D. **Left Posterior Fascicular Block (LPFB):** This is a diagnosis of exclusion (see criteria above).

Right Superior Axis Deviation

This category is rare. Causes include RVH, apical myocardial infarction, VT, and hyperkalemia. Right superior axis deviation may rarely be seen as an atypical form of LAFB.

G. VENTRICULAR HYPERTROPHY

1. LEFT VENTRICULAR HYPERTROPHY

The ECG is very insensitive as a screening tool for LVH, but electrocardiographic criteria are usually specific. Echocardiography is the major resource for this diagnosis.

The best electrocardiographic criterion for the diagnosis of LVH is the Cornell voltage, the sum of the R-wave amplitude in lead aVL and the S-wave depth in lead V_3, adjusted for sex:

1. RaVL + SV_3 >20 mm (females), >25 mm (males). The R-wave height in aVL alone is a good place to start.
2. RaVL >9 mm (females), >11 mm (males).

Alternatively, application of the following criteria will diagnose most cases of LVH.

3. Sokolow-Lyon criteria: SV_1 + RV_5 or RV_6 (whichever R wave is taller) >35 mm (in patients age >35).
4. Romhilt-Estes criteria: Points are scored for QRS voltage (1 point), the presence of LAE (1 point), typical repolarization abnormalities in the absence of digitalis (1 point), and a few other findings. The combination of LAE (see above) and typical repolarization abnormalities (see below) (score ≥5 points) will suffice for the diagnosis of LVH even when voltage criteria are not met.
5. RV_6 > RV_5 (usually occurs with dilated LV). First exclude anterior myocardial infarction and establish that the R waves in V_5 are >7 mm tall and that in V_6 they are >6 mm tall before using this criterion.

Repolarization Abnormalities

Typical repolarization abnormalities in the presence of LVH are an ominous sign of end-organ damage. In repolarization abnormalities in LVH, the ST segment and T wave are directed opposite to the dominant QRS waveform in all leads. However, this directional rule does not apply either in the transitional lead (defined as a lead having an R-wave height equal to the S wave depth) or in the transitional zone (defined as leads adjacent to the transitional lead) or one lead to the left in the precordial leads.

Spectrum of Repolarization Abnormalities

The waveforms below, usually seen in leads I, aVL, V₅, and V₆ but more specifically in leads with dominant R waves, represent hypothetical stages in the progression of LVH.

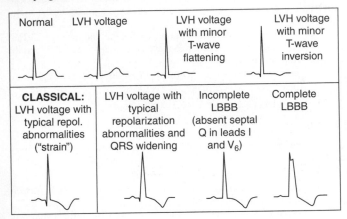

Normal	LVH voltage	LVH voltage with minor T-wave flattening	LVH voltage with minor T-wave inversion
CLASSICAL: LVH voltage with typical repol. abnormalities ("strain")	LVH voltage with typical repolarization abnormalities and QRS widening	Incomplete LBBB (absent septal Q in leads I and V₆)	Complete LBBB

2. RIGHT VENTRICULAR HYPERTROPHY (RVH)

The ECG is insensitive for the diagnosis of RVH. In 100 cases of RVH from one echocardiography laboratory, only 33% had RAD because of the confounding effects of LV disease. Published electrocardiographic criteria for RVH are listed below, all of which have ≥97% specificity.

With rare exceptions, right atrial enlargement is synonymous with RVH.

Diagnostic Criteria

Recommended criteria for the electrocardiographic diagnosis of RVH are as follows:

1. Right axis deviation (>90 degrees), or
2. An R/S ratio ≥1 in lead V₁ (absent posterior myocardial infarction [MI] or RBBB), or
3. An R wave >7 mm tall in V₁ (not the R′ of RBBB), or
4. An rsR′ complex in V₁ (R′ ≥10 mm), with a QRS duration of <0.12 s (incomplete RBBB), or
5. An S wave >7 mm deep in leads V₅ or V₆ (in the absence of a QRS axis more negative than +30 degrees), or
6. RBBB with RAD (axis derived from first 60 ms of the QRS). (Consider RVH in RBBB if the R/S ratio in lead I is <0.5.)

A variant of RVH (type C loop) may produce a false-positive sign of an anterior myocardial infarction.

Repolarization Abnormalities

The morphology of repolarization abnormalities in RVH is identical to those in LVH, when a particular lead contains tall R waves reflecting the hypertrophied RV or LV. In RVH, these typically occur in leads V_{1-2} or V_3 and in leads aVF and III. This morphology of repolarization abnormalities due to ventricular hypertrophy is illustrated earlier (p. 448). In cases of RVH with massive dilation, all precordial leads may overlie the diseased RV and may exhibit repolarization abnormalities.

H. LOW VOLTAGE OF THE QRS COMPLEX

Low-Voltage Limb Leads Only

Defined as peak-to-peak QRS voltage <5 mm in all limb leads.

Low-Voltage Limb and Precordial Leads

Defined as peak-to-peak QRS voltage <5 mm in all limb leads and <10 mm in all precordial leads. Primary myocardial causes include multiple or massive infarctions; infiltrative diseases such as amyloidosis, sarcoidosis, or hemochromatosis; and myxedema. Extracardiac causes include pericardial effusion, COPD, pleural effusion, obesity, anasarca, and subcutaneous emphysema. When there is COPD, expect to see low voltage in the limb leads as well as in leads V_5 and V_6.

I. PROGRESSION OF THE R WAVE IN THE PRECORDIAL LEADS

The normal R-wave height increases from V_1 to V_5. The normal R-wave height in V_5 is always taller than that in V_6 because of the attenuating effect of the lungs. The normal R-wave height in lead V_3 is usually >2 mm.

Poor R-Wave Progression

The term "poor R-wave progression" (PRWP) is a nonpreferred term because most physicians use this term to imply the presence of an anterior myocardial infarction, although it may not be present. Other causes of small R waves in the right precordial leads include LVH, LAFB, LBBB, cor pulmonale (with the type C loop of RVH), and COPD.

Reversed R-Wave Progression (RRWP)

Reversed R-wave progression is defined as a loss of R-wave height between leads V_1 and V_2 or between leads V_2 and V_3 or between leads V_3 and V_4. In the absence of LVH, this finding suggests anterior myocardial infarction or precordial lead reversal.

J. TALL R WAVES IN THE RIGHT PRECORDIAL LEADS

Etiology

Causes of tall R waves in the right precordial leads include the following:

A. **Right Ventricular Hypertrophy:** This is the most common cause. There is an R/S ratio ≥ 1 or an R-wave height >7 mm in lead V_1.

B. **Posterior Myocardial Infarction:** There is an R wave ≥ 6 mm in lead V_1 or ≥ 15 mm in lead V_2. One should distinguish the tall R wave of RVH from the tall R wave of posterior myocardial infarction in lead V_1. In RVH, there is a downsloping ST segment and an inverted T wave, usually with right axis deviation. In contrast, in posterior myocardial infarction, there is usually an upright, commonly tall T wave and, because posterior myocardial infarction is usually associated with concomitant inferior myocardial infarction, a left axis deviation.

C. **Right Bundle Branch Block:** The QRS duration is prolonged, and typical waveforms are present (see p. 433).

D. **The WPW Pattern:** Left-sided accessory pathway locations produce prominent R waves with an R/S ratio ≥ 1 in V_1, with an absent PR segment and initial slurring of the QRS complex, usually best seen in lead V_4.

E. **Rare or Uncommon Causes:** The normal variant pattern of early precordial QRS transition (not uncommon); the reciprocal effect of a deep Q wave in leads V_{5-6} (very rare); Duchenne muscular dystrophy; dextrocardia (very rare); chronic constrictive pericarditis (very rare); and reversal of the right precordial leads.

K. MYOCARDIAL INJURY, ISCHEMIA, AND INFARCTION

Definitions

A. **Myocardial Infarction:** Pathologic changes in the QRS complex reflect ventricular activation away from the area of infarction.

B. **Myocardial Injury:** Injury always points *outward* from the surface that is injured.
  1. **Epicardial injury:** ST elevation in the distribution of an acutely occluded artery.
  2. **Endocardial injury:** Diffuse ST-segment depression, which is really reciprocal to the primary event, reflected as ST elevation in aVR.

C. **Myocardial Ischemia:** Diffuse ST-segment depression, usually with associated T-wave inversion. It usually reflects subendocardial injury, reciprocal to ST elevation in lead aVR. In ischemia, there may only be inverted T waves with a symmetric, sharp nadir.

D. **Reciprocal Changes:** Passive electrical reflections of a primary event viewed from either the other side of the heart, as in epicardial injury, or the other side of the ventricular wall, as in subendocardial injury.

Steps in the Diagnosis of Myocardial Infarction

The following pages contain a systematic method for the electrocardiographic diagnosis of myocardial injury or infarction, arranged in seven steps. Following the steps will achieve the diagnosis in most cases.

Step 1: Identify the presence of myocardial injury by ST-segment deviations.
Step 2: Identify areas of myocardial injury by assessing lead groupings.
Step 3: Define the primary area of involvement and identify the culprit artery producing the injury.
Step 4: Identify the location of the lesion in the artery to risk stratify the patient.
Step 5: Identify any electrocardiographic signs of infarction found in the QRS complexes.
Step 6: Determine the age of the infarction by assessing the location of the ST segment in leads with pathologic QRS abnormalities.
Step 7: Combine all observations into a final diagnosis.

STEPS ONE AND TWO

Identify presence of and areas of myocardial injury.

The GUSTO study of patients with ST-segment elevation in two contiguous leads defined four affected areas as set out in Table 7–3.

TABLE 7–3. GUSTO STUDY DEFINITIONS.

Area of ST-Segment Elevation	Leads Defining This Area
Anterior (Ant)	V_{1-4}
Apical (Ap)	V_{5-6}
Lateral (Lat)	I, aVL
Inferior (Inf)	II, aVF, III

Two other major areas of possible injury or infarction were not included in the GUSTO categorization because they do not produce ST elevation in two contiguous standard leads. These are:

1. **Posterior Injury:** The most commonly used sign of posterior injury is ST depression in leads V_{1-3}, but posterior injury may best be diagnosed by obtaining posterior leads V_7, V_8, and V_9.

2. **Right Ventricular Injury:** The most sensitive sign of right ventricular injury, ST-segment elevation ≥ 1 mm, is found in lead V_4R. A very specific—but insensitive—sign of right ventricular injury or infarction is ST elevation in V_1, with concomitant ST-segment depression in V_2 in the setting of ST elevation in the inferior leads.

STEP THREE

Identify the primary area of involvement and the culprit artery.

Primary Anterior Area

ST elevation in two contiguous V_{1-4} leads defines a primary anterior area of involvement. The left anterior descending coronary artery (LAD) is the culprit artery. Lateral (I and aVL) and apical (V_5 and V_6) areas are contiguous to anterior (V_{1-4}), so ST elevation in these leads signifies more myocardium at risk and more adverse outcomes.

Primary Inferior Area

ST-segment elevation in two contiguous leads (II, aVF, or III) defines a primary inferior area of involvement. The right coronary artery (RCA) is usually the culprit artery. Apical (V_5 and V_6), posterior (V_{1-3} or V_{7-9}), and right ventricular ($V_4 R$) areas are contiguous to the inferior (II, aVF, and III) area, so ST elevation in these contiguous leads signifies more myocardium at risk and more adverse outcomes.

The Culprit Artery

In the GUSTO trial, 98% of patients with ST-segment elevation in any two contiguous V_{1-4} leads, either alone or with associated changes in leads V_{5-6} or I and aVL, had LAD obstruction. In patients with ST-segment elevation only in leads II, aVF, and III, there was RCA obstruction in 86%.

PRIMARY ANTERIOR PROCESS

Acute occlusion of the LAD produces a sequence of changes in the anterior leads (V_{1-4}).

Earliest Findings

A. **"Hyperacute" Changes:** ST elevation with loss of normal ST-segment concavity, commonly with tall, peaked T waves.

rS complex   V$_2$

B. **Acute Injury:** ST elevation, with the ST segment commonly appearing as if a thumb has been pushed up into it.

rS complex   V$_2$

Evolutionary Changes

A patient who presents to the emergency department with chest pain and T-wave inversion in leads with pathologic Q waves is most likely to be in the evolutionary or completed phase of infarction. Successful revascularization usually causes prompt resolution of the acute signs of injury or infarction and results in the electrocardiographic signs of a fully evolved infarction. The tracing below shows QS complexes in lead V$_2$.

A. **Development of Pathologic Q Waves (Infarction):** Pathologic Q waves develop within the first hour after onset of symptoms in at least 30% of patients.

QS complexes
V$_2$ shown

day 1

B. **ST-Segment Elevation Decreases:** T-wave inversion usually occurs in the second 24-hour period after infarction.

day 2

C. **Fully Evolved Pattern:** Pathologic Q waves, ST segment rounded upward, T waves inverted.

chronic

PRIMARY INFERIOR PROCESS

A primary inferior process usually develops after acute occlusion of the RCA, producing changes in the inferior leads (II, III, and aVF).

Earliest Findings

The earliest findings are of acute injury (ST-segment elevation). The J point may "climb up the back" of the R wave (a), or the ST segment may rise up into the T wave (b).

aVF

Evolutionary Changes

ST-segment elevation decreases and pathologic Q waves develop. T-wave inversion may occur in the first 12 hours of an inferior myocardial infarction—in contrast to that in anterior myocardial infarction.

aVF

Right Ventricular Injury or Infarction

With right ventricular injury, there is ST-segment elevation, best seen in lead V_4R. With right ventricular infarction, there is a QS complex.

For comparison, the normal morphology of the QRS complex in lead V_4R is shown below. The normal J point averages +0.2 mm.

POSTERIOR INJURY OR INFARCTION

Posterior injury or infarction is commonly due to acute occlusion of the left circumflex coronary artery, producing changes in the posterior leads (V_7, V_8, V_9) or reciprocal ST-segment depression in leads V_{1-3}.

Acute Pattern

Acute posterior injury or infarction is shown by ST-segment depression in V_{1-3} and perhaps also V_4, usually with upright (often prominent) T waves.

Chronic Pattern

Chronic posterior injury or infarction is shown by pathologic R waves with prominent tall T waves in leads V_{1-3}.

STEP FOUR

Identify the location of the lesion within the artery to risk stratify the patient.

Primary Anterior Process

Aside from an acute occlusion of the left main coronary artery, occlusion of the proximal LAD conveys the most adverse outcomes. Four electrocardiographic signs indicate proximal LAD occlusion:

1. ST elevation >1 mm in lead I, in lead aVL, or in both
2. New RBBB
3. New LAFB
4. New first-degree AV block

If the occlusion occurs in a more distal portion of the LAD (after the first diagonal branch and after the first septal perforator), ST-segment elevation is observed in the anterior leads but the four criteria described above are not seen. In patients with occlusion of the left main coronary artery, diffuse endocardial injury leads to ST-segment elevation in aVR, because this is the only lead that "looks" directly at the ventricular endocardium, and diffuse ST-segment depression is observed in the anterior and inferior leads.

Primary Inferior Process

Nearly 50% of patients with inferior myocardial infarction have distinguishing features that may produce complications or adverse outcomes unless successfully managed:

1. Precordial ST-segment depression in V_{1-3} (suggests concomitant posterior wall involvement);
2. Right ventricular injury or infarction (identifies a proximal RCA lesion);
3. AV block (implies a greater amount of involved myocardium);
4. The sum of ST-segment depressions in leads V_{4-6} exceeds the sum of ST-segment depressions in leads V_{1-3} (suggests multivessel disease).

Reciprocal Changes in the Setting of Acute Myocardial Infarction

ST depressions in leads remote from the primary site of injury are felt to be a purely reciprocal change. With successful reperfusion, the ST depressions usually resolve. If they persist, patients more likely have significant three-vessel disease and so-called ischemia at a distance. Mortality rates are higher in such patients.

STEP FIVE

Identify Electrocardiographic Signs of Infarction in the QRS Complexes

The 12-lead ECG shown below contains numbers corresponding to pathologic widths for Q waves and R waves for selected leads (see Table 7–4 for more complete criteria).

One can memorize the above criteria by mastering a simple scheme of numbers that represent the durations of pathological Q waves or R waves. Begin with lead V_1 and repeat the numbers in the box below in the following order. The numbers increase from "any" to 50.

Any Q wave in lead V_1, for anterior MI
Any Q wave in lead V_2, for anterior MI
Any Q wave in lead V_3, for anterior MI

20 Q wave ≥ 20 ms in lead V_4, for anterior MI
30 Q wave ≥ 30 ms in lead V_5, for apical MI
30 Q wave ≥ 30 ms in lead V_6, for apical MI
30 Q wave ≥ 30 ms in lead I, for lateral MI
30 Q wave ≥ 30 ms in lead aVL, for lateral MI
30 Q wave ≥ 30 ms in lead II, for inferior MI
30 Q wave ≥ 30 ms in lead aVF, for inferior MI

R40 R wave ≥ 40 ms in lead V_1, for posterior MI
R50 R wave ≥ 50 ms in lead V_2, for posterior MI

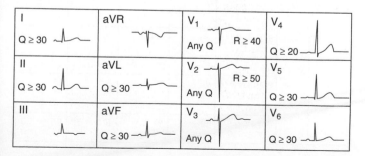

I	aVR	V_1	V_4
Q ≥ 30		Any Q R ≥ 40	Q ≥ 20
II	aVL	V_2	V_5
Q ≥ 30	Q ≥ 30	R ≥ 50 Any Q	Q ≥ 30
III	aVF	V_3	V_6
	Q ≥ 30	Any Q	Q ≥ 30

TABLE 7–4. DIAGNOSIS OF MYOCARDIAL INFARCTION.

Infarct Location	ECG Lead	Criterion	Sensitivity	Specificity	Likelihood Ratio (+)	Likelihood Ratio (−)
Inferior	II	$Q \geq 30$ ms	45	98	22.5	0.6
	aVF	$Q \geq 30$ ms	70	94	11.7	0.3
		$Q \geq 40$ ms	40	98	20.0	0.6
		$R/Q \leq 1$	50	98	25.0	0.5
Anterior	V_1	Any Q	50	97	16.7	0.5
	V_2	Any Q, or $R \leq$ 0.1 mV and $R \leq 10$ ms, or $RV_2 \leq RV_1$	80	94	13.3	0.2
	V_3	Any Q, or $R \leq$ 0.2 mV, or $R \leq 20$ ms	70	93	10.0	0.3
	V_4	$Q \geq 20$ ms	40	92	5.0	0.9
		$R/Q \leq 0.5$, or $R/S \leq 0.5$	40	97	13.3	0.6
Anterolateral (lateral)						
	I	$Q \geq 30$ ms	10	98	5.0	0.9
		$R/Q \leq 1$, or $R \leq 2$ mm	10	97	3.3	0.9
	aVL	$Q \geq 30$ ms	7	97	0.7	1.0
		$R/Q \leq 1$	2			
Apical	V_5	$Q \geq 30$	5	99	5.0	1.0
		$R/Q \leq 2$, or $R \leq 7$ mm, or $R/S \leq 2$, or notched R	60	91	6.7	0.4
		$R/Q \leq 1$, or $R/S \leq 1$	25	98	12.5	0.8
	V_6	$Q \leq 30$	3	98	1.5	1.0
		$R/Q \leq 3$, or $R \leq 6$ mm, or $R/S \leq 3$, or notched R	40	92	25.0	0.7
		$R/Q \leq 1$, or $R/S \leq 1$	10	99	10.0	0.9

TABLE 7–4. DIAGNOSIS OF MYOCARDIAL INFARCTION. (*CONTINUED*)

Infarct Location	ECG Lead	Criterion	Sensitivity	Specificity	Likelihood Ratio (+)	Likelihood Ratio (−)
Posterolateral						
	V₁	R/S ≤ 1	15	97	5.0	0.9
		R ≥ 6 mm, or R ≥ 40 ms	20	93	2.9	0.9
		S ≤ 3 mm	8	97	2.7	0.9
	V₂	R ≥ 15 mm, or R ≥ 50 ms	15	95	3.0	0.9
		R/S ≥ 1.5	10	96	2.5	0.9
		S ≤ 4 mm	2	97	0.7	1.0

Notched R = a notch that begins within the first 40 ms of the R wave; **Q** = Q wave; **R/Q** = ratio of R-wave height to Q-wave depth; **R** = R wave; **R/S ratio** = ratio of R-wave height to S-wave depth; **RV₂ ≤ RV₁** = R-wave height in V₂ less than or equal to that in V₁; **S** = S wave. (Reproduced, with permission, from Haisty WK Jr et al. Performance of the automated complete Selvester QRS scoring system in normal subjects and patients with single and multiple myocardial infarctions. J Am Coll Cardiol 1992;19:341.)

Test Performance Characteristics for Electrocardiographic Criteria in the Diagnosis of Myocardial Infarction

Haisty and coworkers studied 1344 patients with normal hearts documented by coronary arteriography and 837 patients with documented myocardial infarction (366 inferior, 277 anterior, 63 posterior, and 131 inferior and anterior) (Table 7–4). (Patients with LVH, LAFB, LPFB, RVH, LBBB, RBBB, COPD, or WPW patterns were excluded from analysis because these conditions can give false-positive results for myocardial infarction.) Shown above are the sensitivity, specificity, and likelihood ratios for the best-performing infarct criteria. Notice that leads III and aVR are not listed: lead III may normally have a Q wave that is both wide and deep, and lead aVR commonly has a wide Q wave.

Mimics of Myocardial Infarction

Conditions that can produce pathologic Q waves, ST-segment elevation, or loss of R-wave height in the absence of infarction are set out in Table 7–5.

TABLE 7–5. MIMICS OF MYOCARDIAL INFARCTION.

Condition	Pseudoinfarct Location
WPW pattern	Any, most commonly inferoposterior or lateral
Hypertrophic cardiomyopathy	Lateral apical (18%), inferior (11%)
LBBB	Anteroseptal, anterolateral, inferior
RBBB	Inferior, posterior (using criteria from leads V_1 and V_2), anterior
LVH	Anterior, inferior
LAFB	Anterior (may cause a tiny Q in V_2)
COPD	Inferior, posterior, anterior
RVH	Inferior, posterior (using criteria from leads V_1 and V_2), anterior, or apical (using criteria for R/S ratios from leads V_{4-6})
Acute cor pulmonale	Inferior, possibly anterior
Cardiomyopathy (nonischemic)	Any, most commonly inferior (with IVCD pattern), less commonly anterior
Chest deformity	Any
Left pneumothorax	Anterior, anterolateral
Hyperkalemia	Any
Normal hearts	Posterior, anterior

COPD = chronic obstructive pulmonary disease; *LAFB* = left anterior fascicular block; *LBBB* = left bundle branch block; *LVH* = left ventricular hypertrophy; *RBBB* = right bundle branch block; *RVH* = right ventricular hypertrophy.

STEP SIX

Determine the Age of the Infarction

An **acute infarction** manifests ST-segment elevation in a lead with a pathologic Q wave. The T waves may be either upright or inverted.

An **old** or **age-indeterminate infarction** manifests a pathologic Q wave, with or without slight ST-segment elevation or T-wave abnormalities.

Persistent ST-segment elevation ≥1 mm after a myocardial infarction is a sign of dyskinetic wall motion in the area of infarct. Half of these patients have ventricular aneurysms.

STEP SEVEN

Combine Observations into a Final Diagnosis

There are two possibilities for the major electrocardiographic diagnosis: myocardial infarction or acute injury. If there are pathologic changes in the QRS complex, one should make a diagnosis of myocardial infarction—beginning with the primary area, followed by any contiguous areas—and state the age of the infarction. If there are no pathologic changes in the QRS complex, one should make a diagnosis of acute injury of the affected segments—beginning with the primary area and followed by any contiguous areas.

L. ST SEGMENTS

Table 7–6 summarizes major causes of ST-segment elevations. Table 7–7 summarizes major causes of ST-segment depressions or T-wave inversions. The various classes and morphologies of ST–T waves as seen in lead V_2 are shown in Table 7–8.

M. U WAVES

Normal U Waves

In many normal hearts, low-amplitude positive U waves <1.5 mm tall that range from 160–200 ms in duration are seen in leads V_2 or V_3. Leads V_2 and V_3 are close to the ventricular mass and small-amplitude signals may be best seen in these leads.

Cause: Bradycardias.

Abnormal U Waves

Abnormal U waves have increased amplitude or merge with abnormal T waves and produce T–U fusion. Criteria include an amplitude ≥1.5 mm or a U wave that is as tall as the T wave that immediately precedes it.

Causes: Hypokalemia, digitalis, antiarrhythmic drugs.

Inverted U Waves

These are best seen in leads V_{4-6}.

Causes: LVH, acute ischemia.

Table 7–9 summarizes various classes and morphologies of ST–T–U abnormalities as seen in lead V_4.

N. QT INTERVAL

A prolonged QT interval conveys adverse outcomes. The QT interval is inversely related to the heart rate. QT interval corrections for heart rate often use Bazett's formula, defined as the observed QT interval divided by the square root of the R–R interval in seconds. A corrected QT interval of ≥440 ms is abnormal.

TABLE 7–6. MAJOR CAUSES OF ST-SEGMENT ELEVATION.

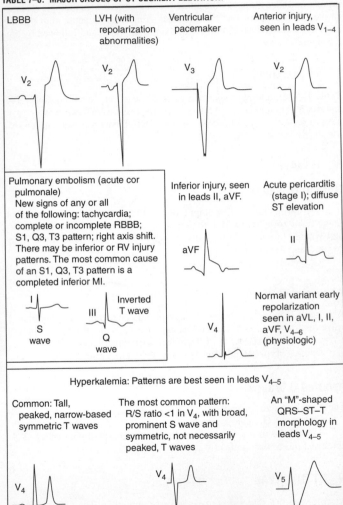

LBBB

LVH (with repolarization abnormalities)

Ventricular pacemaker

Anterior injury, seen in leads V_{1-4}

V_2

V_2

V_3

V_2

Pulmonary embolism (acute cor pulmonale)
New signs of any or all of the following: tachycardia; complete or incomplete RBBB; S1, Q3, T3 pattern; right axis shift. There may be inferior or RV injury patterns. The most common cause of an S1, Q3, T3 pattern is a completed inferior MI.

I
S wave

III
Inverted T wave
Q wave

Inferior injury, seen in leads II, aVF.

aVF

Acute pericarditis (stage I); diffuse ST elevation

II

V_4

Normal variant early repolarization seen in aVL, I, II, aVF, V_{4-6} (physiologic)

Hyperkalemia: Patterns are best seen in leads V_{4-5}

Common: Tall, peaked, narrow-based symmetric T waves

V_4

The most common pattern: R/S ratio <1 in V_4, with broad, prominent S wave and symmetric, not necessarily peaked, T waves

V_4

An "M"-shaped QRS–ST–T morphology in leads V_{4-5}

V_5

TABLE 7–7. MAJOR CAUSES OF ST-SEGMENT DEPRESSION OR T-WAVE INVERSION.

Whenever the ST segment or the T wave is directed counter to an expected repolarization abnormality, consider ischemia, healed MI, or drug or electrolyte effect.	In RBBB, there is an obligatory inverted T wave in right pre-cordial leads with an R' (usually only in V₁) or its equivalent (a qR complex in septal MI). An upright T in these leads suggests completed posterior MI.	Altered depolarization RBBB V₁

LBBB	LVH (with repolarization abnormality)	Subarachnoid hemorrhage	RVH
V₅	V₆	V₄	RVH V₁₋₃

Inferior subendocardial injury	Posterior subepicardial injury	Anterior subendocardial injury or non-Q wave MI	
II 	V₂ 	V₅ 	V₄

Hypokalemia	Digitalis	Antiarrhythmics	J point depression secondary to catecholamines
V₄ 	V₄ 	V₄ 	II
When K⁺ ≤ 2.8, 80% have ECG changes			PR interval and ST segment occupy the same curve

TABLE 7–8. VARIOUS CLASSES AND MORPHOLOGIES OF ST–T WAVES AS SEEN IN LEAD V₂.

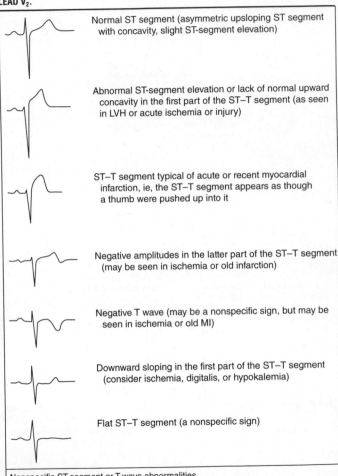

	Normal ST segment (asymmetric upsloping ST segment with concavity, slight ST-segment elevation)
	Abnormal ST-segment elevation or lack of normal upward concavity in the first part of the ST–T segment (as seen in LVH or acute ischemia or injury)
	ST–T segment typical of acute or recent myocardial infarction, ie, the ST–T segment appears as though a thumb were pushed up into it
	Negative amplitudes in the latter part of the ST–T segment (may be seen in ischemia or old infarction)
	Negative T wave (may be a nonspecific sign, but may be seen in ischemia or old MI)
	Downward sloping in the first part of the ST–T segment (consider ischemia, digitalis, or hypokalemia)
	Flat ST–T segment (a nonspecific sign)

Nonspecific ST-segment or T-wave abnormalities
By definition, nonspecific abnormalities of either the ST segment (ones that are only slightly depressed or abnormal in contour) or T wave (ones that are either 10% the height of the R wave that produced it, or are either flat or slightly inverted) do not conform to the characteristic wave-forms found above or elsewhere.

TABLE 7–9. VARIOUS CLASSES AND MORPHOLOGIES OF ST–T–U ABNORMALITIES AS SEEN IN LEAD V$_4$.

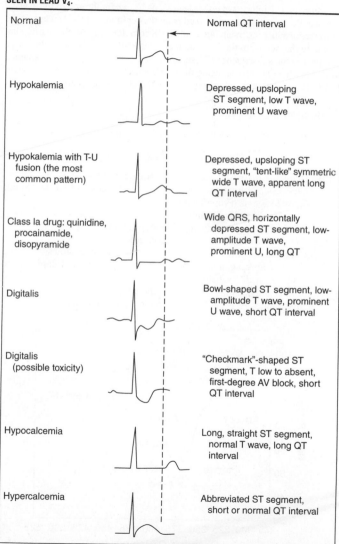

Normal	Normal QT interval
Hypokalemia	Depressed, upsloping ST segment, low T wave, prominent U wave
Hypokalemia with T-U fusion (the most common pattern)	Depressed, upsloping ST segment, "tent-like" symmetric wide T wave, apparent long QT interval
Class Ia drug: quinidine, procainamide, disopyramide	Wide QRS, horizontally depressed ST segment, low-amplitude T wave, prominent U, long QT
Digitalis	Bowl-shaped ST segment, low-amplitude T wave, prominent U wave, short QT interval
Digitalis (possible toxicity)	"Checkmark"-shaped ST segment, T low to absent, first-degree AV block, short QT interval
Hypocalcemia	Long, straight ST segment, normal T wave, long QT interval
Hypercalcemia	Abbreviated ST segment, short or normal QT interval

Use of the QT Nomogram (Hodges Correction)

Measure the QT interval in either lead V_2 or V_3, where the end of the T wave can usually be clearly distinguished from the beginning of the U wave. If the rate is regular, use the mean rate of the QRS complexes. If the rate is irregular, calculate the rate from the immediately prior R–R cycle, because this cycle determines the subsequent QT interval. Use the numbers you have obtained to classify the QT interval using the nomogram below. Or remember that at heart rates of ≥ 40 bpm, an observed QT interval ≥ 480 ms is abnormal.

Prolonged QT Interval

The four major causes of a prolonged QT interval are as follows:

- **A. Electrolyte Abnormalities:** Hypokalemia, hypocalcemia

- **B. Drugs:** Also associated with **torsade de pointes.**
  Class Ia antiarrhythmic agents: Quinidine, procainamide, disopyramide
  Class Ic agents: Propafenone
  Class III agents: Amiodarone, N-acetylprocainamide, sotalol
  Antibiotics: Erythromycin, trimethoprim-sulfamethoxazole
  Antifungals: Ketoconazole, itraconazole
  Chemotherapeutics: Pentamidine, perhaps anthracyclines
  Psychotropic agents: Tricyclic and heterocyclic antidepressants, phenothiazines, haloperidol
  Toxins and poisons: Organophosphate insecticides
  Miscellaneous: Prednisone, probucol, chloral hydrate

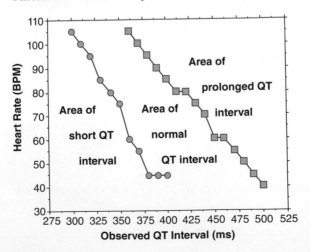

C. Congenital Long QT Syndromes: Though rare, a congenital long QT syndrome should be considered in any young patient who presents with syncope or presyncope.

D. Miscellaneous Causes:
Third-degree and sometimes second-degree AV block
At the cessation of ventricular pacing
LVH (usually minor degrees of lengthening)
Myocardial infarction (in the evolutionary stages where there are marked repolarization abnormalities)
Significant active myocardial ischemia
Cerebrovascular accident (subarachnoid hemorrhage)
Hypothermia

Short QT Interval

The five causes of a short QT interval are hypercalcemia, digitalis, thyrotoxicosis, increased sympathetic tone, and genetic abnormality.

O. MISCELLANEOUS ABNORMALITIES

Right-Left Arm Cable Reversal versus Mirror Image Dextrocardia

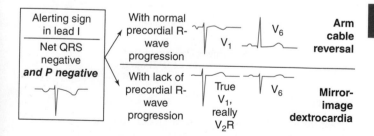

Misplacement of the Right Leg Cable

This error should not occur but it does occur nevertheless. It produces a "far field" signal when one of the bipolar leads (I, II, or III) records the signal between the left and right legs. The lead appears to have no signal except for a tiny deflection representing the QRS complex. There are usually no discernible P waves or T waves. RL–RA cable reversal is shown here.

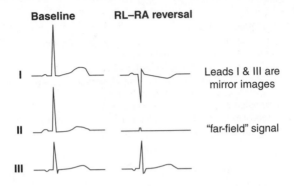

Baseline **RL–RA reversal**

I   Leads I & III are mirror images

II   "far-field" signal

III

Early Repolarization Normal Variant ST–T Abnormality

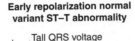

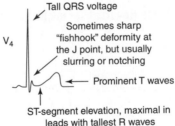

Early repolarization normal variant ST–T abnormality

Tall QRS voltage

Sometimes sharp "fishhook" deformity at the J point, but usually slurring or notching

V₄

Prominent T waves

ST-segment elevation, maximal in leads with tallest R waves

Hypothermia

Hypothermia is usually characterized on the ECG by a slow rate, a long QT, and muscle tremor artifact. An Osborn wave is typically present.

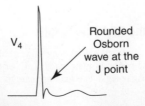

V₄

Rounded Osborn wave at the J point

Acute Pericarditis: Stage I (With PR-Segment Abnormalities)

There is usually widespread ST-segment elevation with concomitant PR-segment depression in the same leads. The PR segment in aVR protrudes above the baseline like a knuckle, reflecting atrial injury.

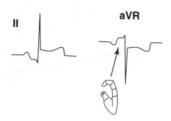

Differentiating Pericarditis From Early Repolarization

Only lead V_6 is used. If the indicated amplitude ratio A/B is ≥25%, suspect pericarditis (shown on left side). If A/B <25%, suspect early repolarization (shown on right side).

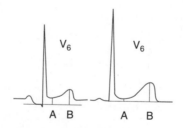

Wolff-Parkinson-White Pattern

The WPW pattern is most commonly manifest as an absent PR segment and initial slurring of the QRS complex in any lead. The lead with the best sensitivity is V_4.

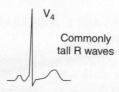

Commonly
tall R waves

A. Left Lateral Accessory Pathway: This typical WPW pattern mimics lateral or posterior myocardial infarction.

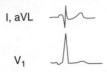

B. Posteroseptal Accessory Pathway: This typical WPW pattern mimics inferoposterior myocardial infarction.

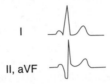

COPD Pattern, Lead II

The P-wave amplitude in the inferior leads is equal to that of the QRS complexes.

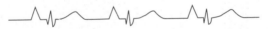

Prominent P waves with low QRS voltage

II. BASIC ECHOCARDIOGRAPHY

Over the last 30 years, echocardiography has arguably transformed cardiology more dramatically than any diagnostic test since the development of the electrocardiogram. With echocardiography, direct visualization of cardiac structures such as the atria, ventricles, valves, great vessels, and pericardium became possible. With the additional application of Doppler principles, besides structural information, echocardiography can now accurately estimate intracardiac blood flow and pressures.

PHYSICAL PRINCIPLES AND STANDARD VIEWS OF ECHOCARDIOGRAPHY

In echocardiography, low-intensity, high-frequency signals are produced and, since different tissues have different reflective properties, analysis of the return signals can be collated into a real-time image that can be evaluated by the clinician (Figure 7–6). In addition to providing a two-dimensional image of the heart, application of Doppler principles (named in honor of Christian Johann Doppler, who originally described these principles more than 150 years ago) provides additional information on blood flow. If a sound source is stationary, the wavelength and frequency of the reflected sound are constant, but if the sound source is moving, the wavelength and frequency change. The best everyday example is a siren or train whistle that increases in pitch as it comes toward you and then decreases as it moves away. By evaluating the changes in frequency of the ultrasound sound signal, information on the motion of blood within the cardiac chambers can be obtained.

In transthoracic echocardiography, a hand-held probe that emits and receives the echocardiographic signals is used. Since bone does not allow efficient passage of signals, the heart is best visualized when the transducer is placed between the ribs. As shown in Figure 7–7, two general positions are used: the first, on the anterior chest along the left edge of the sternum

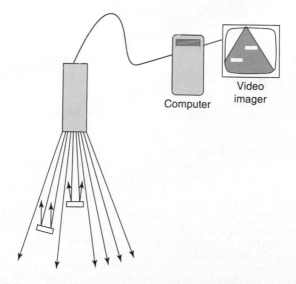

Figure 7–6. Schematic drawing of how echocardiographic images are obtained. A transducer emits sound signals in a pie-slice–shaped pattern. Different types of tissues reflect the signal with varying intensities (eg, blood allows complete transmission of the signal, calcified tissues reflect almost all of the signal, and myocardium has an intermediate value), and the return signal is processed and then displayed on a monitor. (*Adapted, with permission, from Kusumoto FM.* Cardiovascular Pathophysiology. *Hayes Barton Press, 2004.*)

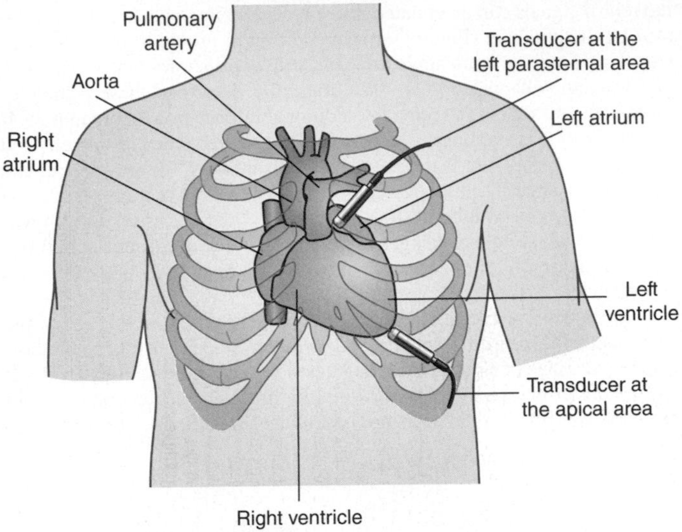

Figure 7–7. For transthoracic echocardiography, two standard transducer positions or windows are used. In the left parasternal view, the transducer is placed just to the left of the sternum in the third or fourth interspace, depending on which interspace provides the best view. In the apical view, the transducer is placed on the anterior left chest below the nipple at the point where the heart can best be palpated (apical impulse). (*Adapted, with permission, from Kusumoto FM.* Cardiovascular Pathophysiology. *Hayes Barton Press, 2004.*)

(left parasternal view) and the second, lower and more laterally just below the left nipple (called the apical view because when correctly aligned the ventricular apex will be the first cardiac structure visualized). The two views are complementary, since they provide roughly perpendicular imaging planes of the heart.

Figure 7–8 illustrates how a transthoracic echocardiographic image is acquired from the apical position. The probe emits the signal in a pie-slice–shaped plane that is directed to the heart. If the plane is oriented horizontally, the left- and right-sided chambers will be imaged. This view is called the four-chamber view because all four cardiac chambers are observed in the image. The plane can also be oriented vertically (Figure 7–9). In this case, the plane "cuts" the anterior wall and the inferior wall. This view is often called a two-chamber view because the left atrium and the left ventricle are imaged. The right atrium and the right ventricle are no longer in the imaging plane, so they are not seen. Similarly, from the parasternal position, the imaging plane can be oriented to encompass the apex (called

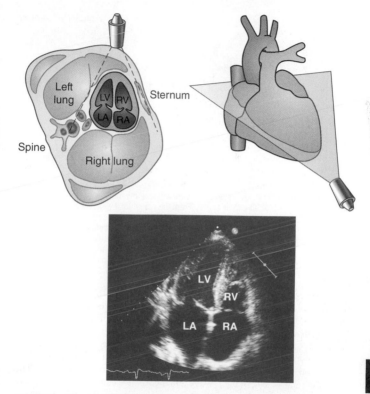

Figure 7–8. Schematic drawing showing the acquisition of a four-chamber view. The transducer is oriented horizontally from the apical position (top right), the imaging plane encompasses all four chambers of the heart (top left) and can be displayed as an echocardiographic image (bottom). ***LA*** = left atrium; ***LV*** = left ventricle; ***RA*** = right atrium; ***RV*** = right ventricle. (Adapted, with permission, from Kusumoto FM. Cardiovascular Pathophysiology. Hayes Barton Press, 2004.)

the parasternal long-axis view because it follows the axis formed by the mitral valve and the left ventricular apex) or perpendicularly to "cut" the heart like a loaf of bread (short-axis view). In the short-axis view, the left ventricle looks like a doughnut.

An extensive discussion of Doppler flows within the heart is beyond the scope of this introduction to echocardiography, but an example is shown in Figure 7–10. In this example, flow at the mitral valve is evaluated and displayed relative to time. The mitral valve is open only during diastole, so

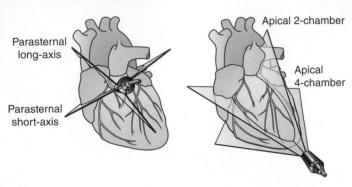

Figure 7–9. From either the parasternal or apical window, the transducer can be oriented with the imaging plane at 90-degree angles. From the parasternal view, the plane can be oriented to simultaneously evaluate the left atrium and the left ventricle (the parasternal long-axis view) or to "cut" the heart like a loaf of bread (the short-axis view). From the apical position, the plane can be horizontal and image all four cardiac chambers simultaneously (also called the four-chamber view) or can be vertical and image only the left ventricle and the left atrium (also called the two-chamber view). (*Used, with permission, from Armstrong WF, Ryan T.* Feigenbaum's Echocardiography, *7th edition. Lea & Febiger, 2009.*)

no signal is recorded during systole. During diastole, mitral flow has two peaks. The first peak is called the E wave (for early filling) and is due to the first rush of blood from the atrium into the left ventricle. (Remember that the left atrium was filling but not emptying during systole.) A second surge of blood flow into the left ventricle is due to left atrial contraction. The second peak is called the A wave because it is due to atrial contraction. The shape and relative size of the E wave and the A wave can be used to evaluate the filling properties of the left ventricle and estimate left atrial pressure.

Normally, the E wave is larger than the A wave, but patients with non-compliant left ventricles and higher left atrial pressures who depend on left atrial filling often have a smaller E wave and a larger A wave. Although only Doppler flow across the mitral valve is described here, it is important to remember that Doppler can be used to evaluate flow across any of the cardiac valves.

VENTRICULAR ANATOMY AND FUNCTION

Transthoracic echocardiography is extremely useful for evaluating left ventricular geometry and function. Figure 7–11 shows parasternal short axis and four-chamber views during systole and diastole in a normal heart. During systole, the left ventricle becomes smaller and the walls thicken. Comparison of systole and diastole provides a visual estimate of overall

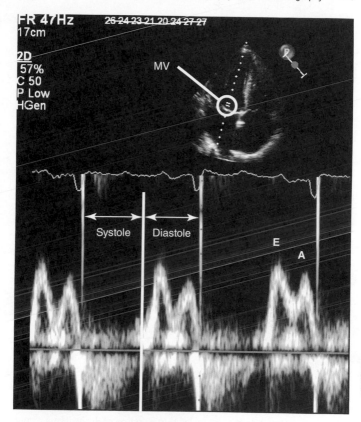

Figure 7–10. Doppler display of normal mitral inflow. During systole, the mitral valve (MV) is closed so that while the left atrium continues to fill from pulmonary venous flow, no blood flows into the left ventricle. During diastole, the mitral valve opens and there is a sudden surge of blood flow into the left ventricle producing the E wave. Filling of the left ventricle slows until left atrial contraction leads to second surge of blood flow and produces an A wave. (*By permission of Mayo Foundation for Medical Education and Research.*)

left ventricular function and also can identify any regional wall motion abnormalities that may be due to coronary artery disease. Overall cardiac function is usually expressed as the ejection fraction—ie, the portion of blood pumped by the left ventricle with each heartbeat. Although methods for quantifying the ejection fraction have been developed, most laboratories estimate the ejection fraction visually by examining the left ventricle in different projections.

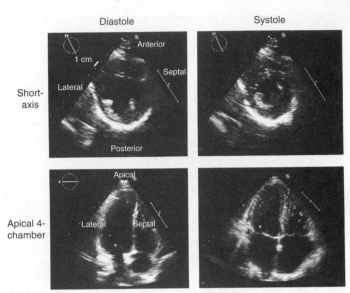

Diastole   Systole

Short-axis

Apical 4-chamber

Figure 7–11. Short-axis and apical four-chamber views during systole and diastole in a patient with a normal heart. During systole, the left ventricular cavity shrinks and the left ventricular walls thicken. The four-chamber view during systole shows that the mitral valve (*) is closed and during diastole the mitral valve is open. All echocardiographic displays show 1-cm marks to the side of the image to allow the clinician to estimate ventricular size. (*By permission of Mayo Foundation for Medical Education and Research.*)

In the United States, abnormal left ventricular function is most frequently due to a myocardial infarction from coronary artery disease. In myocardial infarction, reduction in blood flow leads to a portion of the heart not receiving enough blood supply, and this in turn leads to decreased muscle function. A regional wall motion abnormality develops, which can be identified as a region of the left ventricle that does not contract and thicken normally.

In some cases, myocardial infarction can lead to a left ventricular aneurysm. Figure 7–12 shows a two-chamber view of a patient with a very large ventricular aneurysm of the inferior wall due to a prior inferior myocardial infarction.

When left ventricular structure or function is abnormal, the term **cardiomyopathy** is usually used. As previously mentioned, myocardial infarction due to coronary artery disease is the most common cause of reduced left ventricular function in the US, and this condition is specifically described as an ischemic cardiomyopathy. In some cases, reduced left ventricular function is due to causes other than coronary artery disease, such as a viral

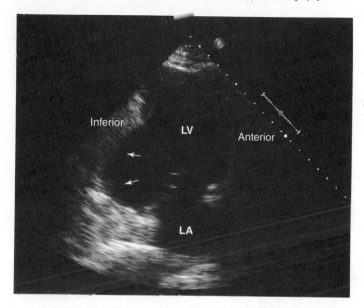

Figure 7–12. A two-chamber view in a patient with an inferior wall left ventricular aneurysm. To obtain a two-chamber view, the imaging plane is vertically oriented (Figure 7–9) so that the anterior wall and inferior wall of the left ventricle are both imaged. The right-sided chambers are not seen because they are out of the imaging plane. In this patient, a prior inferior wall myocardial infarction led to the development of a left ventricular aneurysm (*arrows*). In an aneurysm, development of scar tissue leads to a bulging region in the left ventricle that does not contract. **LA** = *left atrium;* **LV** = *left ventricle.* (*By permission of Mayo Foundation for Medical Education and Research.*)

infection or drug toxicity, although most often no specific cause can be identified (this condition is often called **idiopathic dilated cardiomyopathy**). When the heart is enlarged and has reduced function and the patient has no evidence of coronary artery disease, the term **nonischemic cardiomyopathy** is often used. In advanced cases of nonischemic cardiomyopathy, the left ventricle is often enlarged and has a more spherical shape (Figure 7–13).

In hypertrophic cardiomyopathy, a genetic abnormality (usually involving one of the components of the sarcomere) leads to abnormal thickening of the left ventricle (Figure 7–14). Although the ejection fraction is usually normal in patients with hypertrophic cardiomyopathy, abnormal filling of the left ventricle can lead to fluid accumulation in the lungs and shortness of breath. Normally, the left ventricle is less than 1 cm thick. As shown in Figure 7–14, echocardiography is extremely useful for identifying patients with abnormally thick ventricular walls.

Short-axis

4-Chamber

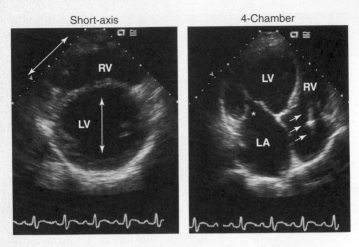

Figure 7–13. Short-axis and four-chamber views of a patient with a nonischemic cardio-myopathy are shown. Double-headed arrows in the short-axis view emphasize the enlarged left ventricular chamber size (almost 6 cm in diameter) and in the four-chamber view, the spherical shape of the left ventricle (LV) can be observed (compare with Figure 7–11). Also in the four-chamber view, a defibrillator lead can be observed in the right ventricle (RV; *arrows*). The (*) marks the mitral valve. **LA** = *left atrium*. (*By permission of Mayo Foundation for Medical Education and Research.*)

4-Chamber

Parasternal long-axis

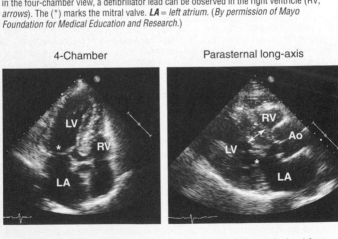

Figure 7–14. An echocardiogram (four-chamber and parasternal long-axis views) from a patient with a hypertrophic cardiomyopathy. The interventricular septum separating the left ventricle (LV) and right ventricle (RV) is abnormally thick (*double headed arrow*). The (*) marks the mitral valve. **LA** = *left atrium;* **Ao** = *aorta.* (*By permission of Mayo Foundation for Medical Education and Research.*)

The echocardiogram also can be used to identify a pericardial effusion, a condition in which fluid accumulates in the pericardial space (Figure 7–15). If the effusion is large enough or accumulates rapidly, the elevated intrapericardial pressure can prevent normal filling of the left and right ventricles. This condition is called **pericardial tamponade**. Even if the ventricles contract normally, inadequate filling can lead to extreme reduction in the amount of blood expelled by the ventricles with each heartbeat (stroke volume), which can lead to profound hypotension. Echocardiography has emerged as the best test for rapidly determining whether a significant pericardial effusion is present.

VALVULAR ANATOMY AND FUNCTION

The echocardiogram is an excellent diagnostic test to evaluate the valves of the heart. In general, abnormal valve function can be classified as **stenosis,** in which forward flow of blood through the valve is restricted, or **regurgitation,** in which blood "leaks backward" because the valve leaflets do not

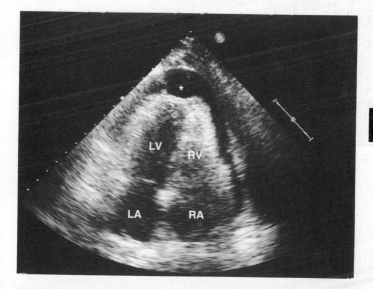

Figure 7–15. A four-chamber view in a patient with a pericardial effusion. The pericardial effusion (*) is identified as a dark echo-free area surrounding the heart due to abnormal fluid accumulation. *LA* = left atrium; *LV* = left ventricle; *RA* = right atrium; *RV* = right ventricle. (*By permission of Mayo Foundation for Medical Education and Research.*)

come together and close normally. Generally, the severity of valve stenosis or regurgitation is assessed by echocardiography Doppler evaluation. Valvular regurgitation produces a high-velocity jet that can be identified within the chamber into which the blood leaks back. For example, **mitral regurgitation** can be identified by a high-velocity jet within the left atrium and the area of the high-velocity jet correlates roughly with the severity of the valvular abnormality.

Aortic Valve

Narrowing of the aortic valve is one of the most common valvular abnormalities encountered clinically. Normally, the aortic valve has three leaflets, but in some patients only two leaflets are present. During childhood and early adulthood, the valve functions normally, but a harsh murmur due to turbulent blood flow during ventricular contraction (systole) is often heard. However, in the fifth or sixth decade of life, progressive turbulent flow often leads to thickening of the aortic valve leaflets, stenosis of the aortic valve, and reduction in stroke volume.

Aortic stenosis can also develop in patients with trileaflet aortic valves. In this case, progressive calcification of the leaflets presents as aortic stenosis in the seventh or eighth decade. On echocardiography, the aortic valve appears "bright" or echogenic as a result of calcium deposition that almost completely reflects the ultrasound signal (Figure 7–16). Aortic stenosis produces a high-velocity jet across the aortic valve into the

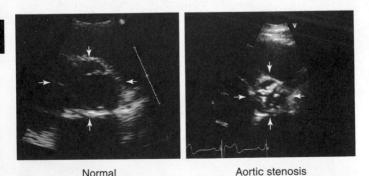

Normal   Aortic stenosis

Figure 7–16. Echocardiographic images of a normal aortic valve and an aortic valve associated with severe aortic stenosis. Although both aortic valves have three leaflets, in the patient with aortic stenosis the leaflets are calcified. In both examples, the aortic valve is outlined by the four arrows. (*By permission of Mayo Foundation for Medical Education and Research.*)

aorta (caused by blood being forcefully expelled across the narrow opening), which can be identified by Doppler echocardiography. The velocity of the jet can be used to estimate the severity of the gradient; the normal velocity of blood at the aortic valve is 1 m/s, but in severe aortic stenosis, velocities of 4–5 m/s can be measured at the aortic valve. In general, the higher the velocity recorded across the aortic valve, the larger the pressure gradient between the left ventricle and the aorta and the more severe the aortic stenosis.

If the aortic valve does not close normally, blood from the aorta can leak back into the left ventricle. This condition is called **aortic regurgitation,** in which blood flows backward from the aorta into the left ventricle. Aortic regurgitation can develop with infection of the aortic valve (endocarditis), in the presence of a bicuspid aortic valve, or with any process that causes enlargement of the aortic root (and consequent enlargement of the ring that provides the support for the valve leaflets). The turbulent flow from aortic regurgitation occurs in diastole, and consequently a murmur is heard during diastole. Doppler echocardiography is useful for evaluating the severity of aortic regurgitation. Aortic regurgitation is recorded as a turbulent jet within the left ventricle, emanating from the aortic valve during diastole (Figure 7–17).

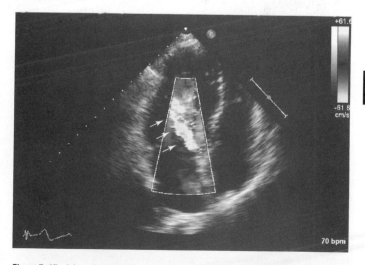

Figure 7–17. A four-chamber view of a patient with severe aortic regurgitation. During diastole, a large turbulent jet is present (*arrows*), emanating from the aortic valve. (*By permission of Mayo Foundation for Medical Education and Research.*)

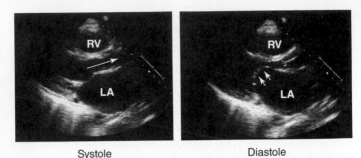

Systole   Diastole

Figure 7–18. A parasternal long-axis view of a patient with severe mitral stenosis due to rheumatic heart disease. During systole, the mitral valve is closed and blood is expelled through the open aortic valve (*single arrow*). During diastole, opening of the mitral valve is restricted, and a characteristic bowing of the mitral valve (*arrows*) is observed. **LA** = *left atrium;* **RV** = *right ventricle.* (*By permission of Mayo Foundation for Medical Education and Research.*)

Mitral Valve

The mitral valve can be easily evaluated by transthoracic echocardiography. Abnormal function can be due to either mitral stenosis or mitral regurgitation.

Mitral stenosis is almost always due to rheumatic heart disease related to untreated streptococcal infections (see Chapter 5) and can be identified by restricted opening of the mitral valve leaflets on echocardiography (Figure 7–18). Of all the valvular lesions, mitral stenosis is the least commonly encountered in developed countries but still remains a common problem in many parts of the developing world.

Mitral regurgitation is much more commonly observed than mitral stenosis and can be due to severe mitral valve prolapse, endocarditis of the mitral valve, myocardial ischemia, or rheumatic valvular disease. Like aortic regurgitation, Doppler techniques are used to identify the high-velocity turbulent jet. However, in mitral regurgitation, the high-velocity jet is observed in the left atrium, emanates from the mitral valve, and occurs during ventricular contraction (systole). An example of an echocardiogram from a patient with mitral regurgitation is shown in Figure 7–19. A wide-necked jet that encompasses a larger portion of the left atrium is characteristic of severe mitral regurgitation.

Tricuspid Valve

In tricuspid regurgitation, a regurgitant jet is present in the right atrium, emanating from the tricuspid valve (Figure 7–20). Like mitral regurgitation,

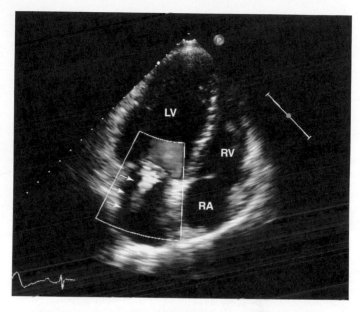

Figure 7–19. A four-chamber view of a patient with mitral regurgitation. A high-velocity jet is observed in the left atrium (*arrows*), emanating from the mitral valve. A wide-necked jet that fills a large portion of the left atrium suggests severe mitral regurgitation. ***LV*** = left ventricle; ***RA*** = right atrium; ***RV*** = right ventricle. (*By permission of Mayo Foundation for Medical Education and Research.*)

the jet is observed during systole. Doppler evaluation of the tricuspid valve is frequently used to assess right-sided cardiac pressures. The relative pressure difference between two chambers can be estimated by using a simplified formula of the Bernoulli equation:

$$\Delta P = 4V^2$$

where ΔP is the pressure difference in mm Hg and V is the velocity between two cardiac chambers in m/s. Figure 7–21 shows a Doppler signal from the tricuspid valve in a patient with severe tricuspid regurgitation. Using the simplified Bernoulli equation, the difference between right atrial pressure and right ventricular pressure reaches 56 mm Hg during systole.

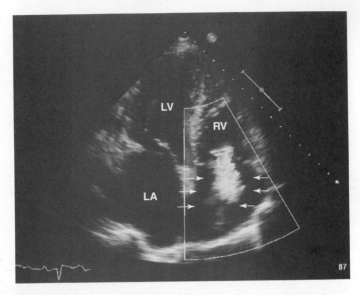

Figure 7–20. A four-chamber view of a patient with severe tricuspid regurgitation. The high-velocity jet (*arrows*) emanates from the tricuspid valve. *LA* = left atrium; *LV* = left ventricle; *RV* = right ventricle. (*By permission of Mayo Foundation for Medical Education and Research.*)

Since normal right ventricular peak systolic pressure ranges from 15 to 30 mm Hg, the presence of elevated right-sided cardiac pressure can thus be readily identified.

TRANSESOPHAGEAL ECHOCARDIOGRAPHY AND INTRACARDIAC ECHOCARDIOGRAPHY

In transthoracic echocardiography, the ultrasound transducers are mounted on a hand-held probe that is manipulated on the surface of the chest to obtain the desired images. In transesophageal echocardiography, the transducer can be placed on a probe designed to enter the esophagus. In intracardiac echocardiography, the transducer can be placed on a catheter designed to enter the heart itself via one of the central veins (usually the femoral vein) and advanced via the inferior vena cava into the heart. Imaging from a transducer located adjacent to the heart (transesophageal echocardiography) or from inside the heart (intracardiac echocardiography) produces images with exquisite detail and resolution.

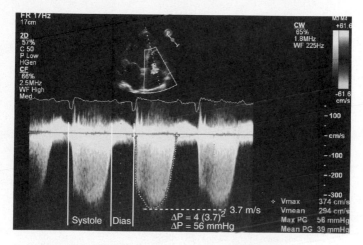

Figure 7–21. A Doppler signal due to the severe tricuspid regurgitation shown in Figure 7–20. In tricuspid regurgitation, the high-velocity flow is recorded during systole and not in diastole (Dias). Since the jet of tricuspid regurgitation is flowing away from the transducer, a negative signal is recorded (contrast this to the normal mitral inflow signal shown in Figure 7–10). The simplified Bernoulli equation can be used to estimate the pressure difference between the right ventricle and right atrium from the peak velocity recorded from the tricuspid regurgitation signal (3.74 m/s or 374 cm/s).

REFERENCES

Bernath P, Kusumoto FM. *ECG Interpretation for Everyone: An On-The-Spot Guide.* Wiley-Blackwell, in press.

Colucci RA et al. Common types of supraventricular tachycardia: diagnosis and management. Am Fam Physician 2010;82:942. [PMID: 20949888]

Couderc JP et al. Short and long QT syndromes: does QT length really matter? J Electrocardiol 2010;43:396. [PMID: 20728018]

Dhar S et al. Current concepts and management strategies in atrial flutter. South Med J 2009;102:917. [PMID: 19668035]

Escárcega RO et al. The Brugada syndrome. Acta Cardiol 2009;64:795. [PMID: 20128157]

Estes EH Jr et al. The electrocardiogram in left ventricular hypertrophy: past and future. J Electrocardiol 2009;42:589. [PMID: 19643433]

Haqqani HM et al. Using the 12-lead ECG to localize the origin of atrial and ventricular tachycardias: part 2—ventricular tachycardia. J Cardiovasc Electrophysiol 2009;20:825. [PMID: 19302478]

Hudaverdi M et al. Echocardiography for the clinician: a practical update. Intern Med J 2010;40:476. [PMID: 20059600]

Johnson JN et al. QTc: how long is too long? Br J Sports Med 2009;43:657. [PMID: 19734499]

Kumar A et al. Acute coronary syndromes: diagnosis and management, part I. Mayo Clin Proc 2009;84:917. [PMID: 19797781]

Kumar A et al. Acute coronary syndromes: diagnosis and management, part II. Mayo Clin Proc 2009;84:1021. [PMID: 19880693]

Kusumoto FM. *ECG Interpretation: From Pathophysiology to Clinical Application.* Springer Science, 2009.

Linton NW et al. Narrow complex (supraventricular) tachycardias. Postgrad Med J 2009;85:546. [PMID: 19789194]

Medi C et al. Supraventricular tachycardia. Med J Aust 2009;190:255. [PMID: 19296791]

Nikus K et al. Electrocardiographic classification of acute coronary syndromes: a review by a committee of the International Society for Holter and Non-Invasive Electrocardiology. J Electrocardiol 2010;43:91. [PMID: 19913800]

Oh JE, Seward JB, Tajik AJ. *The Echo Manual*, 3rd ed. Wolters Kluwer, 2007.

Sawhney NS et al. Diagnosis and management of typical atrial flutter. Cardiol Clin 2009;27:55. [PMID: 19111764]

Scirica BM. Acute coronary syndrome: emerging tools for diagnosis and risk assessment. J Am Coll Cardiol 2010;55:1403. [PMID: 20359589]

Srivathsan K et al. Ventricular tachycardia and ventricular fibrillation. Expert Rev Cardiovasc Ther 2009;7:801. [PMID: 19589116]

St John Sutton MG et al. Assessment of left ventricular systolic function by echocardiography. Heart Fail Clin 2009;5:177. [PMID: 19249687]

Thavendiranathan P et al. Does this patient with palpitations have a cardiac arrhythmia? JAMA 2009;302:2135. [PMID: 19920238]

8

Diagnostic Tests in Differential Diagnosis

Stephen J. McPhee, MD, Chuanyi Mark Lu, MD, Diana Nicoll, MD, PhD, MPA, and Michael Pignone, MD, MPH

HOW TO USE THIS SECTION

This section shows how diagnostic tests can be used in differential diagnosis and difficult diagnostic challenges. Material is presented in tabular format, and contents are listed in alphabetical order by disease topic.

Abbreviations used throughout this section include the following:

N	=	Normal
Abn	=	Abnormal
Pos	=	Positive
Neg	=	Negative
↑	=	Increased or high
↓	=	Decreased or low
Occ	=	Occasional

Contents (Tables)   *Pages*

TABLE 8-1. ACID–BASE DISTURBANCE: LABORATORY CHARACTERISTICS OF PRIMARY OR SINGLE ACID–BASE DISTURBANCE.

Disturbance	Acute Primary Change	Partial Compensatory Response	Arterial pH	Serum [K⁺] (meq/L)	Unmeasured Anions (Anion Gap[1])	Clinical Features
Normal	None	None	7.35–7.45	3.5–5.0	12–18	None
Respiratory acidosis	Pco₂ ↑ (CO₂ retention)	↑ HCO₃⁻	↓	↑	N	Dyspnea, polypnea, respiratory outflow obstruction, ↑ anterior-posterior chest diameter, rales, wheezes. In severe cases, stupor, disorientation, coma.
Respiratory alkalosis	Pco₂ ↓ (CO₂ depletion)	↓ HCO₃⁻	↑	↓	N or ↓	Anxiety, occasional complaint of breathlessness, frequent sighing, lungs usually clear to examination, positive Chvostek and Trousseau signs.
Metabolic acidosis	HCO₃⁻ depletion	↓ Pco₂	↓	↑ or ↓	N or ↑	Weakness, air hunger, Kussmaul respiration, dry skin and mucous membranes, poor skin turgor. In severe cases, coma, hypotension, death.
Metabolic alkalosis	HCO₃⁻ retention	↑ Pco₂	↑	↓	N	Weakness, positive Chvostek and Trousseau signs, hyporeflexia.

[1]Anion gap = $([Na^+] + [K^+]) - (HCO_3^- + [Cl^-]) = 12–18$ meq/L normally.
Reproduced, with permission, from Stobo JD et al (editors): The Principles and Practice of Medicine, 23rd ed. Originally published by Appleton & Lange. Copyright © 1996 by Appleton & Lange.

TABLE 8–2. ANEMIA: DIAGNOSIS OF COMMON ANEMIAS BASED ON RED CELL INDICES.

Type of Anemia	MCV (fL)	MCHC (g/dL)	Common Causes	Common Laboratory Abnormalities	Other Clinical Findings
Microcytic, hypochromic	<80	<32	Iron deficiency	Hypochromic red cells, elliptocytes, low reticulocyte count, low serum ferritin, low serum and bone marrow iron, high TIBC, high serum/plasma soluble transferrin receptor (sTfR).	Mucositis, brittle nails, bleeding (eg, positive fecal occult blood), esophageal webs, pica.
		Variable, but usually <32	Thalassemias	Abnormal red cell morphology, normal to high RBC count, elevated reticulocyte count, normal serum iron parameters, abnormal hemoglobin electrophoresis, high hemoglobin A_2 in β-thalassemia minor.	Asian, African, or Mediterranean descent. Splenomegaly, growth failure, bony deformities.
		<32	Chronic lead poisoning	Basophilic stippling of RBCs, elevated blood lead and free erythrocyte protoporphyrin levels.	Peripheral neuropathy (eg, wrist drop), abdominal pain, learning disorders (in children), headache, history of exposure to lead.
		Variable, but usually < 32	Sideroblastic anemia	High serum iron, high transferrin saturation, erythroid hyperplasia with ring sideroblasts in bone marrow.	Dimorphic red cell population with hypochromic red cells on blood smear.

(continued)

TABLE 8–2. ANEMIA: DIAGNOSIS OF COMMON ANEMIAS BASED ON RED CELL INDICES. *(CONTINUED)*

Type of Anemia	MCV (fL)	MCHC (g/dL)	Common Causes	Common Laboratory Abnormalities	Other Clinical Findings
Normocytic, normochromic	80–100	32–36	Acute blood loss	Fecal occult blood test positive if GI bleeding is the underlying cause. High reticulocyte count, thrombocytosis (variable).	Recent blood loss.
		32–36	Hemolysis	Haptoglobin low or absent, high reticulocyte count, high indirect bilirubin, high serum LDH, spherocytes, schistocytes, or "bite" cells on smear.	Hemoglobinuria, splenomegaly.
		32–36	Chronic disease[1]	Low serum iron, TIBC low or low normal, normal s TfR, normal or high ferritin, low reticulocyte count, normal or high bone marrow iron stores with rare or no sideroblasts.	Depends on cause, typically chronic inflammatory conditions.

Macrocytic, normochromic	>10¹ [2]	32–36	Vitamin B₁₂ deficiency	Hypersegmented PMNs, macro-ovalocytes, neutropenia and/or thrombocytopenia, low serum vitamin B₁₂ levels, high serum/urine MMA, achlorhydria and high serum gastrin, and high serum LDH.	Peripheral neuropathy, glossitis, anorexia and diarrhea.
		32–36	Folate deficiency	Hypersegmented PMNs, macro-ovalocytes, neutropenia and/or thrombocytopenia, low serum and red cell folate levels, high homocysteine level.	Alcoholism, tropical sprue, malnutrition, antifolate agents (eg, trimethoprim-sulfamethoxazole, methotrexate, others).
		32–36	Liver disease	Decreased platelets; MCV usually <120 fL; normal serum vitamin B₁₂ and folate levels.	Signs of liver disease, alcohol abuse.
		Usually 32–36	Myelodysplastic syndrome	MCV usually <120 fL, low reticulocyte count, may have neutropenia and/or thrombocytopenia, pseudo-Pelgeroid neutrophils, unilineage or multilineage dysplasia in the marrow.	Chronic anemia with or without pancytopenia.
		32–36 or >36	Reticulocytosis	Marked (>15%) reticulocytosis.	Variable, including acute hemorrhage or hemolysis.

[1] May be microcytic, hypochromic.
[2] If MCV >120–130, vitamin B₁₂ or folate deficiency is likely.
MCV = mean corpuscular volume; **MMA** = methylmalonic acid; **PMN** = polymorphonuclear cell; **TIBC** = total iron-binding capacity, serum.

TABLE 8–3. MICROCYTIC ANEMIA: LABORATORY EVALUATION OF MICROCYTIC, HYPOCHROMIC ANEMIAS.

Diagnosis	MCV (fL)	Serum Iron (mcg/dL)	Iron-binding Capacity (mcg/dL)	Transferrin Saturation (%)	Serum Ferritin (mcg/L)	Free Erythrocyte Protoporphyrin (mcg/dL)	Basophilic Stippling	Bone Marrow Iron Stores
Normal	80–100	50–175	250–460	16–55	50–300	<35	Absent	Present
Iron deficiency anemia	↓	<30	↑	<16	<45[1]	↑	Absent	Absent
Anemia of chronic disease	N or ↓	↓	N or ↓	N or ↓	N or ↑	↑	Absent	Present
Thalassemia minor	↓	N	N	N	N	N	Usually present	Present

[1] Ferritin levels of 25–45 have a likelihood ratio of 2.0 for iron deficiency anemia.

Data from Stobo JD et al (editors). The Principles and Practice of Medicine, 23rd ed. Originally published by Appleton & Lange. Copyright © 1996 by Appleton & Lange.

TABLE 8–4. ARTHRITIS: EXAMINATION AND CLASSIFICATION OF SYNOVIAL (JOINT) FLUID.

Type of Joint Fluid	Volume (mL)	Clarity, Color	WBC (per mcL)	PMNs	Gram Stain and Culture	Fluid Glucose (mg/dL)	Differential Diagnosis	Comments
Normal	<3.5	Transparent, clear	<200	<25%	Neg	Equal to serum glucose		
Non-inflammatory (Group I)	Often >3.5	Transparent, yellow	<2000	<25%	Neg	Equal to serum glucose	Degenerative joint disease, trauma, avascular necrosis, osteochondritis dissecans, osteochondromatosis, neuropathic arthropathy, subsiding or early inflammation, hypertrophic osteoarthropathy, pigmented villonodular synovitis.	

(continued)

TABLE 8-4. ARTHRITIS: EXAMINATION AND CLASSIFICATION OF SYNOVIAL (JOINT) FLUID. (CONTINUED)

Type of Joint Fluid	Volume (mL)	Clarity, Color	WBC (per mcL)	PMNs	Gram Stain and Culture	Fluid Glucose (mg/dL)	Differential Diagnosis	Comments
Inflammatory (Group II)	Often >3.5	Translucent to opaque, yellow to opalescent	2000–75,000 (occasionally >75,000 but rarely >100,000)	≥50%	Neg	>25, but lower than serum glucose	Rheumatoid arthritis, acute crystal-induced synovitis (gout, pseudogout), reactive arthritis, ankylosing spondylitis, psoriatic arthritis, sarcoidosis, arthritis accompanying ulcerative colitis and Crohn disease, rheumatic fever, systemic lupus erythematosus, scleroderma; tuberculous, viral, or mycotic infections.	Crystals are diagnostic of gout or pseudogout: gout crystals (urate) are needle-shaped and show negative birefringence; pseudogout crystals (calcium pyrophosphate) are more rectangular and show positive birefringence when red compensator filter is used with polarized light microscopy. Phagocytic inclusions in PMNs suggest rheumatoid arthritis (RA cells).

Purulent (Group III)	Often >3.5	Opaque, yellow to green	>100,000	≥75%	Usually positive (gonococci seen in only about 25% of cases)	<25, much lower than serum glucose	Mostly pyogenic bacterial infections (eg, *Staphylococcus aureus*, *Neisseria gonorrhoeae*).	WBC count and % PMN lower with infections caused by organisms of low virulence (eg, *N. gonorrhoeae*) or if antibiotic therapy already started.
Hemorrhagic (Group IV)	Often >3.5	Cloudy, pink to red	Usually >2000; many RBCs.	<30%	Neg	Equal to serum glucose	Trauma with or without fracture, hemophilia or other hemorrhagic diathesis, neuropathic arthropathy, pigmented villonodular synovitis, synovioma, hemangioma and other benign neoplasms.	Fat globules strongly suggest intra-articular fracture

Modified, with permission, from McPhee SJ, Papadakis MA, Rabow MW (editors). Current Medical Diagnosis & Treatment 2012, 51st ed., McGraw-Hill, 2011.

TABLE 8–5. ASCITES: ASCITIC FLUID PROFILES IN VARIOUS DISEASE STATES.

Diagnosis	Appearance	Fluid Protein (g/dL)	Serum Albumin-Ascites Gradient (SAAG)	Fluid Glucose (mg/dL)	WBC and Differential (per mcL)	RBC (per mcL)	Gram Stain and Culture	Cytology	Comments
Normal	Clear	<3.0		Equal to plasma glucose	<250	Few or none	Neg	Neg	
HIGH SAAG									
Cirrhosis	Clear	<3.0	≥1.1	N	<250, MN	Few	Neg	Neg	Occasionally turbid, rarely bloody.
Congestive heart failure	Clear	<2.5	≥1.1	N	<250, MN	Few	Neg	Neg	
LOW SAAG									
Nephrotic syndrome	Clear	<2.5	<1.1	N	<250, MN	Few	Neg	Neg	
Bacterial peritonitis	Cloudy	>3.0	<1.1	<50 with perforated viscus	>500, PMN	Few	Pos	Neg	Blood cultures frequently positive.
Tuberculous peritonitis	Clear	>3.0	<1.1	<60	>500, MN	Few, occasionally many	Stain Pos in 25%; culture Pos in 65%	Neg	Occasionally chylous. Peritoneal biopsy positive in 65%.

Malignancy	Clear or bloody	>3.0	<1.1	<60	>500, MN, PMN	Many	Neg	Pos in 60–90%	Occasionally chylous. Peritoneal biopsy diagnostic.
Pancreatitis	Clear or bloody	>2.5	<1.1	N	>500, MN, PMN	Many	Neg	Neg	Occasionally chylous. Fluid amylase >1000 IU/L, sometimes >10,000 IU/L. Fluid amylase > serum amylase.
OTHER									
Chylous ascites	Turbid	Varies, often >2.5		N	Few	Few	Neg	Neg	Fluid TG >400 mg/dL (turbid). Fluid TG > serum TG.
Pseudomyxoma peritonei	Gelatinous	<2.5		N	<250	Few	Neg	Occ Pos	

*IU = international units; **MN** = mononuclear cells; **PMN** = polymorphonuclear cells; **SAAG** = serum-ascites albumin gradient; **TG** = triglycerides.*

TABLE 8–6. AUTOANTIBODIES: FREQUENCY (%) OF IN RHEUMATIC DISEASES.[1]

	ANA	Anti-dsDNA	Rheumatoid Factor	Anti-Sm	Anti-SS-A	Anti-SS-B	Anti-SCL-70	Anti-Centromere	Anti-Jo-1	ANCA
Rheumatoid arthritis	30–60	0–5	70	0	0–5	0–2	0	0	0	0
Systemic lupus erythematosus	95–100	60	20	10–25	15–20	5–20	0	0	0	0–1
Sjögren syndrome	95	0	75	0	65	65	0	0	0	0
Diffuse scleroderma	80–95	0	30	0	0	0	33	1	0	0
Limited scleroderma (CREST syndrome)	80–95	0	30	0	0	0	20	50	0	0
Polymyositis/dermatomyositis	80–95	0	33	0	0	0	0	0	20–30	0
Polyangiitis with granulomatosis	0–15	0	50	0	0	0	0	0	0	93–96[1]

[1]Frequency for generalized, active disease.
Anti-dsDNA = anti-double-stranded DNA antibody; **ANA** = antinuclear antibodies; **Anti-Sm** = anti-Smith antibody; anti-SCL-70, anti-scleroderma antibody; **ANCA** = antineutrophil cytoplasmic antibody; **CREST** = calcinosis cutis, Raynaud phenomenon, esophageal motility disorder, sclerodactyly, and telangiectasia.

TABLE 8–7. BLEEDING DISORDERS: LABORATORY EVALUATION.

Suspected Diagnosis	Platelet Count	PT	PTT	TT	Further Diagnostic Tests
Idiopathic thrombocytopenic purpura (ITP), drug effect, bone marrow suppression	↓	N	N	N	Platelet antibodies, bone marrow examination.
Disseminated intravascular coagulation (DIC)	↓	↑	↑	↑	Fibrinogen (functional), D-dimers.
Platelet function defect, salicylates, or uremia	N	N	N	N	Bleeding time or PFA-100 CT, platelet aggregation, blood urea nitrogen, creatinine.
von Willebrand disease	N	N	↑ or N	N	Bleeding time or PFA-100 CT, factor VIII assay, vWF antigen and activity, vWF multimer analysis.
Factor VII deficiency or inhibitor	N	↑	N	N	Factor VII assay (normal plasma should correct PT if no inhibitor is present).
Factor V, X, II, I deficiencies as in liver disease or with anticoagulants	N	↑	↑	N or ↑	Liver function tests.
Factor VIII (hemophilia), IX, or XI deficiencies or inhibitor	N	N	↑	N	Inhibitor screen (mixing study), individual factor assays, Bethesda assay.
Factor XIII deficiency	N	N	N	N	5M urea solubility test (screen test), factor XIII assay.
Increase in fibrinolytic activity	N	N	N	N	Euglobulin clot lysis time (screening test), α_2-antiplasmin, plasminogen activator inhibitor-1 (PAI-1), renal function test (eg, eGFR)

Note: In approaching patients with bleeding disorders, try to distinguish clinically between platelet disorders (eg, patient has petechiae, bruises, gingival bleeding, nosebleeds) and factor deficiency states (eg, patient has deep tissue hematoma and/or hemarthrosis).
eGFR = estimated glomerular filtration rate; **PFA-100 CT** = platelet function analyzer-100 closure time; **PT** = prothrombin time; **PTT** = activated partial thromboplastin time; **TT** = thrombin time.
Modified, with permission, from Stobo JD et al. (editors): The Principles and Practice of Medicine, 23rd ed. Originally published by Appleton & Lange. Copyright © 1996 by Appleton & Lange.

TABLE 8–8. CEREBROSPINAL FLUID (CSF): CSF PROFILES IN CENTRAL NERVOUS SYSTEM DISEASES.

Diagnosis	Appearance	Opening Pressure (mm H$_2$O)	RBC (per mcL)	WBC and Diff (per mcL)	CSF Glucose (mg/dL)	CSF Protein (mg/dL)	Smears	Culture	Comments
Normal	Clear, colorless	70–200	0	≤5 MN, 0 PMN	45–85	15–45	Neg	Neg	
Bacterial meningitis	Cloudy	↑↑↑	0	200–20,000, mostly PMN	<45	>50	Gram stain Pos	Pos	
Tuberculous meningitis	N or cloudy	↑↑↑	0	100–1000, mostly MN	<45	>50	AFB stain Pos	±|	PMN predominance may be seen early in course.
Fungal meningitis	N or cloudy	N or ↑	0	100–1000, mostly MN	<45	>50		±|	Counterimmunoelectrophoresis or latex agglutination may be diagnostic. CSF and serum cryptococcal antigen positive in cryptococcal meningitis.
Viral (aseptic) meningitis	N	N or ↑	0	100–1000, mostly MN	45–85	N or ↑	Neg	Neg	RBC count may be elevated in herpes simplex encephalitis. Glucose may be decreased in herpes simplex or mumps infections. Viral cultures may be helpful.

Parasitic meningitis	N or cloudy	N or ↑	0	100–1000, mostly MN, E	<45	N or ↑	Amebae may be seen on wet smear	±	
Carcinomatous meningitis	N or cloudy	N or ↑	0	N or 100–1000, mostly MN	<45	N or ↑	Cytology Pos	Neg	
Cerebral lupus erythematosus	N	N or ↑	0	N or ↑, mostly MN	N	N or ↑	Neg	Neg	
Subarachnoid hemorrhage	Pink-red, supernatant yellow	↑	↑ crenated or fresh	N or 100–1000, mostly PMN	N or ↓	N or ↑	Neg	Neg	Blood in all tubes equally. Pleocytosis and low glucose sometimes seen several days after subarachnoid hemorrhage, reflecting chemical meningitis caused by subarachnoid blood.
"Traumatic" tap	Bloody, supernatant clear	N	↑↑↑ fresh	↑	N	↑	Neg	Neg	Most blood in tube #1; least blood in tube #4.

(continued)

TABLE 8–8. CEREBROSPINAL FLUID (CSF): CSF PROFILES IN CENTRAL NERVOUS SYSTEM DISEASES. (CONTINUED)

Diagnosis	Appearance	Opening Pressure (mm H$_2$O)	RBC (per mcL)	WBC and Diff (per mcL)	CSF Glucose (mg/dL)	CSF Protein (mg/dL)	Smears	Culture	Comments
Spirochetal, early, acute syphilitic meningitis	Clear to turbid	↑	0	N or ↑	15–75	>50	Neg	Neg	PMN may predominate early. Positive serum RPR or VDRL. CSF VDRL insensitive. If clinical suspicion is high, institute treatment despite negative CSF VDRL.
Late CNS syphilis	Clear	Usually N	0	N or ↑	N	N or ↑	Neg	Neg	CSF VDRL insensitive.
"Neighborhood" meningeal reaction	Clear or turbid, often xanthochromic	Variable, usually N	Variable	↑	N	N or ↑	Neg	Usually Neg	May occur in mastoiditis, brain abscess, sinusitis, septic thrombophlebitis, brain tumor, intrathecal drug therapy.
Hepatic encephalopathy	N	N	0	N or ↑	N	N	Neg	Neg	CSF glutamine >15 mg/dL.
Uremia	N	Usually ↑	0	N or ↑	N or ↑	N or ↑	Neg	Neg	
Diabetic coma	N	Low	0	N or ↑	↑	N	Neg	Neg	

CNS = central nervous system; **E** = eosinophils; **MN** = mononuclear cells (lymphocytes or monocytes); **PMN** = polymorphonuclear cells; **WBC** = white

TABLE 8–9. CIRRHOSIS: CHILD-TURCOTTE-PUGH STAGES AND MODEL FOR END-STAGE LIVER DISEASE (MELD) SCORING SYSTEM.

Numerical Score Child-Turcotte-Pugh scoring system			
Parameter	1	2	3
Ascites	None	Slight	Moderate to severe
Encephalopathy	None	Slight to moderate	Moderate to severe
Bilirubin, mg/dL (mcmol/L)	<2.0 (<34.2)	2–3 (34.2–51.3)	>3.0 (>51.3)
Albumin, g/dL (g/L)	>3.5 (>35)	2.8–3.5 (28–35)	<2.8 (<28)
Prothrombin time (seconds increased)	1–3	4–6	>6.0
	Total Numerical Score and Corresponding Child Class Score Class 5–6 A 7–9 B 10–15 C		

MELD scoring system

MELD = $11.2 \times \log_e (INR) + 3.78 \times \log_e (\text{bilirubin [mg/dL]}) + 9.57 \times \log_e (\text{creatinine [mg/dL]}) + 6.43$. (Range 6–40).

INR = *international normalized ratio.*

Reproduced with permission, from McPhee SJ, Papadakis MA, Rabow MW (editors). Current Medical Diagnosis & Treatment 2012. 51st ed. McGraw-Hill Companies, Inc., 2012

TABLE 8–10. GENETIC DISEASES: MOLECULAR DIAGNOSTIC TESTING.

Test/Range/Collection	Physiologic Basis	Interpretation	Comments
Breast cancer BRCA1 and BRCA2 mutations Blood Lavender $$$$	Mutations in two genes, BRCA1 and BRCA2, are the major cause of familial early-onset breast cancer. A mutation in either gene confers an increased risk of breast and ovarian cancer. Although many mutations have been reported in BRCA1 and BRCA2, three mutations found in Ashkenazi Jews have carrier frequencies high enough to warrant a preliminary screen before comprehensive and expensive testing such as DNA sequencing.	This assay detects the 185 del AG and 5382 ins C mutations in BRCA1 and the 6174 del T mutation in BRCA2. These three mutations have a combined carrier frequency of approximately 1.7% in the Ashkenazi Jewish population.	Euhus DM. New insights into the prevention and treatment of familial breast cancer. J Surg Oncol 2011;103:294. [PMID: 21337561] Surbone A. Social and ethical implications of BRCA testing. Ann Oncol 2011;22(Suppl 1):i60. [PMID: 21285154]
Cystic fibrosis mutation PCR + reverse dot blot Blood Lavender $$$$	Cystic fibrosis is caused by a mutation in the cystic fibrosis transmembrane regulator gene (CFTR). Over 800 mutations have been found, with the most common being ΔF508, present in 70% of cases. Approximately 90% persons with cystic fibrosis carry at least one ΔF508 mutation. Another mutation, G551D, accounts for 5% of CFTR mutations and identifies a select subgroup of patients for treatment with an agent that targets the specific mutant protein.	Test specificity approaches 100%, so a positive result should be considered diagnostic of a cystic fibrosis mutation. Because of the wide range of mutations, an assay for the ΔF508 mutation alone is 68% sensitive. Screening for 64 mutations provides a sensitivity of 70–95% in all US ethnic groups except Asians, and >81% when the US population is considered as a whole. The test can distinguish between heterozygous carriers and homozygous patients.	Cystic fibrosis is the most common inherited disease in North American Caucasians, affecting 1 in 2500 births. Caucasians have a carrier frequency of 1 in 25. The disease is autosomal recessive. Carrier screening might be offered to individuals and couples in high-risk groups (eg, Ashkenazi Jews, central or northern Europeans, one partner with cystic fibrosis, and individuals with a family history of cystic fibrosis) who seek preconception counseling, infertility care, or prenatal care. Accurso FJ et al. Effect of VX-770 in persons with cystic fibrosis and the G551D-CFTR mutation. N Engl J Med 2010;363:1991. [PMID: 21083385] Lommatzsch ST et al. Genetics of cystic fibrosis. Semin Respir Crit Care Med 2009;30:531. [PMID: 19760540]

Duchenne muscular dystrophy (DMD) PCR, sequencing Blood (lavender) $$$$	DMD is a rare, X-linked disease. It occurs as a result of mutations (mainly deletions) in the dystrophin gene at locus Xp21.2. Mutations lead to an absence of or defect in dystrophin, causing progressive muscle degeneration and loss of independent ambulation by the age of 13–16 years.	The multiplex PCR-based genetic testing may not detect all mutations, and dystrophin gene sequencing may be necessary.	Testing for a DMD mutation is necessary for confirming the diagnosis even if muscle biopsy demonstrates the absence of dystrophin protein expression. Bushby K et al. Diagnosis and management of Duchenne muscular dystrophy. Part 1: diagnosis, and pharmacological and psychological management. Lancet Neurol 2010;9:77. [PMID: 19945913]
Familial adenomatous polyposis (FAP) PCR, Sequencing Lavender $$$$	Familial adenomatous polyposis is an autosomal dominant condition, which predisposes the mutation carrier to colorectal cancer in early adulthood. The condition is characterized by hundreds to thousands of adenomatous polyps in the colon that usually develop in the second to third decade of life. A milder condition, termed Attenuated FAP (AFAP), lacks the classical features of FAP, with patients having fewer polyps and an older age of onset. FAP has been linked to germline mutations of the APC gene.	A PCR-based assay is used to amplify all exons of the APC gene, and direct sequence analysis of PCR products corresponding to the entire APC coding region is performed. The testing is used only to confirm clinical diagnosis of FAP and AFAP and to identify asymptomatic but affected family members in FAP/AFAP families in which a familial mutation has been identified.	Numerous germline mutations have been located between codons 156 and 2011 of the APC gene. Mutations spanning the region between codons 543 and 1309 are strongly associated with congenital hypertrophy of retinal pigment epithelium. Mutations between codons 1310 and 2011 are associated with increased risk of desmoid tumors. Mutations at codon 1309 are associated with early development of colorectal cancer. Mutations between codons 976 and 1067 are associated with increased risk of duodenal adenomas. The cumulative frequency of extracolonic manifestations is highest for mutations between codons 976 and 1067. Jasperson KW et al. Hereditary and familial colon cancer. Gastroenterology 2010;138:2044. [PMID: 20420945] Pineda M et al. Detection of genetic alterations in hereditary colorectal cancer screening. Mutat Res 2010;693:19. [PMID: 19931546]

(continued)

TABLE 8–10. GENETIC DISEASES: MOLECULAR DIAGNOSTIC TESTING. *(CONTINUED)*

Test/Range/Collection	Physiologic Basis	Interpretation	Comments
Fragile X syndrome PCR, Southern blot Blood, cultured amnio-cytes Lavender $$$$	Fragile X syndrome results from a mutation in the familial mental retardation–1 gene *(FMRI)*, located at Xq27.3. Fully symptomatic patients have abnormal methylation of the gene (which blocks transcription) during oogenesis. The gene contains a variable number of repeating CGG sequences and, as the number of abnormal methylation increases, the probability of sequences increases with subsequent genera-tions so that women who are unaffected carri-ers may have offspring who are affected.	Normal patients have 6–52 CGG repeat sequences. Patients with 52–200 repeat sequences are asymptomatic carriers (premuta-tion). Patients with more than 200 repeat sequences (full mutation) are very likely to have abnormal methylation and to be symp-tomatic.	Fragile X syndrome is the most common cause of inherited mental retardation, occurring in 1 in 1000–1500 men and 1 in 2000–2500 women. Full mutations can show variable penetration in females, but most such women will be at least mildly retarded. Chonchaiya W et al. Fragile X: a family of disorders. Adv Pediatr 2009;56:165. [PMID: 19968948] Hill MK et al. A systematic review of population screen-ing for fragile X syndrome. Genet Med 2010;12:396. [PMID: 20548240]
Hemochromatosis, hereditary Blood Lavender $$$$	Hereditary hemochromatosis is an autosomal recessive disorder of iron metabolism that varies in clinical severity. Three *HFE* gene mutations (C282Y, H63D, and S65C) have been described in most patients with hemo-chromatosis. Mutations in genes encoding other iron regu-lation proteins (hepcidin, ferroportin, hemo-juvelin, transferrin receptor 2) account for rare cases of hereditary hemochromatosis.	Homozygosity for the C282Y muta-tion is responsible for up to 90% of hemochromatosis patients. The estimated penetrance is 80% for men and 35% for women over 40. Compound heterozygosity (C282Y/H63D or C282Y/S65C) may cause hemochromatosis, but the penetrance is very low. Homo-zygous H63D genotypes (H63D/H63D) rarely show symptoms of hemochromatosis. Heterozygotes for C282Y (C282Y/WT), H63D (H63D/WT), or S65C (S65C/WT) are not significantly associated with hemochromatosis.	Pietrangelo A. Hereditary hemochromatosis: patho-genesis, diagnosis, and treatment. Gastroenterology 2010;139:393. [PMID: 20542038] Van Bokhoven MA et al. Diagnosis and management of hereditary haemochromatosis. BMJ 2011;342:c7251. [PMID: 21248018]

Diagnostic Tests in Differential Diagnosis 509

Hemophilia A Southern blot Blood, cultured amniocytes Lavender $$$$	Approximately half of severe hemophilia A cases are caused by a recurrent mutation, ie, an inversion mutations within intron 22 of the factor VIII gene. Methods are available for rapid detection of the intron 22 inversions.	Test specificity approaches 100%, so a positive result should be considered diagnostic of a hemophilia A mutation. Because of a variety of mutations, however, test sensitivity for hemophilia A is only about 50%.	Hemophilia A is one of the most common X-linked diseases in humans, affecting 1 in 5000 men. De Brasi CD et al. Molecular characteristics of the intron 22 homologs of the coagulation factor VIII gene: an update. J thromb Haemost 2008;6:1822. [PMID: 19647227] Shetty S et al. Challenges of multiple mutations in individual patients with haemophilia. Eur J Haematol 2011;86:185. [PMID: 21175850]
Hereditary nonpolyposis colorectal cancer PCR, sequencing Blood (EDTA) and tumor tissue block $$$$	Hereditary nonpolyposis colorectal cancer (HNPCC) (also called Lynch syndrome) accounts for 3–4% of all colorectal cancers. It is caused by inactivation of DNA mismatch repair genes (eg, MLH1, MSH2, MSH6), resulting in accumulation of spontaneous mutations in short repetitive DNA sequences termed microsatellites.	Initial screening includes microsatellite instability (MSI) and immunohistochemistry (IHC) analysis. If MSI is scored as high (MSI-H) and IHC demonstrates the absence of one of the three mismatch repair protein in tumor tissue, then direct sequencing of MLH1, MSH2, or MSH6 is performed to identify the mutation(s).	Testing is used to confirm clinical diagnosis in those with colorectal cancer who meet Amsterdam and/or Bethesda criteria for diagnosis of HNPCC. Once the familial mutation is identified, testing at-risk family members for the specific mutation can be performed. Jasperson KW et al. Hereditary and familial colon cancer. Gastroenterology 2010;138:2044. [PMID: 20420945] Pineda M et al. Detection of genetic alterations in hereditary colorectal cancer screening. Mutat Res 2010;693:19. [PMID: 19931546]
Huntington disease PCR + Southern blot Blood, cultured amniocytes, or buccal cells Lavender $$$$	Huntington disease is an inherited neurodegenerative disorder associated with an autosomal dominant mutation on chromosome 4. The disease is highly penetrant, but symptoms (disordered movements, cognitive decline, and emotional disturbance, are often not expressed until middle age. The mutation results in the expansion of a CAG trinucleotide repeat sequence within the gene that encodes Huntington protein.	Normal patients have fewer than 34 CAG repeats, whereas patients with disease usually have more than 37 repeats and may have 80 or more. Occasional affected patients can be seen with "high normal" (32–34) numbers of repeats. Tests showing 34–37 repeats are indeterminate.	Huntington disease testing involves ethical dilemmas. Counseling is recommended before testing. Ross CA et al. Huntington's disease: from molecular pathogenesis to clinical treatment. Lancet Neurol 2011;10:83. [PMID: 21163446] Roze E et al. Huntington's disease. Adv Exp Med Biol 2010;685:45. [PMID: 20687494]

(continued)

TABLE 8–10. GENETIC DISEASES: MOLECULAR DIAGNOSTIC TESTING. *(CONTINUED)*

Test/Range/Collection	Physiologic Basis	Interpretation	Comments
Kennedy disease/ spinal and bulbar muscular atrophy (KD/SBMA) PCR, Southern blot, sequencing Lavender $$$$	The disease is a degenerative neuromuscular disorder. Familial and sporadic cases are caused by expansion of a CAG trinucleotide tandem repeat in exon 1 of the androgen receptor gene on chromosome Xq11-12.	Normal individuals have up to 30 CAG repeats; patients with KD/SBMA have ≥ 40 CAG repeats (sensitivity >99%).	Finsterer J. Perspective of Kennedy's disease. J Neurol Sci 2010;298:1. [PMID: 20846673]
Myotonic dystrophy (MD) PCR, Southern blot, sequencing Lavender $$$$	The disease is caused by expansions of microsatellite repeats. The most common mutation associated with DM1 is expansion of the trinucleotide repeat CTG in the *DMPK* gene, and for DM2, the expansion of the CCTG repeat in the *ZNF9* gene.	Affected individuals have 50 to several thousands repeats.	Radvansky J et al. The expanding world of myotonic dystrophies: how can they be detected? Genet Test Mol Biomarkers 2010;14:733. [PMID: 20933737] Turner C et al. The myotonic dystrophies: diagnosis and management. J Neurol Neurosurg Psychiatry 2010;81:358-67. [PMID: 20176601]
Neurofibromatosis (NF): von Reckling-hausen disease (NF1) and bilateral acoustic NF (NF2) PCR, Southern blot Lavender $$$$	NF1 is one of the most common genetic disorders of humans (1 in 3500). The *NF1* gene is located at chromosome region 17q11.2 and codes for the neurofibromin protein. Mutations in the *merlin* gene are responsible for NF2, which is characterized by bilateral schwannomas.	The mutations tested by the DNA analysis are laboratory-dependent. Clinical correlation is important.	Ferner RE. The neurofibromatosis. Pract Neurol 2010;10:82. [20308235] Lu-Emerson C et al. The neurofibromatosis. Part 1: NF1. Rev Neurol Dis 2009;6:E47. [PMID: 19587630] Lu-Emerson C et al. The neurofibromatosis. Part 2: NF2 and schwannomatosis. Rev Neurol Dis 2009;6:E81. [PMID: 19898272]

Niemann-Pick disease PCR, sequencing Lavender $$$$	The disease is rare autosomal recessive lysosomal storage disorder. Three mutations (c.911T>C, c.996delC, c.1493G>T) in the acid sphingomyelinase (*SMPD1*) gene account for >94% of cases of type A disease that results in severe neurologic impairment in infancy and childhood. For type C disease, mutational analysis (*NPC1* or *NPC2*/*HE1* gene) is also available.	The combination of DNA and biochemical (sphingomyelinase activity) analyses improves the detection rate of the disease.	Rosenbaum AI et al. Niemann–Pick type C disease: molecular mechanisms and potential therapeutic approaches. J Neurochem 2011;116:789. [PMID: 20807315] Schuchman EH. The pathogenesis and treatment of acid sphingomyelinase-deficient Niemann–Pick disease. Int J Clin Pharmacol Ther 2009;47(Suppl 1):S48. [PMID: 20040312]
Phenylketonuria (PKU) PCR, sequencing, Southern blot Lavender $$$$	The severity of the disease correlates with extent of mutations of the phenylalanine hydroxylase (*PAH*) gene. Little or no enzyme activity results in the classic PKU. Phenylalanine hydroxylase activity determines the type of replacement therapy.	More than 400 point mutations in the PAH gene have been reported, and thus direct sequencing the entire coding regions of the gene may be necessary.	Blau N et al. Phenylketonuria. Lancet 2010;376:1417. [PMID: 20971365]

(continued)

TABLE 8–10. GENETIC DISEASES: MOLECULAR DIAGNOSTIC TESTING. *(CONTINUED)*

Test/Range/Collection	Physiologic Basis	Interpretation	Comments
Prader-Willi syndrome (PWS), Angelman syndrome (AS) FISH, chromosomal analysis Blood Green $$$$	Prader-Willi syndrome and Angelman syndrome are clinically different diseases related at the molecular level. They are caused by loss of function mutations in two chromosomal regions located close to each other on chromosome 15. An interstitial deletion of 15q11-13 is found in about 70% of patients with PWS or AS. PWS results when the deletion affects the paternal chromosome, and AS occurs when it affects the maternal chromosome. A DNA probe from the affected region is used to determine the origin of the deletion by Southern blot analysis. In about 33% of patients with PWS and 20–30% with AS, no deletion can be found. Instead, uniparental disomy (UPD) may be found resulting in either two maternal or two paternal copies of chromosome 15. In 1–2% of patients with PWS and 20% of patients with AS, neither a deletion nor UPD can be found.	This test detects both the deletion and the UPD defects in PWS and AS.	Buiting K. Prader-Willi syndrome and Angelman syndrome. Am J Med Genet C Semin Med Genet 2010;154C:365. [PMID: 20803659]
Tay-Sachs disease PCR, Sequencing Lavender $$$$	Tay-Sachs disease is an autosomal recessive disease caused by a deficiency of β-hexosaminidase A. Mutations in the α-subunit of hexosaminidase A are responsible for the enzyme deficiency. More than 75 mutations of the α-subunit gene have been described.	The mutations tested by the DNA analysis are laboratory-dependent. The combination of DNA and biochemical analyses improves the detection rate of the disease.	Norton ME. Genetic screening and counseling. Curr Opin Obstet Gynecol 2008;20:157. [PMID: 18388816]

α-Thalassemia PCR + Southern blot Blood, cultured amniocytes, chorionic villi Lavender $$$$	A deletion mutation in the α-globin gene region of chromosome 16 due to unequal crossing-over events can lead to defective synthesis of the α-globin chain of hemoglobin. Normally, there are two copies of the α-globin gene on each chromosome 16, and the severity of disease increases with the number of defective genes.	This assay is highly specific (approaches 100%). Sensitivity, however, can vary because detection of different mutations may require the use of different probes. α-Thalassemia due to point mutations may not be detected.	Patients with one deleted gene are usually normal or very slightly anemic; patients with two deletions usually have hypochromic microcytic anemia; patients with three deletions have elevated hemoglobin H and moderately severe hemolytic anemia (Hb H disease); patients with four deletions generally die in utero with hydrops fetalis. The most clinically significant situations arise when both parents are carriers for a deletion that encompasses both α-globin genes (*cis* deletion), as seen mostly in Southeast Asian and Filipino populations. Each offspring of such carriers has a 25% risk of hydrops fetalis. Less deleterious effects arise from chromosomes of Mediterranean and black ancestries. These chromosomes usually carry one α-globin gene deletion per chromosome. Offspring of carriers of a two α-globin gene deletion and single α-gene deletion are at risk for Hb H disease. Higgs DR et al: The molecular basis of alpha thalassemia: a model for understanding human molecular genetics. Hematol Oncol Clin North Am 2010;24:1033. [PMID: 21075279] Lal A et al: Heterogeneity of hemoglobin H disease in childhood. N Engl J Med 2011;364:710. [PMID: 21345100]

(continued)

TABLE 8–10. GENETIC DISEASES: MOLECULAR DIAGNOSTIC TESTING. *(CONTINUED)*

Test/Range/Collection	Physiologic Basis	Interpretation	Comments
β-Thalassemia PCR + reverse dot blot Blood, chorionic villi, cultured amniocytes Lavender $$$$	β-Thalassemia results from a mutation in the gene encoding the β-globin subunit of hemoglobin A (which is composed of a pair of α chains and a pair of β chains). A relative excess of α-globin chains precipitates within red blood cells, causing hemolysis and anemia. Over 300 different mutations have been described; testing usually covers a panel of the more common mutations. The test can distinguish between heterozygous and homozygous individuals.	Test specificity approaches 100%, so a positive result should be considered diagnostic of a thalassemia mutation. Because of the large number of mutations, sensitivity can be poor. A panel with the 43 most common mutations has a sensitivity that approaches 95%.	β-Thalassemia is very common; about 3% of the world's population are carriers. The incidence is increased in persons of Mediterranean, African, and Asian descent. The mutations may vary from population to population, and different testing panels may be needed for patients of different ethnicities. Cousens NE et al. Carrier screening for beta-thalassemia: a review of international practice. Eur J Hum Genet 2010;18:1077. [PMID: 20571509] Galanello R et al. Beta-thalassemia. Orphanet J Rare Dis 2010;5:11. [PMID: 20492708]

PCR (polymerase chain reaction) *is a method for amplifying a particular DNA sequence in a specimen, facilitating mutation detection by hybridization-based assay (eg, Southern blot, reverse dot blot, FISH) and direct DNA sequencing;* ***Southern blot*** *is a molecular hybridization technique whereby DNA is extracted from the sample and digested by different restriction enzymes, and the resulting fragments are separated by electrophoresis and identified by labeled probes;* ***Reverse dot blot*** *is a molecular hybridization technique in which a specific oligonucleotide probe is bound to a solid membrane prior to reaction with PCR-amplified DNA.*

TABLE 8–11. HEPATITIS B VIRUS INFECTION: COMMON SEROLOGIC TEST PATTERNS AND THEIR INTERPRETATION.

HBsAg	Anti-HBs	Anti-HBc	HBeAg	Anti-HBe	Interpretation
+	−	IgM	+	−	Acute hepatitis B
+	−	IgG[1]	+	−	Chronic hepatitis B with active viral replication
+	−	IgG	−	+	Chronic hepatitis B with low viral replication
+	+	IgG	+ or −	+ or −	Chronic hepatitis B with heterotypic anti-HBs (about 10% of cases)
−	−	IgM	+ or −	−	Acute hepatitis B
−	+	IgG	−	+ or −	Recovery from hepatitis B (immunity)
−	+	−	−	−	Vaccination (immunity)
−	−	IgG	−	−	False-positive; less commonly, infection in the remote past

[1]Low levels of IgM anti-HBc may also be detected.

TABLE 8–12. HYPERLIPIDEMIA: RISK FACTOR ASSESSMENT FOR CORONARY HEART DISEASE (CHD).

Risk Score Sheet for Men[1]

Age (years)	Points
30–34	−1
35–39	0
40–44	1
45–49	2
50–54	3
55–59	4
60–64	5
65–69	6
70–74	7

Diabetes	Points
No	0
Yes	2

Smoker	Points
No	0
Yes	2

LDL-C (mg/dL)	LDL-C (mmol/L)	Points
<100	<2.59	−3
100–129	2.60–3.36	0
130–159	3.37–4.14	0
160–190	4.50–4.92	1
>190	>4.92	2

HDL-C (mg/dL)	HDL-C (mmol/L)	Points
<35	<0.9	2
35–44	0.01–1.16	1
45–49	1.17–1.29	0
50–59	1.30–1.55	0
≥60	≥1.56	−1

BP (mm Hg) Systolic	Diastolic <80	Diastolic 80–84	Diastolic 85–89	Diastolic 90–99	Diastolic ≥100
<120	0	0	1	2	3
120–129	0	0	1	2	3
130–139	1	1	1	2	3
140–159	2	2	2	2	3
≥160	3	3	3	3	3

TABLE 8–12. HYPERLIPIDEMIA: RISK FACTOR ASSESSMENT FOR CORONARY HEART DISEASE (CHD). (*CONTINUED*)

Total CHD Risk Points	10-year CHD Risk (%)
<+3	1
−2	2
−1	2
0	3
1	4
2	5
3	6
4	7
5	9
6	11
7	14
8	18
9	22
10	27
11	33
12	40
13	47
≥14	56

(continued)

TABLE 8–12. HYPERLIPIDEMIA: RISK FACTOR ASSESSMENT FOR CORONARY HEART DISEASE (CHD). (CONTINUED)

Risk Score Sheet for Women[1]

Age (years)	Points
30–34	–9
35–39	–4
40–44	0
45–49	3
50–54	6
55–59	7
60–64	8
65–69	8
70–74	8

Diabetes	Points
No	0
Yes	4

Smoker	Points
No	0
Yes	2

LDL-C (mg/dL)	LDL-C (mmol/L)	Points
<100	<2.59	–2
100–129	2.60–3.36	0
130–159	3.37–4.14	0
160–190	4.50–4.92	2
>190	>4.92	2

HDL-C (mg/dL)	HDL-C (mmol/L)	Points
<35	<0.9	5
35–44	0.01–1.16	2
45–49	1.17–1.29	1
50–59	1.30–1.55	0
≥60	≥1.56	–2

| Risk Score Sheet for Women[1] | | | | | |
BP (mm Hg) Systolic	Diastolic <80	Diastolic 80–84	Diastolic 85–89	Diastolic 90–99	Diastolic ≥100
<120	-3	0	0	2	3
120–129	0	0	0	2	3
130–139	0	0	0	2	3
140–159	2	2	2	2	3
≥160	3	3	3	3	3

Total CHD Risk Points	10-year CHD risk (%)
≤-2	1
-1	2
0	2
1	2
2	3
3	3
4	4
5	5

(continued)

TABLE 8–12. HYPERLIPIDEMIA: RISK FACTOR ASSESSMENT FOR CORONARY HEART DISEASE (CHD). *(CONTINUED)*

6	6
7	7
8	8
9	9
10	11
11	13
12	15
13	17
14	20
15	24
16	27
≥17	32

[1] The score sheet uses age, LDL-cholesterol (LDL-C), HDL-cholesterol (HDL-C), blood pressure (BP), diabetes, and smoking. To calculate the Framingham risk estimate, add points for age, presence of diabetes, smoking status, LDL-C, HDL-C, and BP. Find the total point score on the bottom table to determine the 10-year risk of CHD. The score is used to calculate the risk of developing clinical CHD in men and women who do not have known CHD. Adapted with permission from Wilson PW et al. Prediction of coronary heart disease using risk factor categories. Circulation 1998;97:1837. Copyright © 1998 Lippincott Williams & Wilkins.

TABLE 8–13. LEUKEMIAS AND LYMPHOMAS: CLASSIFICATION AND IMMUNOPHENOTYPING.

Disease	Typical Immunophenotype	Comments
Acute Myeloid Leukemias (AML)		
AML with t (8;21) (q22;q22), (*AML1/ETO*)	Blasts express CD34, HLA-DR, CD13, CD33, CD15, MPO, and CD117. CD19 is often expressed.	AML with t (8;21) is usually associated with good response to chemotherapy and high rate of complete remission with long-term disease-free survival.
AML with inv (16) (p13;q22) or t (16;16) (p13;q22), (CBFβ/ *MYH11*)	Blasts express CD13, CD33, MPO, CD117, as well as CD14, CD4, CD11b, CD11c, CD64, and CD36.	AML with inv (16) or t (16;16) typically shows myeloid and monocytic differentiation and the presence of eosinophilia, referred to as AMML–Eo. The disease usually responds well to chemotherapy with high rate of complete remission.
AML with t (15;17) (q22;q12), (*PML/RARα*) and variants	Leukemic cells express CD13, CD33, MPO, and CD117, but not CD34 and HLA-DR.	AML with t (15;17), known as acute promyelocytic leukemia (APL), is sensitive to all-*trans* retinoic acid (ATRA) treatment. APL is frequently associated with DIC.
AML with t(9;11)(p22;q23), (*MLLT3/MLL*)	Leukemic cells variably express HLA-DR, CD33, CD117, MPO, and monocytic markers (CD4, CD14, CD11b, CD11c, CD64, and lysozyme). CD34 is often absent.	AML with 11q23 (MLL) abnormalities is usually associated with monocytic features. AML with 11q23 abnormalities has an intermediate survival.
AML with t(6;9)(p23;q34) *DEK/ NUP214*	Blasts often express MPO, CD13, CD33, HLA-DR, CD117, CD34, and CD15. Some cases also express CD64 or TdT	AML with t(6;9) may have monocytic features, and is often associated with basophilia and multilineage dysplasia. Disease in both adults and children has a poor prognosis.
AML with inv(3)(q21q26) or t(3;3) (q21;q26), (*RPN1/EVI1*)	Blasts often express CD13, CD33, HLA-DR, CD34. Some case may also express CD7 (aberrant), CD41 or CD61.	AML with inv(3) or t(3;3) is an aggressive disease with poor prognosis.
AML with t(1;22)(p13;q13) (RBM15/ MKL1) (megakaryocytic)	Blasts often express CD41, CD61, CD36, and may also express CD13 and CD33.	Disease most commonly occurs in infants without Down syndrome. Outcome is generally poor, but may respond to intensive chemotherapy with long survival.

(continued)

TABLE 8–13. LEUKEMIAS AND LYMPHOMAS: CLASSIFICATION AND IMMUNOPHENOTYPING. (CONTINUED)

AML with myelodysplasia-related changes	Blasts often express CD34, HLA-DR, CD13, CD33, MPO, CD117. Aberrant expression of Cd7 and/or CD56 may occur.	AML with myelodysplasia-related changes including AML arising from prior MDS or MDS/MPN, AML with an MDS-related cytogenetic abnormality, and AML with multilineage dysplasia. The disease has poor prognosis with low rate of achieving remission.
AML, therapy-related (t-AML)	Alkylating agent/radiation related: Blasts express CD34, HLA-DR, CD13, CD33, MPO, and CD117. Topoisomerase II inhibitor related: Same as AML with 11q23 abnormalities.	Alkylating agent/radiation related AML is generally refractory to chemotherapy and is associated with short survival. Topoisomerase II inhibitor-related AML often show monocytic differentiation. Therapy-related myelodysplastic syndrome (t-MDS) has similar prognosis as t-AML.
AML, minimally differentiated (also known as AML-M0)	Blasts express CD13, CD33, CD117, CD34, HLA-DR, but not MPO.	Flow cytometric immunophenotyping is required for the confirmation of myeloid differentiation.
AML without maturation (also known as AML-M1)	Blasts express CD13, CD33, CD117, and MPO. CD34 is often positive.	Blasts constitute >90% of the nonerythroid nucleated cells in the marrow, and at least 3% of the blasts are positive for MPO.
AML with maturation (also known as AML-M2)	Blasts express CD13, CD33, CD15, CD117, and MPO. CD34 and HLA-DR are often positive.	Blasts constitute 20–89% of nonerythroid cells, and monocytes comprise <20% of the bone marrow cells.
Acute myelomonocytic leukemia (also known as AML-M4)	Leukemic cells variably express CD13, CD33, CD117, HLA-DR, CD14, CD4, CD11b, CD11c, and CD64. CD34 may be positive.	Monocytic component (monoblasts to monocytes) comprises 20–79% of bone marrow cells.
Acute monoblastic/monocytic leukemia (also known as AML-M5)	Leukemic cells variably express CD13, CD33, CD117, HLA-DR, CD14, CD4, CD11b, CD11c, CD64, and CD68. CD34 is typically negative.	Monocytic component (monoblasts to monocytes) comprises >80% of bone marrow cells.

Acute erythroid leukemia (also known as AML-M6) and pure erythroid leukemia	Erythroblasts generally lack myeloid markers, but are positive for CD36 and glycophorin A (CD235). Myeloblasts express CD13, CD33, CD117, and MPO with or without CD34 and HLA-DR. The erythroid cells in pure erythroid leukemia express CD36 and glycophorin A with the more immature forms expressing CD34 and HLA-DR.	The diagnostic criteria for acute erythroid leukemia: erythroblasts constitute >50% of the marrow cells, and myeloblasts comprise >20% of the nonerythroid cells. Pure erythroid leukemia is a neoplastic proliferation of erythroid precursors (>80% of nucleated marrow cells) without a significant myeloblastic component.
Acute megakaryocytic leukemia (known as AML-M7)	Blasts express one or more of the platelet glycoproteins (CD41, CD61, CD42), and variably express HLA-DR, CD34, CD117, CD13, and CD33.	Flow cytometric immunophenotyping is required for confirmation of megakaryocytic differentiation.
Blastic plasmacytoid dendritic cell neoplasm (formerly known as blastic NK-cell lymphoma)	Neoplastic cells express CD4, CD43, CD45RA, CD56, and plasmacytoid dendritic cell-associated antigens CD123 CD303, TCL1. May also express CD68 and TdT.	The disease is also called agranular CD4+/CD56+ hematodermic tumor. Besides marrow involvement, skin lesions are present. The disease is aggressive with short survival.
Acute leukemia of ambiguous lineage	Undifferentiated acute leukemia: Blasts express HLA-DR, CD34, CD38, and may express TdT, but lack lineage-specific markers such as CD79a, CD22, strong CD19, igM, CD3, and MPO. Bilineal acute leukemia: There is a dual population of blasts with each population expressing markers of a distinct lineage, such as myeloid and lymphoid, or B and T. Biphenotypic acute leukemia: The blasts co-express myeloid and T or B lineage-specific antigens, or concurrent B and T antigens.	Cases of bilineal and biphenotypic acute leukemia usually present with cytogenetic abnormalities. The common abnormalities include Philadelphia chromosome, t (4;11)(q 21;q 23) or other 11q23 abnormalities. The prognosis of acute leukemia of ambiguous lineage is poor.

(continued)

TABLE 8–13. LEUKEMIAS AND LYMPHOMAS: CLASSIFICATION AND IMMUNOPHENOTYPING. *(CONTINUED)*

Acute Lymphoblastic Leukemias/Lymphomas (ALL/LBL)		
Precursor B-lymphoblastic leukemia/lymphoblastic lymphoma (B-ALL/LBL) (also known as B-cell acute lymphoblastic leukemia)	Early precursor B-ALL/LBL: TdT+, HLA-DR+, CD34(−/+), CD10−, CD19+, cCD22+, CD20−, CD15+, clg−, sIg−. Common B-ALL/LBL: TdT+, HLA-DR+, CD34+, CD10+, CD45+(weak), CD19+, CD20+, clg−, sIg−. Pre-B-ALL/LBL: TdT(−/+), CD34(−/+), HLA-DR+, CD45+(weak), CD19+, CD20+, clgM+, sIg−.	Cytogenetic abnormalities in B-ALL/LBL include several groups: hypodiploid, low hyperdiploid (<50), high hyperdiploid (>50), translocations, and pseudodiploid. The commonly seen translocations include t (9;22), t (12;21), t (5;14), t (1;19), t (17;19), t (4;11), and other translocations involving 11q23. The cytogenetic findings are prognostically important.
Precursor T-lymphoblastic leukemia/lymphoblastic lymphoma (T-ALL/LBL)	T-ALL/LBL often has an immunophenotype that corresponds to the common thymocyte stage of differentiation. The blasts are positive for TdT and often CD10, and variably express CD1a, CD2, CD3, CD4, CD5, CD7, and CD8. CD4 and CD8 are frequently co-expressed on the blasts. Some T-ALL/LBL has an immunophenotype that corresponds to prothymocyte stage of differentiation. The blasts are negative for both CD4 and CD8.	In about one-third of T-ALL/LBL translocations have been detected involving the α and δ T-cell receptor (TCR) loci at 14q11.2, the β locus at 7q35, and the γ locus at 7p14-15, with a variety of partner genes. T-ALL/LBL can be part of a unique disease entity known as the 8p11 myeloproliferative syndrome caused by constitutive activation of FGFR1. The disease is characterized by chronic myeloproliferative disorder that frequently presents with eosinophilia and associated T-cell lymphoblastic lymphoma.
Mature B-cell Neoplasms		
Chronic lymphocytic leukemia/ small lymphocytic lymphoma (CLL/SLL)	Lymphoma cells are light chain restricted and express CD5, CD19, CD20 (weak), CD22 (weak), CD79a, CD23, CD43, and are negative for CD10, Bcl-1 (cyclin D1), and FMC-7. A subset of cases expresses CD11c (weak). Cases with unmutated Ig variable region genes have been reported to be positive for CD38 and ZAP-70.	The clinical course is often indolent but incurable. The disease may progress/transform to prolymphocytic leukemia (PLL) or large B-cell lymphoma (Richter syndrome). CD38 and/or ZAP-70 positivity is associated with worse prognosis, and both have been used as prognostic markers for the disease. Trisomy 12 is reported in ~20% of cases, and deletions at 13q14 in up to 50% of cases. Trisomy 12 in CLL/SLL correlates with a worse prognosis.

B-cell prolymphocytic leukemia (B-PLL)	The cells of B-PLL strongly express surface IgM and B-cell antigens CD19, CD20, CD22, CD79a, CD79b, and FMC-7. CD5 is present in about one-third of cases and CD23 is typically negative.	B-PLL can be divided into CD5+ B-PLL (arising in CLL/SLL) and CD5– B-PLL (de novo PLL). CD5+ B-PLL has a longer median survival than CD5– B-PLL.
Lymphoplasmacytic lymphoma/Waldenström macroglobulinemia (LPL)	The cells express strong surface immunoglobulin, usually of IgM type, and express B-cell antigens (CD19, CD20, CD22, CD79a) and are CD5–, CD10–, CD23–, CD43±, and CD38+. Lack of CD5 and strong immunoglobulin expression are useful in distinction from CLL/SLL.	Characteristic features include IgM monoclonal gammopathy; spectrum of small lymphocytes, plasmacytoid lymphocytes and plasma cells; interstitial, nodular, or diffuse pattern of bone marrow involvement; and typical immunophenotype (sIgM+, CD19+, CD20+, CD5–, CD23–, CD10–).
Splenic marginal zone lymphoma (SMZL)	The tumor cells express surface IgM, and are positive for CD19, CD20, CD79a, and are negative for CD5, CD10, CD23, CD25, CD43, CD103, and Bcl-1 (cyclin D1).	Circulating lymphoma cells are usually characterized by the presence of short polar villi (villous lymphocytes). The clinical course is indolent, but the disease is incurable.
Hairy cell leukemia (HCL)	Leukemic cells express surface immunoglobulin, B-cell markers (CD19, CD20, CD22, CD79a), and are often positive for CD11c, CD25, FMC-7, and CD103, but negative for CD5, CD10, and CD23.	Patients often present with splenomegaly, pancytopenia (monocytopenia is characteristic), and may have circulating hairy leukemic cells. Bone marrow reticulin fibers are characteristically increased, resulting in "dry tap" during aspirate procedure. Interferon-alpha, deoxycoformycin (pentostatin), or 2-chlorodeoxyadenosine (2-CdA, cladribine) can induce long-term remissions.
Plasma cell myeloma/plasmacytoma	The malignant cells express monoclonal cytoplasmic immunoglobulin, lack CD45 and pan-B cell antigens (CD19, CD20, CD22), but CD79 is often positive. The cells are typically positive for CD38, CD138, and often express CD56, CD43, and rarely CD10. The phenotype of plasma cell leukemia is similar to that of myeloma, but CD56 is negative.	Plasma cells do not express surface immunoglobulin. For clonality (or light chain restriction) determination by flow cytometry analysis, cell permeabilization procedure is necessary. The procedure gives antibodies access to intracellular structures/molecules.

(continued)

TABLE 8–13. LEUKEMIAS AND LYMPHOMAS: CLASSIFICATION AND IMMUNOPHENOTYPING. *(CONTINUED)*

Extranodal marginal zone B-cell lymphoma of mucosa-associated lymphoid tissue (MALT lymphoma)	Lymphoma cells typically express surface immunoglobulin with light chain restriction. The cells are positive for CD19, CD20, CD79a, CD43, and negative for CD5, CD10, CD23, and Bcl-1.	Trisomy 3 is found in ~60% and t (11;18) (q21;q21) has been detected in 25–50% of MALT lymphoma cases. Neither t (14;18) nor t (11;14) is present. Cases with t (11;18) appear to be resistant to *H. pylori* eradication therapy.
Nodal marginal zone B-cell lymphoma (NMZL)	The immunophenotype of most cases is similar to that of extranodal MALT lymphoma.	NMZL is a primary nodal B-cell neoplasm that morphologically resembles lymph nodes involved by marginal zone lymphomas of extranodal or splenic types, but without evidence of extranodal or splenic disease.
Follicular lymphoma (FL)	Lymphoma cells are usually positive for pan–B-cell antigens (CD19, CD20), surface immunoglobulin, CD10, Bcl-2, Bcl-6, and negative for CD5. Bcl-2 is expressed in the majority of cases, ranging from nearly 100% in grade 1 to 75% in grade 3 FL.	All cases have cytogenetic abnormalities. The t (14;18) (q32;q21) translocation, involving rearrangement of the *Bcl-2* gene and *IgH* gene, is present in 80–95% of FL. FL may transform into high-grade B-cell lymphoma with features intermediate between DLBCL and Burkitt lymphoma, and c-*myc* (8q24) rearrangement is often involved. Bcl-2 is useful in distinguishing reactive follicular hyperplasia (Bcl-2 negative) and FL (Bcl-2-positive).
Mantle cell lymphoma (MCL)	Lymphoma cells express surface immunoglobulin, pan–B-cell antigens (CD19, CD20), Bcl-1, FMC-7, CD5, CD43, and are typically negative for CD10, CD23, and Bcl-6.	MCL and CLL/SLL are the two common CD5-positive B-cell lymphoproliferative disorders. But unlike CLL/SLL, MCL cells express bright surface immunoglobulin, bright CD20 and FMC-7, and are CD23 negative. Virtually all cases express Bcl-1 (cyclin D1) due to gene rearrangement.
Diffuse large B-cell lymphoma (DLBCL)	DLBCL cells typically express various pan–B-cell antigens (CD19, CD20, CD22, CD79a), surface and/or cytoplasmic immunoglobulin with light chain restriction, Bcl-6, and CD10. Bcl-2 is positive in 30–50% of cases.	Morphologic variants of DLBCL include centroblastic, immunoblastic, T-cell/histiocyte rich, anaplastic, and plasmablastic DLBCL. Bcl-2 expression has been reported to be associated with an adverse disease-free survival, while expression of Bcl-6 appears to be associated with a better prognosis.

Mediastinal (thymic) large B-cell lymphoma (Med-DLBCL)	Lymphoma cells express CD45 and B-cell antigen (CD19, CD20). Immunoglobulin and HLA-DR are often absent. The cells do not express CD5 and CD10, and lack Bcl-2, Bcl-6, and c-myc rearrangements.
	Med-DLBCL is a subtype of DLBCL arising in the mediastinum of putative thymic B-cell origin with distinct clinical, immunophenotypic, and genotypic features. Tissue sections usually show diffuse lymphoid proliferation, compartmentalized into groups by fine/delicate fibrotic bands.
Intravascular large B-cell lymphoma	Lymphoma cells express pan–B-cell antigens (CD19, CD20).
	The disease is a rare subtype of extranodal DLBCL characterized by the presence of lymphoma cells only in the lumina of small vessels, particularly capillaries. Brain and skin are the common sites of involvement.
Primary effusion lymphoma (PEL)	Lymphoma cells express CD45, but are usually negative for pan–B-cell markers (CD19, CD20). Surface and cytoplasmic immunoglobulin is often absent. Activation and plasma cell-related markers such as CD30, CD38, and CD138 are usually positive.
	PEL is a neoplasm of large B cells usually presenting as serous effusions without detectable tumor masses. It is universally associated with human herpes virus 8 (HHV-8), most often occurring in the setting of immunodeficiency.
Lymphomatoid granulomatosis (LYG)	Lymphoma cells express CD20, and are variably positive for CD30, but negative for CD15. The cells lack immunoglobulin expression. The background small lymphocytes are CD3–positive T cells.
	LYG is an angiocentric and angiodestructive lymphoproliferative disease involving extranodal sites, composed of Epstein-Barr virus (EBV)-positive B cells admixed with reactive T cells, which usually numerically predominate. LYG may progress to an EBV-positive DLBCL. The common sites of involvement are lung, kidney, brain, liver, and skin.
Burkitt lymphoma (BL)	Lymphoma cells express surface immunoglobulin with light chain restriction, pan–B-cell antigens (CD19, CD20), CD10, and Bcl-6. The cells are negative for CD5, CD23, CD34, and TdT. Nearly 100% of the cells are positive for Ki-67, a proliferation marker.
	All BL cases show a translocation of c-myc gene at chromosome 8q24 to the IgH gene at 14q32 or less commonly to light chain loci at 2p12 or 22q11. Genetic abnormalities involving the c-myc gene play an essential role in BL pathogenesis. The expression of CD10 and Bcl-6 indicates a germinal center origin of the tumor cells. BL is highly aggressive but potentially curable.

(continued)

TABLE 8–13. LEUKEMIAS AND LYMPHOMAS: CLASSIFICATION AND IMMUNOPHENOTYPING. *(CONTINUED)*

Mature T-cell and NK-cell Neoplasms

T-cell prolymphocytic leukemia (T-PLL)	Leukemic cells express CD2, CD3, CD7, but not TdT and CD1a. The cells can be CD4+/CD8–(60%), CD4+/CD8+ (25%), or CD4–/CD8+ (15%).	T-PLL is an aggressive T-cell leukemia characterized by the proliferation of small to medium sized prolymphocytes with a mature post-thymic T-cell phenotype involving the blood, bone marrow, lymph nodes, spleen, and skin.
T-cell large granular lymphocyte leukemia (T-LGL)	T-LGL cells have a mature T-cell immunophenotype. Approximately 80% of cases are CD3+, TCR α, β+, CD4–, and CD8+.	T-LGL is a heterogeneous disorder characterized by a persistent (>6 months) increase in peripheral blood large granular lymphocytes (LGLs), without a clearly identified cause. Severe neutropenia with or without anemia is a characteristic clinical feature. Pure red cell hypoplasia has been reported in association with T-LGL leukemia. Splenomegaly, rheumatoid arthritis, and the presence of autoantibodies are commonly seen in patients with T-LGL.
Aggressive NK-cell leukemia	Leukemic cells are CD2+, surface CD3–, cytoplasmic CD3e+, CD56+, and positive for cytotoxic molecules (TIA–1, granzyme B, and/or perforin). This immunophenotype is identical to that of extranodal NK/T-cell lymphoma, nasal type.	Aggressive NK-cell leukemia is characterized by a systemic proliferation of NK cells. The disease has an aggressive clinical course. T-cell receptor (TCR) genes are in germline configuration.
Adult T-cell leukemia/lymphoma (ATLL)	Tumor cells express T-cell antigens (CD2, CD3, CD5), but usually lack CD7. Most cases are CD4+, CD8– Rare cases are CD4–, CD8+, or double negative for CD4 and CD8. CD25 is expressed in virtually all cases.	ATLL is a peripheral T-cell neoplasm most often composed of highly pleomorphic lymphoid cells. The disease is usually widely disseminated, and is caused by the human T-cell leukemia virus type 1 (HTLV-1). ATLL is endemic in Japan, the Caribbean basin, and parts of Central Africa.

Extranodal NK/T-cell lymphoma, nasal type	The typical immunophenotype is CD2+, CD56+, surface CD3−, and cytoplasmic CD3 ε+. Most cases are positive for cytotoxic molecules (TIA-1, granzyme B, perforin).	The disease entity is designated NK/T (rather than NK) cell lymphoma because while most cases appear to be NK-cell neoplasms (EBV+, CD56+), rare cases show an EBV+, CD56− cytotoxic T-cell phenotype. T-cell receptor and immunoglobulin genes are in germline configuration in a majority of cases. EBV can be demonstrated in the tumor cells in nearly all cases. The prognosis is variable.
Enteropathy-type T-cell lymphoma	Tumor cells are CD3+, CD5−, CD7+, CD8∓, CD4−, CD1C3+, and contain cytotoxic molecules.	The tumor occurs most commonly in the jejunum or ileum, and there is a clear association with celiac disease. The prognosis is usually poor.
Hepatosplenic T-cell lymphoma	Tumor cells are CD3+, CD4−, CD8−, CD5−, CD56±. The cells are usually TCR γδ+ and TCR α β−.	Hepatosplenic T-cell lymphoma is an extranodal and systemic neoplasm derived from cytotoxic T cells usually of γδ T-cell receptor type, demonstrating marked sinusoidal infiltration of spleen, liver, and bone marrow. The clinical course is aggressive.
Subcutaneous panniculitis-like T-cell lymphoma (SPTCL)	Tumor cells are usually CD3+, TCR α β +, CD5−, CD4−, CD8−, and express cytotoxic molecules.	SPTCL is a cytotoxic T-cell lymphoma, which preferentially infiltrates subcutaneous tissue. Some patients may present with a hemophagocytic syndrome with pancytopenia. The clinical course is aggressive.
Mycosis fungoides and Sézary syndrome (MF/SS)	The typical phenotype is CD2+, CD3+, TCR β +, CD5−, CD4+/CD8− (rarely CD4−/CD8+). Virtually all cases are negative for CD26 (a marker for treatment monitoring). CD7 is usually negative.	MF is a mature T-cell lymphoma, presenting in the skin with patches/plaques and characterized by epidermal and dermal infiltration of small to medium-sized T cells with cerebriform nuclei. SS is a generalized mature T-cell lymphoma characterized by the presence of erythroderma, lymphadenopathy, and neoplastic T lymphocytes in the blood.

(continued)

TABLE 8–13. LEUKEMIAS AND LYMPHOMAS: CLASSIFICATION AND IMMUNOPHENOTYPING. *(CONTINUED)*

Primary cutaneous CD30-positive T-cell lymphoproliferative disorders	Primary cutaneous anaplastic large cell lymphoma (C-ALCL): Tumors cells express T-cell antigens (CD2, CD3, CD5, CD7) and are usually positive for CD4. CD30 is expressed in >75% of the cells. Aberrant T-cell phenotype with loss of one or more T-cell antigens is common. Lymphomatoid papulosis (LyP): The atypical T cells are CD4+, CD8−. The cells often express aberrant phenotypes with variable loss of pan–T-cell antigens (eg, CD2, CD5, or CD7). CD30 is positive in a LyP subtype (type A).	LyP and C-ALCL constitute a spectrum of related conditions originating from transformed or activated CD30-positive T lymphocytes. They may coexist in individual patients, they can be clonally related and they often show overlapping clinical and/or histologic features.
Angioimmunoblastic T-cell lymphoma (AITL)	Neoplastic cells express T cell antigens (CD2, CD3, CD5, CD7), usually without aberrant antigen loss, and are CD4+ and CD8−. The neoplastic T cells are positive for CD10 and/or Bcl-6. CD21 stain highlights the intact or disrupted follicular dendritic meshwork.	AITL is a T-cell lymphoma characterized by systemic disease and a polymorphous infiltrate involving lymph nodes. TCR genes are rearranged in the majority (>75%) of cases. Secondary EBV-related B-cell lymphoma may occur. Almost all cases are positive for CD10 and/or Bcl-6, suggesting a germinal center derivation of the tumor cells. The clinical course is very aggressive.
Peripheral T-cell lymphoma, unspecified	Neoplastic cells express T cell antigens (CD2, CD3, CD5, CD7), but aberrant T-cell pheno-types with antigen loss are frequent. Most nodal cases are CD4+, CD8−, CD30, and CD56 may be positive.	The diseases are among the most aggressive of the non-Hodgkin lymphomas.
Anaplastic large cell lymphoma (ALCL)	The tumor cells express one or more T-cell antigens (CD2, CD3, CD5, CD7). The cells usually express CD30 (membrane and in the Golgi region). ALK (cytoplasmic and/or nuclear), EMA, cytotoxic molecules, CD43, and CD45.	Expression of ALK in ALCL is due to genetic alteration of the ALK locus on chromosome 2. The most common alteration is t(2;5)(p23;q35), resulting in fusion of the ALK gene and nucleophosmin (NPM) gene on 5q35. ALK-positive ALCL has a favorable prognosis.

For details, see Swerdlow SH, et al (editors). *WHO Classification of Tumors of Haematopoietic and Lymphoid Tissues.* IARC Press: Lyon 2008.
ALK = anaplastic large cell lymphoma kinase; **CD** = cluster of differentiation; **EMA** = epithelial membrane antigen; **MPO** = myeloperoxidase.

TABLE 8–14. LIVER FUNCTION TESTS.

Clinical Condition	Direct Bilirubin (mg/dL)	Indirect Bilirubin (mg/dL)	Urine Bilirubin	Serum Albumin and Total Protein (g/dL)	Alkaline Phosphatase (IU/L)	Prothrombin Time (seconds)	ALT, AST (IU/L)
Normal	0.1–0.3	0.2–0.7	None	Albumin, 3.4–4.7 Total protein, 6.0–8.0	30–115 (lab-specific)	11–15 seconds. After vitamin K, 15% increase within 24 hours.	ALT, 5–35; AST, 5–40 (lab-specific)
Hepatocellular jaundice (eg, viral, alcoholic hepatitis; drug or other toxicity [acetaminophen, *Amanita* sp. mushroom poisoning], shock liver, hepatic vein thrombosis)	↑↑	↑	↑	↓ Albumin	N to ↑	Prolonged if damage is severe. Does not respond to parenteral vitamin K.	Increased in hepatocellular damage. Modestly increased in alcoholic hepatitis in which AST/ALT ratio often >2:1; markedly increased (>1000 IU/L) in viral hepatitides, drug or other toxicity, shock liver, hepatic vein thrombosis.
Uncomplicated obstructive jaundice (eg, common bile duct obstruction)	↑↑	↑	↑	N	↑	Prolonged if obstruction marked but responds to parenteral vitamin K.	N to minimally ↑
Hemolysis	N	↑	None	N	N	N	N

(continued)

TABLE 8–14. LIVER FUNCTION TESTS. (*CONTINUED*)

Clinical Condition	Direct Bilirubin (mg/dL)	Indirect Bilirubin (mg/dL)	Urine Bilirubin	Serum Albumin and Total Protein (g/dL)	Alkaline Phosphatase (IU/L)	Prothrombin Time (seconds)	ALT, AST (IU/L)
Gilbert syndrome	N	↑	None	N	N	N	N
Intrahepatic cholestasis (drug-induced)	↑↑	↑	↑	N	↑↑	N	AST N or ↑; ALT N or ↑
Primary biliary cirrhosis	↑↑	↑	↑	N ↑ globulin	↑↑	N or ↑	↑

ALT = alanine aminotransferase; **AST** = aspartate aminotransferase

Data from Tierney LM Jr, McPhee SJ, Papadakis MA (editors). Current Medical Diagnosis & Treatment 1996. *Originally published by Appleton & Lange. Copyright © 1996 by The McGraw-Hill Companies, Inc.;* and from Harvey AM et al (editors): The Principles and Practice of Medicine, 22nd ed. *Originally published by Appleton & Lange. Copyright © 1988 by The McGraw-Hill Companies, Inc.*

TABLE 8–15. OSMOL GAP: CALCULATION AND APPLICATION IN CLINICAL TOXICOLOGY.

The osmol gap (Δ osm) is determined by subtracting the calculated serum osmolality from the measured serum osmolality.

Calculated

$$osmolality\ (oms) = 2(Na^+[meq/L]) + \frac{Glucose\ (mg/dL)}{18} + \frac{BUN\ (mg/dL)}{2.8}$$

osmol gap (Δoms) = Measured osmolality – Calculated osmolality

Serum osmolality may be increased by contributions of circulating alcohols and other low-molecular-weight substances. Since these substances are not included in the calculated osmolality, there will be a gap proportionate to their serum concentration and inversely proportionate to their molecular weight:

$$Serum\ concentration\ (mg/dL) = \Delta osm \times \frac{Molecular\ weight\ of\ toxin}{10}$$

For ethanol (the most common cause of Δ osm), a gap of 30 mosm/L indicates an ethanol level of:

$$30 \times \frac{46}{10} = 138\ mg/dL$$

See the following for toxic concentrations of alcohols and their corresponding osmol gaps.

TOXIC CONCENTRATIONS OF ALCOHOLS AND THEIR CORRESPONDING OSMOL GAPS

	Molecular Weight	Toxic Concentration (mg/dL)	Approximate Corresponding Δ osm (mosm/L)
Ethanol	46	300	65
Methanol	32	100	16
Ethylene glycol	60	100	16
Isopropanol	60	150	25

Note: The normal osmol gap may vary by as much as $\pm$ 10 mosm/L; thus, small osmol gaps may be unreliable in the diagnosis of poisoning. **BUN** = blood urea nitrogen; **Na**$^+$ = sodium.

Modified with permission from Stone CK, Humphries RL (editors): Current Emergency Diagnosis & Treatment, 6th ed. McGraw-Hill, 2008.

TABLE 8–16. RANSON CRITERIA FOR ASSESSING SEVERITY OF ACUTE PANCREATITIS.

Three or more of the following predict a severe course complicated by pancreatic necrosis with a sensitivity of 60–80%:

    Age >55 years
    White blood cell count > 16×10^3/mcL (16×10^9/L)
    Blood glucose > 200 mg/dL (11 mmol/L)
    Serum lactic dehydrogenase >350 units/L (7 mkat/L)
    Aspartate aminotransferase >250 units/L (5 mkat/L)

Development of the following in the first 48 hours indicates a worsening prognosis:

    Hematocrit drop of >10 percentage points
    Blood urea nitrogen rise >5 mg/dL (1.8 mmol/L)
    Arterial PO_2 <60 mm Hg (7.8 kPa)
    Serum calcium <8 mg/dL (0.2 mmol/L)
    Base deficit >4 meq/L
    Estimated fluid sequestration of >6 L

MORTALITY RATES CORRELATE WITH THE NUMBER OF CRITERIA PRESENT[1]

Number of Criteria	Mortality Rate
0–2	1%
3–4	16%
5–6	40%
7–8	100%

[1]*An Acute Physiology and Chronic Health Evaluation (APACHE) II score ≥ 8 also correlates with mortality.*

TABLE 8–17. SEVERITY INDEX FOR ACUTE PANCREATITIS.

CT Grade	Points	Pancreatic Necrosis	Additional Points	Severity Index[1]	Mortality Rate[2]
A Normal pancreas	0	0%	0	0	0%
B Pancreatic enlargement	1	0%	0	1	0%
C Pancreatic inflammation and/or peripancreatic fat	2	<30%	2	4	<3%
D Single acute peripancreatic fluid collection	3	30–50%	4	7	6%
E Two or more acute peripancreatic fluid collections or retroperitoneal air	4	>50%	6	10	>17%

[1]Severity index = CT Grade Points + Additional Points.
[2]Based on the severity index.
Adapted with permission from Balthazar EJ. Acute pancreatitis: assessment of severity with clinical and CT evaluation. Radiology. 2002;223(3):603.

TABLE 8–18. PLEURAL EFFUSION: PLEURAL FLUID PROFILES IN VARIOUS DISEASE STATES.

Diagnosis	Gross Appearance	Protein (g/dL)	Glucose[1] (mg/dL)	WBC and Differential (per mcL)	RBC (per mcL)	Microscopic Exam	Culture	Comments
Normal	Clear	1.0–1.5	Equal to serum	≤1000, mostly MN	0 or Few	Neg	Neg	
TRANSUDATES[2]								
Congestive heart failure	Serous	<3: some-times ≥3	Equal to serum	<1000	<10,000	Neg	Neg	Most common cause of pleural effusion. Effusion right-sided in 55–70% of patients.
Nephrotic syndrome	Serous	<3	Equal to serum	<1000	<1000	Neg	Neg	Occurs in 20% of patients. Cause is low protein osmotic pressure.
Hepatic cirrhosis	Serous	<3	Equal to serum	<1000	<1000	Neg	Neg	From movement of ascites across diaphragm. Treatment of underlying ascites usually sufficient.
EXUDATES[3]								
Tuberculosis	Serous to serosan-guineous	>4; may exceed 5 g/dL	Equal to serum; Occ <60	5000–10,000, mostly MN	<10,000	Concentrate Pos for AFB in <50%	May yield MTb	PPD usually positive; pleural biopsy positive; eosinophils (>10%) or mesothelial cells (>5%) make diagnosis unlikely.

	Appearance		Glucose	WBC	RBC	Cytology	Culture	Comments
Malignancy	Turbid to bloody; Occ serous	≥3 in 90%	Equal to serum; <60 in 15% of cases	1000 to <100,000 mostly MN	100–>100,000	Pos cytology in >50%	Neg	Eosinophils uncommon; fluid tends to reaccumulate after removal.
Empyema	Turbid to purulent	≥3	Less than serum; often <20	25,000–100,000, mostly PMN	<5000	Pos	Pos	Drainage necessary; putrid odor suggests anaerobic infection.
Parapneumonic effusion, uncomplicated	Clear to turbid	≥3	Equal to serum	5000–25,000, mostly PMN	<5000	Neg	Neg	Tube thoracostomy unnecessary; associated infiltrate on chest x-ray; fluid pH ≥7.2.
Pulmonary embolism, infarction	Serous to grossly bloody	≥3	Equal to serum	1000–50,000, MN or PMN	100–>100,000	Neg	Neg	Variable findings; no pathognomonic features; 25% are transudates.
Rheumatoid	Turbid or yellow-green	≥3	Very low (<40 in most)	1000–20,000, mostly MN	<1000	Neg	Neg	Secondary empyema common; high LDH, low complement, high rheumatoid factor, cholesterol crystals are characteristic.
Pancreatitis	Turbid to serosanguineous	≥3	Equal to serum	1000–50,000, mostly PMN	1000–10,000	Neg	Neg	Effusion usually left-sided; high amylase level.

(continued)

TABLE 8–18. PLEURAL EFFUSION: PLEURAL FLUID PROFILES IN VARIOUS DISEASE STATES. *(CONTINUED)*

Diagnosis	Gross Appearance	Protein (g/dL)	Glucose[1] (mg/dL)	WBC and Differential (per mcL)	RBC (per mcL)	Microscopic Exam	Culture	Comments
Esophageal rupture	Turbid to purulent; red-brown	≥3	Equal to serum	<5000–>50,000, mostly PMN	1000–10,000	Pos	Pos	Usually left-sided; high fluid amylase level (salivary); pneumothorax in 25% of cases; pH <6.0 strongly suggests diagnosis.

[1]Glucose of pleural fluid in comparison to serum glucose.

[2]Transudative effusions also occur in myxedema and sarcoidosis.

[3]Exudative pleural effusions meet at least one of the following criteria: (1) pleural fluid protein/serum protein ratio >0.5; (2) pleural fluid LDH/serum LDH ratio >0.6; and (3) pleural fluid LDH >2/3 upper normal limit for serum LDH. Transudative pleural effusions meet none of these criteria.
AFB = acid-fast bacilli; **LDH** = lactate dehydrogenase; **MN** = mononuclear cells (lymphocytes or monocytes); **MTb** = Mycobacterium tuberculosis; **PMN** = polymorphonuclear cells.

Data from Therapy of pleural effusion. A statement by the Committee on Therapy. Am Rev Respir Dis 1968;97:479; Way LW (editor). Current Surgical Diagnosis & Treatment. 10th ed. Originally published by Appleton & Lange. Copyright © 1994 by The McGraw-Hill Companies, Inc McPhee SJ, Papadakis MA, Rabow MW (editors): Current Medical Diagnosis & Treatment 2012, 51st ed. McGraw Hill, 2012.

TABLE 8–19. PRENATAL DIAGNOSTIC METHODS: AMNIOCENTESIS AND CHORIONIC VILLUS SAMPLING.

Method	Procedure	Laboratory Analyses	Waiting Time for Results	Advantages	Disadvantages
Amniocentesis	Between the 15th and 20th weeks, and by the transabdominal approach, 20–30 mL of amniotic fluid is removed for analysis. Preceding ultrasound locates the placenta and identifies twinning and missed abortion.	**1. Amniotic fluid** • α-Fetoprotein, acetylcholinesterase • Biochemical analysis (metabolic diseases) • Virus isolation studies **2. Amniotic cell culture** • Chromosomal analysis (cytogenetic [karyotyping], molecular, certain gene mutation analyses)	2–4 weeks	Over 50 years of experience.	Therapeutic abortion, if indicated, must be done in the second trimester. (RhoGam should be given to Rh-negative mothers to prevent sensitization.) Risks: • Fetal: abortion (0.06–0.3%). • Maternal: transient vaginal spotting or amniotic fluid leakage (1.2%) or chorioamnionitis (<0.1%). Risks are somewhat higher if amniocentesis is performed earlier (11th to 14th weeks).
Chorionic villus sampling	Between the 10th and 12th week, and with constant ultrasound guidance, the trophoblastic cells of the chorionic villi are obtained by transcervical or transabdominal endoscopic needle biopsy or aspiration.	**1. Direct cell analysis** • Chromosomal and DNA analysis (cytogenetic, certain gene mutations) **2. Cell culture** • Biochemical analyses (as above)	1–10 days	Over 40 years of experience. Therapeutic abortion, if indicated, can be done in the first trimester.	Chromosomal abnormalities detected by this technique may be confined to the placenta (confined placental mosaicism) and thus CVS may be less informative than amniocentesis. Risks • Fetal: abortion (0.06–0.3%). • Maternal: spotting or infection (<0.5%).

TABLE 8–20. PULMONARY EMBOLISM: THE REVISED GENEVA SCORE FOR PROBABILITY ASSESSMENT.[1]

A. PROGNOSTIC MODEL FOR PULMONARY EMBOLISM (PESI SCORE).

Risk factor	Points
Age	No. of years of age
Male sex	10
Cancer	30
Heart failure	10
Chronic lung disease	10
Heart rate >110 bpm	20
Systolic blood pressure <100 mm Hg	20
Respiratory rate > 30 breaths per minute	20
Temperature < 36°C	20
Change in mental status	60
Oxygen saturation <90%	20

Severity class	Points	30-day mortality
I	0–65	<1.6%
II	66–85	<3.5%
III	86–105	<7.1%
IV	106–125	4–11.4%
V	>125	10–24.5%

[1]A comparison of different prediction rules can be found in Ceriani E et al. Clinical prediction rules for pulmonary embolism: a systematic review and meta-analysis.
J Thromb Haemost 2010;8:957. [PMID: 20149072]

Adapted with permission from Aujesky D et al: Derivation and validation of a prognostic model for pulmonary embolism. Am J Respir Crit Care Med 2005;Oct 15:172(8):1041-1046.

TABLE 8–20. PULMONARY EMBOLISM: THE REVISED GENEVA SCORE FOR PROBABILITY ASSESSMENT. (*CONTINUED*)

B. RISK STRATIFICATION IN PULMONARY EMBOLISM.

PE-related early mortality	Hypotension	ECHO/CTA/ Biomarkers	PESI Scale Score	Treatment
High-risk (>15%)	Yes	—	—	Thrombolysis and anticoagulation
Intermediate risk (3–15%)	No	Echo—RV dys-function CTA RV/LV ratio > 1.0	>II	Inpatient treatment Consider throm-bolysis on case-by-case basis
Low-risk (<3%)	No	Echo—No RV dysfunction CTA RV/LV ratio <1.0 No BNP or tro-ponin elevation	I–II	Expedite discharge May consider out-patient treatment

BNP = brain natriuretic peptide; *CTA* = computed tomographic angiography; *Echo* = echocardiogram; *LV* = left ventricle; *PE* = pulmonary embolism; *RV* = right ventricle.

Adapted, with permission, from Torbicki A et al; Task Force for the Diagnosis and Management of Acute Pulmonary Embolism of the European Society of Cardiology. Guidelines on the diagnosis and management of acute pulmonary embolism: the Task Force for the Diagnosis and Management of Acute Pulmonary Embolism of the European Society of Cardiology (ESC). Eur Heart J 2008;29:2276.

TABLE 8–21. PULMONARY FUNCTION TESTS: INTERPRETATION IN OBSTRUCTIVE AND RESTRICTIVE PULMONARY DISEASE.

Tests	Units	Definition	Obstructive Disease	Restrictive Disease
SPIROMETRY				
Forced vital capacity (FVC)	L	The volume that can be forcefully expelled from the lungs after maximal inspiration.	N or ↓	↓
Forced expiratory volume in 1 second (FEV₁)	L	The volume expelled in the first second of the FVC maneuver.	↓	N or ↓
FEV₁/FVC [1]	%		↓	N or ↑
Forced expiratory flow from 25% to 75% of the forced vital capacity (FEF 25–75%)	L/sec	The maximal midexpiratory airflow rate.	↓	N or ↓
Peak expiratory flow rate (PEFR)	L/sec	The maximal airflow rate achieved in the FVC maneuver.	↓	N or ↑
Maximum voluntary ventilation (MVV)	L/min	The maximum volume that can be breathed in 1 minute (usually measured for 15 seconds and multiplied by 4).	↓	N or ↓
LUNG VOLUMES				
Slow vital capacity (SVC)	L	The volume that can be slowly exhaled after maximal inspiration.	N or ↓	↓
Total lung capacity (TLC)	L	The volume in the lungs after a maximal inspiration.	N or ↑	↓
Functional residual capacity (FRC)	L	The volume in the lungs at the end of a normal tidal expiration.	↑	N or ↑
Expiratory reserve volume (ERV)	L	The volume representing the difference between FRC and RV.	N or ↓	N or ↓
Residual volume (RV)	L	The volume remaining in the lungs after maximal expiration.	↑	N or ↑
RV/TLC ratio			↑	N or ↑

N = normal; ↓ = less than predicted; ↑ = greater than predicted. Normal values vary according to subject sex, age, body size, and ethnicity.

[1] Perhaps the most useful single parameter for differentiating obstructive from restrictive lung disease.

Modified, with permission, from Tierney LM Jr, McPhee SJ, Papadakis MA (editors). Current Medical Diagnosis & Treatment 2001. McGraw-Hill, 2001.

TABLE 8–22. RENAL FAILURE: CLASSIFICATION AND DIFFERENTIAL DIAGNOSIS.

Classification	Prerenal Azotemia	Postrenal Azotemia	Acute Tubular Necrosis (Oliguric or Polyuric)	Intrinsic Renal Disease		Acute Interstitial Nephritis
				Acute Glomerulonephritis		
Etiology	Poor renal perfusion (eg, hypovolemia (vomiting, diarrhea), hypotension, severe heart failure	Obstruction of the urinary tract	Ischemia, nephrotoxins	Immune complex-mediated, pauci-immune, anti-GBM related	Allergic reaction; drug reaction; infection; collagen vascular disease
Serum BUN: Cr ratio	>20:1	>20:1	<20:1	>20:1	<20:1
Urinary indices U_{Na^+} (meq/L)	<20	Variable	>20	<20	Variable
FE_{Na^+} (%)	<1	Variable	>1 (when oliguric,	<1	<1; >1
Urine osmolality (mosm/kg)	>500	<400	250–300	Variable	Variable
Urinary sediment	Benign, or hyaline casts	Normal or red cells, white cells, or crystals	Granular (muddy brown) casts, renal tubular casts	Red cells, dysmorphic red cells, and red cell casts	White cells, white cell casts, with or without eosinophils

BUN:Cr = *blood urea nitrogen:creatinine ratio.*

$$FE_{Na^+} = \left(\frac{Urine\ Na^+}{Plasma\ Na^+} \middle/ \frac{Urine\ creatinine}{Plasma\ creatinine} \right) \times 100$$

U_{Na^+} = *urine sodium.*

TABLE 8-23. RENAL TUBULAR ACIDOSIS (RTA): LABORATORY DIAGNOSIS.

Clinical Condition	Renal Defect	GFR	Serum HCO_3^- (meq/L)	Serum K^+ (meq/L)	Minimal Urine pH	Urinary Anion Gap	Associated Disease States	Treatment
Normal	None	N	24–28	3.5–5	4.8–5.2	Absent	None	None
I. Classic distal RTA	Distal H^+ secretion	N	20–23	↓	>5.5	Pos	Various genetic disorders, autoimmune diseases, paraproteinemias, nephrocalcinosis, nephrolithiasis, drugs [amphotericin], toxins, tubulointerstitial diseases.	$NaHCO_3$ (1–3 meq/kg/d).
II. Proximal RTA	Proximal H^+ secretion	N	15–18	↓	<5.5	Pos	Drugs, Fanconi syndrome, various genetic disorders, dysproteinemic states, secondary hyperparathyroidism, toxins (heavy metals), tubulointerstitial diseases, nephrotic syndrome, paroxysmal nocturnal hemoglobinuria.	$NaHCO_3$ or $KHCO_3$ (10–15 meq/kg/d), thiazides.
IV. Hyporeninemic hypoaldosteronemic RTA	Distal Na^+ reabsorption, K^+ secretion, and H^+ secretion	↓	24–28	↑	<5.5	Pos	Hyporeninemic hypoaldosteronism (diabetes mellitus, tubulointerstitial diseases, hypertensive nephrosclerosis, AIDS, drugs [ACE inhibitors, spironolactone, NSAIDs]), primary mineralocorticoid deficiency (eg, Addison disease), salt-wasting mineralocorticoid-resistant hyperkalemia.	Fludrocortisone (0.1–0.5 mg/d), dietary K^+ restriction, furosemide (40–160 mg/d), $NaHCO_3$ (1–3 meq/kg/d).

GFR = glomerular filtration rate.

Adapted from Cogan MG. Fluid & Electrolytes:
Physiology & Pathophysiology. Originally published by Appleton & Lange. Copyright © 1991 by the McGraw-Hill Companies, Inc.

TABLE 8-24. SYPHILIS: CLINICAL AND LABORATORY DIAGNOSIS IN UNTREATED PATIENTS.

	Primary Stage	Secondary Stage	Latent Stage	Late (Tertiary) Stage	
CLINICAL					
Onset After Exposure	21 days (range 10–90)	6 wk–6 mo	Early: <1 yr Late: >1 yr	1 yr until death	
Persistence	2–12 wk	1–3 mo	Early: Up to 1 year Late: Lifelong unless late (tertiary) syphilis appears	Until death	
Clinical Findings	Chancre	Rash, condylomata lata, mucous patches, fever, lymphadenopathy, patchy alopecia	Early: Relapses of secondary syphilis Late: Clinically silent	Dementia, tabes dorsalis, aortitis, aortic aneurysm, gummas	
LABORATORY	Test Sensitivity by stage of infection, % (range)				**Test Specificity, % (range)**
Nontreponemal tests					
VDRL	78 (74–87)	100	96 (88–100)	71 (37–94)	98 (96–99)
RPR	86 (77–99)	100	98 (95–100)	73	98 (93–99)
Early treponemal tests					
TP-PA	88 (86–100)	100	100	NA	96 (95–100)
FTA-ABS	84 (70–100)	100	100	96	97 (94–100)

(continued)

TABLE 8–24. SYPHILIS: CLINICAL AND LABORATORY DIAGNOSIS IN UNTREATED PATIENTS. *(CONTINUED)*

	Primary Stage	Secondary Stage	Latent Stage	Late (Tertiary) Stage
Enzyme immunoassays				
IgG-ELISA	100	100	100	NA
IgM-EIA	93	85	64	NA
ICE	77	100	100	100
Immunochemiluminescence assays				
CLIA	98	100	100	100

CLIA = chemiluminescence assay; **EIA** = enzyme immunoassay; **ELISA** = enzyme-linked immunosorbent assay; **FTA-ABS** = fluorescent treponemal antibody absorption test; **ICE** = immune-capture EIA; **IgG** = immunoglobulin G; **IgM** = immunoglobulin M; **NA** = not available; **RPR** = rapid plasma reagin test; **TPPA** = Treponema pallidum particle agglutination; **VDRL** = Venereal Disease Research Laboratories test.

Data used, with permission, from Sena AC et al. Novel Treponema pallidum serologic tests: a paradigm shift in syphilis screening for the 21st century. Clin Infect Dis 2010;51:700.

TABLE 8–25. THALASSEMIA SYNDROMES: GENETICS AND LABORATORY CHARACTERISTICS.

α-Thalassemia[1]			
Syndrome	α-Globin Genes	Hematocrit	MCV (fL)
Normal	4	N	N
Silent carrier	3	N	N
Thalassemia minor	2	28–40%	60–75
Hemoglobin H disease	1	22–32%	60–70
Hydrops fetalis	0	Fetal death occurs in utero	

[1]Alpha thalassemias are due primarily to deletion of the α-globin genes on chromosome 16.

β-Thalassemia[1]			
Syndrome	β-Globin Genes	Hb A[2]	Hb A$_2$[3]	Hb F[4]
Normal	Homozygous beta	97–99%	1–3%	<1%
Thalassemia minor	Heterozygous beta^0 [5]	80–95%	4–8%	1–5%
	Heterozygous beta$^+$ [6]	80–95%	4–8%	1–5%
Thalassemia intermedia	Homozygous beta$^+$ (mild)	0–30%	0–10%	6–100%
Thalassemia major	Homozygous beta^0	0%	4–10%	90–96%
	Homozygous beta$^+$	0–10%	4–10%	90–96%

[1]β-Thalassemias are usually caused by point mutations in the β-globin gene on chromosome 11 that result in premature chain terminations or defective RNA transcription, leading to reduced or absent β-globin-chain synthesis.

[2]Hb A is composed of two α chains and two β chains: $\alpha_2\beta_2$.

[3]Hb A$_2$ is composed of two α chains and two δ chains: $\alpha_2\delta_2$.

[4]Hb F is composed of two α chains and two γ chains: $\alpha_2\gamma_2$.

[5]β^0 refers to defects that result in absent globin-chain synthesis.

[6]β^+ refers to defects that cause reduced globin-chain synthesis.

Hb = hemoglobin; **MCV** = mean corpuscular volume.

Modified, with permission, from McPhee SJ, Papadakis MA, Rabow MW (editors). Current Medical Diagnosis & Treatment 2012. 51st ed., McGraw-Hill, 2012.

TABLE 8-26. THYROID FUNCTION TESTING AND ITS CLINICAL APPLICATION.

Condition	TSH (mcU/mL)[1]	Free T4 (ng/dL)	Total T4 (mcg/dL)	Total T3 (ng/dL)	Comments and Treatment
Normal[2]	0.35–5.5	Varies with method	5–12	95–190	
Hyperthyroidism	↓	↑	↑	↑	Thyroid scan shows increased diffuse activity (Graves disease) versus "hot" areas (hyperfunctioning nodules). Thyroperoxidase (TPO) and thyroid-stimulating antibody (TSI) elevated in Graves disease.
Hypothyroidism	Usually ↑ (primary[3] hypothyroidism), rarely ↓ (secondary[4] hypothyroidism)	↓	↓	↓	TRH stimulation test shows exaggerated response in primary hypothyroidism. In secondary hypothyroidism, TRH test helps to differentiate pituitary from hypothalamic disorders. In pituitary lesions, TSH fails to rise after TRH; in hypothalamic lesion, TSH rises but response is delayed. Antithyroglobulin and thyroperoxidase (TPO) antibodies elevated in Hashimoto's thyroiditis.
HYPOTHYROIDISM ON REPLACEMENT					
T4 replacement	N or ↓	N	N	∨	TSH ↓ with 0.1–0.2 mg T4 daily.
T3 replacement	N or ↓	↓	↓	∨	TSH ↓ with 50 mcg T3 daily.
Euthyroid following injection of radiocontrast dye	N	N or ↑	N	N	Effects may persist for 2 weeks or longer.

PREGNANCY

					Comments
Hyperthyroid	↓	↑	↑	↑	Effects may persist for 6–10 weeks post-partum
Euthyroid	N	↑	↓	↓	
Hypothyroid	↑	↓	N or ↓	↑	
Oral contraceptives, estrogens, methadone, heroin	N	↑	↓	↑	Increased serum thyroid-binding globulin.
Glucocorticoids, androgens, phenytoin, asparaginase, salicylates (high dose)	N	↓	↑	N or ↓	Decreased serum thyroid-binding globulin.
Nephrotic syndrome	N	↓	↑	N or ↓	Loss of thyroid-binding globulin accounts for serum T$_4$ decrease.
Iodine deficiency	N	↓	N	↑↓	Extremely rare in the United States.
Iodine ingestion	N	N	N	N	Excess iodine may cause hypothyroidism or hyperthyroidism in susceptible individuals.

(continued)

TABLE 8–26. THYROID FUNCTION TESTING AND ITS CLINICAL APPLICATION. (*CONTINUED*)

Laboratory Test Results	Most Common Diagnosis	Other Common Diagnoses
Low TSH, Elevated free T_3 or T_4	Graves disease	Multinodular goiter Toxic nodule Transient thyroiditis
Low TSH, normal free T_3 or T_4	Subclinical hyperthyroidism	Recent thyroxine ingestion for hypothyroidism
Low or normal TSH, low free T_3 or T_4	Nonthyroidal illness[5]	Recent treatment for hyperthyroidism Secondary (pituitary) hypothyroidism
Elevated TSH, low free T_4 or T_3	Chronic autoimmune thyroiditis (Hashimoto disease)	Hypothyroid phase of transient thyroiditis Previous neck irradiation or thyroid surgery Iodine deficiency Drugs (eg, amiodarone)
Elevated TSH, normal free T_4 and T_3	Subclinical autoimmune thyroiditis	Heterophile antibody Incomplete treatment for hypothyroidism
Normal or elevated TSH, elevated free T_4 or T_3	None	Interfering antibodies Intermittent T_4 therapy TSH-secreting pituitary tumor

[1] Thyroid function screening should start with TSH, and a TSH assay with ≤0.02 mcU/mL functional sensitivity is recommended.

[2] Normal values vary with laboratory.

[3] Thyroid (end-organ) failure.

[4] Pituitary or hypothalamic lesions.

[5] Commonly referred to as "euthyroid sick."

N = *normal;* ***V*** = *variable.*

Data from Dayan CM. Interpretation of thyroid function tests. Lancet 2001;357:619. [PMID: 11558500]

TABLE 8-27. TRANSFUSION: SUMMARY CHART OF BLOOD COMPONENT THERAPY.[1]

Component	Major Indications	Action/Benefit	Not Indicated For	Special Precautions	Hazards[1]	Rate/Time of Infusion
Whole blood	Symptomatic anemia with large volume deficit	Increases oxygen-carrying capacity. Increases blood volume	Condition responsive to specific component. Treatment of coagulopathy.	Must be ABO identical	Infectious diseases; hemolytic, septic/toxic, allergic, febrile reactions; TACO, TRALI, TA-GVHD	As fast as patient can tolerate but less than 4 hours
Red blood cells; Red blood cells, low volume; Apheresis red blood cells	Symptomatic anemia	Increases oxygen-carrying capacity	Pharmacologically treatable anemia. Coagulation deficiency. Volume expansion.	Must be ABO-compatible	Infectious diseases; hemolytic, septic/toxic, allergic, febrile reactions; TACO, TRALI, TA-GVHD	As fast as patient can tolerate but less than 4 hours
Red blood cells, leukocyte-reduced[4]	Symptomatic anemia. Reduction of febrile reactions	Increases oxygen-carrying capacity. Reduction of risks of febrile reactions, HLA alloimmunization and CMV infection	Pharmacologically treatable anemia ———— Coagulation deficiency. Volume expansion. Prevention of TA-GVHD.	Must be ABO-compatible	Infectious diseases; hemolytic, septic/toxic, allergic, febrile reactions. TACO, TRALI, TA-GVHD. Hypotensive reaction may occur if bedside leukocyte reduction filter is used.	As fast as patient can tolerate but less than 4 hours

(continued)

TABLE 8–27. TRANSFUSION: SUMMARY CHART OF BLOOD COMPONENT THERAPY.[1] (*CONTINUED*)

Component	Major Indications	Action/Benefit	Not Indicated For	Special Precautions	Hazards[1]	Rate/Time of Infusion
Red blood cells, washed	Symptomatic anemia. IgA deficiency with anaphylactoid reaction. Recurrent severe allergic reactions to unwashed red cell products. Paroxysmal nocturnal hemoglobinuria.	Increases oxygen carrying capacity. Washing reduces plasma proteins. Risk of allergic reactions may be reduced.	Pharmacologically treatable anemia. Coagulation deficiency. Volume expansion.	Must be ABO compatible	Infectious diseases. Hemolytic, septic/ toxic, allergic, febrile reactions. TACO, TRALI, TA-GVHD.	As fast as patient can tolerate but less than 4 hours.
Fresh-frozen plasma (FFP)[2]	Clinically significant plasma protein deficiencies when no specific coagulation factors are available. TTP.	Source of plasma proteins, including all coagulation factors.	Volume expansion. Coagulopathy that can be more effectively treated with specific therapy.	Must be ABO-compatible	Infectious diseases, allergic reactions, TACO, TRALI.	Less than 4 hours.
Cryoprecipitated AHF; Pooled cryo-precipitated AHF	Hemophilia A,[3] von Willebrand's disease,[3] hypofibrinogenemia, factor XIII deficiency.	Provides factor VIII, fibrinogen, von Willebrand factor, factor XIII.	Deficit of any plasma protein other than those enriched in cryo-precipitated AHF.		Infectious diseases; allergic reactions.	Less than 4 hours.

	Bleeding due to thrombocytopenia or platelet function abnormality; prevention of bleeding from marrow hypoplasia.	Improves hemostasis. May be HLA (or other antigen) selected.	Plasma coagulation deficits, some conditions with rapid platelet destruction (eg, ITP, TTP) unless life-threatening hemorrhage.	Should not use some filters (check manufacturer's instructions)	Infectious diseases; Septic/toxic, allergic, febrile reactions, TACO, TA-GVHD, TRALI.	Less than 4 hours.
Apheresis platelets[4], Pooled platelet concentrates						
Apheresis granulocytes	Neutropenia with infection, unresponsive to appropriate antibiotics.	Provides granulocytes with or without platelets.	Infection responsive to antibiotics; eventual marrow recovery not expected.	Must be ABO-compatible. Should not use some filters (check manufacturer's instructions)	Infectious diseases; hemolytic, allergic, febrile reactions, TACO, TRALI, TA-GVHD.	One unit over 2–4 hours. Observe closely for reactions.

[1]For all cellular components, there is a risk that the recipient may become alloimmunized and experience rapid destruction of certain types of blood products. Red cell to containing components and thawed plasma should be stored at 1–6°C. Platelets, granulocytes, and thawed cryoprecipitate should be stored at 20–24°C.

[2]Solvent detergent pooled plasma is an alternative in which some viruses are inactivated, but clotting factor composition is changed.

[3]When virus-inactivated concentrates are not available.

[4]Red blood cells and platelets may be processed in a manner that yields leukocyte-reduced components. The main indications for leukocyte-reduced components are prevention of febrile, nonhemolytic transfusion reactions and prevention of leukocyte alloimmunization. Risks are the same as for standard components except for reduced risk of febrile reactions, HLA alloimmunization and CMV infection. One unit of apheresis platelet is equivalent to 68 units of platelet concentrates.

AHF = antihemophilic factor; **ITP** = idiopathic thrombocytopenic purpura; **TACO** = transfusion-associated circulatory overload; **TA-GVHD** = transfusion-associated graft-versus-host disease; **TRALI** = transfusion-related acute lung injury; **TTP** = thrombotic thrombocytopenic purpura.

Adapted from American Association of Blood Banks, American Red Cross, America's Blood Centers. Circulars of information for the use of human blood and blood components. December 2009 (available at http://www.aabb.org).

TABLE 8–28. URINALYSIS: FINDINGS IN VARIOUS DISEASE STATES.

Disease	Daily Volume	Specific Gravity	Glucose (mg/dL)	Ketones (mg/dL)	Protein (mg/dL)	Esterase (mg/dL)	Nitrite	RBC	WBC	Casts	Other Microscopic Findings
Normal	600–2500 mL	1.001–1.035	Neg	Neg	0–trace (0–15)	Neg	Neg	0 or Occ	0 or Occ	0 or Occ	Hyaline casts
Fever	↓	↑	Neg	Neg	Trace or 1+ (<30)	Neg	Neg	0	Occ	0 or Occ	Hyaline casts, tubular cells
Congestive heart failure	↓	↑ (varies)	Neg	Neg	1–2+ (30–100)	Neg	Neg	None or 1+	0	1+	Hyaline and granular casts
Hypertension	N or ↑	N or ↓	Neg	Neg	None or 1+ (<30)	Neg	Neg	0 or Occ	0 or Occ	0 or 1+	Hyaline and granular casts
Eclampsia	↓	↑	Neg	Neg	3–4+ (300–>2000)	Neg	Neg	None or 1+	0	3–4+	Hyaline casts
Diabetic hyperglycemic coma	↑ or ↓	↑	½–2+ (500–>2000)	Mod–Large (40–≥160)	1+ (30)	Neg	Neg	0	0	0 or 1+	Hyaline casts
Acute glomerulonephritis	↓	↑	Neg	Neg	2–4+ (100–2000)	Pos	Neg	1–4+	1–4+	2–4+	Blood; RBC, cellular, granular, and hyaline casts; renal tubular epithelium

Nephrotic syndrome	N or ↓	N or ↑	Neg	Neg	4+ (>2000)	Neg	Neg	1–2+	0	4+	Granular, waxy, hyaline, and fatty casts; fatty tubular cells
Chronic renal failure	↑ or ↓	Low; invariable	Neg	Neg	1–2+ (30–100)	Neg	Neg	Occ or 1+	0	1–3+	Granular, hyaline, fatty, and broad casts
Connective tissue disorders	N, ↑, or ↓	N or ↓	Neg	Neg	1–4+ (30–>2000)	Neg	Neg	1–4+	0 or Occ	1–4+	Blood, cellular, granular, hyaline, waxy, fatty, and broad casts; fatty tubular cells; "teles-coped" sediment
Pyelonephritis	N or ↓	N or ↓	Neg	Neg	1–2+ (30–100)	Pos	Pos	0 or 1+	4+	0 or 1+	WBC casts and hyaline casts; many pus cells; bacteria

Glucose, ketone, and protein concentrations in mg/dL are listed in parentheses.

TABLE 8–29. VAGINAL DISCHARGE: LABORATORY EVALUATION.

Diagnosis	pH[1]	Odor With KOH (Positive "Whiff" Test)	Epithelial Cells	WBCs	Organisms	KOH Prep	Gram Stain	Comments
Normal	<4.5	No	N	Occ	Variable, large rods not adherent to epithelial cells	Neg	Gram-positive rods	
Candida albicans vaginitis	<4.5	No	N	Occ to slight ↑	Budding yeast or hyphae	Pos	Budding yeast or hyphae	Inspection usually shows a white "cottage cheese" curd. Fungal culture can confirm the diagnosis (see p. 351 [Ch 5])
Bacterial vaginosis (*Gardnerella vaginalis*)	>4.5	Yes	Clue cells[2]	Occ	Coccobacilli adherent to epithelial cells	Neg	Gram-negative coccobacilli	*G. vaginalis* can be isolated on culture as the predominant organism in cases of vaginosis, which is so named because inflammatory cells are not present

Mucopurulent cervicitis (*N. gonorrhoeae*)	Variable	No	N	↑	Variable	Neg	Intracellular gram-negative diplococci	Culture was formerly the gold standard for diagnosis, particularly when Gram stain was negative. Nucleic acid amplification tests for *N. gonorrhoeae* in cervical swab specimens or urine now permit rapid diagnosis, have excellent sensitivity and specificity, and have largely replaced culture (see p. 352 [Ch 5])
Trichomonas vaginalis vaginitis	>4.5	Yes	N	↑	Motile, flagellated organisms	Neg	Flagellated organisms	Parasitic protozoa, *T. vaginalis*, may be isolated in women from vagina, urethra, cervix, Bartholin and Skene glands, and bladder

[1]Nitrazine paper can be used to estimate pH of vaginal secretions.

[2]Epithelial cells covered with bacteria to the extent that cell nuclear borders *are obscured*.

TABLE 8–30. VALVULAR HEART DISEASE: DIAGNOSTIC EVALUATION.

	Mitral Stenosis	Mitral Regurgitation	Aortic Stenosis	Aortic Regurgitation	Tricuspid Stenosis	Tricuspid Regurgitation
Inspection	Malar flush, precordial bulge, and diffuse pulsation in young patients.	Usually prominent and hyperdynamic apical impulse to left of MCL.	Sustained PMI, prominent atrial filling wave.	Hyperdynamic PMI to left of MCL and downward. Visible carotid pulsations. Pulsating nailbeds (Quincke), head bob (deMusset).	Giant *a* wave in jugular pulse with sinus rhythm. Peripheral edema or ascites, or both.	Large *v* wave in jugular pulse; time with carotid pulsation. Peripheral edema or ascites, or both.
Palpation	"Tapping" sensation over area of expected PMI. Right ventricular pulsation left third to fifth ICS parasternally when pulmonary hypertension is present. P_2 may be palpable.	Forceful, brisk PMI; systolic thrill over PMI. Pulse normal, small, or slightly collapsing.	Powerful, heaving PMI to left and slightly below MCL. Systolic thrill over aortic area, sternal notch, or carotid arteries in severe disease. Small and slowly rising carotid pulse. If bicuspid AS check for delay at femoral artery to exclude coarctation.	Apical impulse forceful and displaced significantly to left and downward. Prominent carotid pulses. Rapidly rising and collapsing pulses (Corrigan pulse).	Pulsating, enlarged liver in ventricular systole.	Right ventricular pulsation. Systolic pulsation of liver.

Heart sounds, rhythm, and blood pressure	S₁ loud if valve mobile. Opening snap following S₂. The worse the disease, the closer the S₂-opening snap interval.	S₁ normal or buried in early part of murmur (exception in mitral prolapse where murmur may be late). Prominent third heart sound when severe MR. Atrial fibrillation common. Blood pressure normal. Midsystolic clicks may be present and may be multiple.	A_2 normal, soft, or absent. Prominent S₄. Blood pressure normal with high diastolic pressure.	S₁ normal or reduced, A₂ loud. Wide pulse pressure with diastolic pressure <60 mm Hg. When severe, gentle compression of femoral artery with diaphragm of stethoscope may reveal diastolic flow (Duroziez) and pressure in leg on palpation >40 mm Hg than arm (Hill).	S₁ often loud.	Atrial fibrillation may be present.
			Murmurs			
Location and transmission	Localized at or near apex. Diastolic rumble best heard in left lateral position; may be accentuated by having patient do sit-ups. Rarely, short diastolic murmur along lower left sternal border (Graham Steell) in severe pulmonary hypertension.	Loudest over PMI; posteriorly directed jets (ie, anterior mitral prolapse) transmitted to left axilla, left infrascapular area; anteriorly directed jets (ie, posterior mitral prolapse) heard over anterior precordium. Murmur unchanged after premature beat.	Right second ICS parasternally or at apex, heard in carotid arteries and occasionally in upper interscapular area. May sound like MR at apex (Gallavardin phenomenon), but murmur occurs after S₁ and stops before S₂. The later the peak in the murmur, the more severe the AS	Diastolic: louder along left sternal border in third to fourth interspace. Heard over aortic area and apex. May be associated with low-pitched middiastolic murmur at apex (Austin Flint) due to functional mitral stenosis. If due to an enlarged aorta, murmur may radiate to right sternal border.	Third to fifth ICS along left sternal border out to apex. Murmur increases with inspiration.	Third to fifth ICS along left sternal border. Murmur hard to hear but increases with inspiration. Sit-ups can increase cardiac output and accentuate.

(continued)

TABLE 8–30. VALVULAR HEART DISEASE: DIAGNOSTIC EVALUATION. *(CONTINUED)*

	Mitral Stenosis	Mitral Regurgitation	Aortic Stenosis	Aortic Regurgitation	Tricuspid Stenosis	Tricuspid Regurgitation
Timing	Relation of opening snap to A$_2$ important. The higher the LA pressure, the earlier the opening snap. Presystolic accentuation before S$_1$ if in sinus rhythm. Graham Steell begins with P$_2$ (early diastole) if associated pulmonary hypertension.	Pansystolic: begins with S$_1$ and ends at or after A$_2$. May be late systolic in mitral valve prolapse.	Begins after S$_1$, ends before A$_2$. The more severe the stenosis, the later the murmur peaks.	Begins immediately after aortic second sound and ends before first sound (blurring both); helps distinguish from MR.	Rumble often follows audible opening snap.	At times, hard to hear. Begins with S$_1$ and fills systole. Increases with inspiration.
Character	Low-pitched, rumbling; presystolic murmur merges with loud S$_1$.	Blowing, high-pitched; occasionally harsh or musical.	Harsh, rough.	Blowing, often faint.	As for mitral stenosis.	Blowing, coarse, or musical.
Optimum auscultatory conditions	After exercise, left lateral recumbence. Bell chest piece lightly applied.	After exercise; use diaphragm chest piece. In prolapse, findings may be more evident while standing.	Use stethoscope diaphragm. Patient resting, leaning forward, breath held in full expiration.	Use stethoscope diaphragm. Patient leaning forward, breath held in expiration.	Use stethoscope bell. Murmur usually louder and at peak during inspiration. Patient recumbent.	Use stethoscope diaphragm. Murmur usually becomes louder during inspiration.

Radiography	Straight left heart border from enlarged LA appendage. Elevation of left mainstem bronchus. Large right ventricle and pulmonary artery if pulmonary hypertension is present. Calcification in mitral valve in rheumatic mitral stenosis or in annulus in calcific mitral stenosis.	Enlarged left ventricle and LA.	Concentric left ventricular hypertrophy. Prominent ascending aorta. Calcified aortic valve common.	Moderate to severe left ventricular enlargement. Aortic root often dilated.	Enlarged right atrium with prominent SVC and azygous shadow.	Enlarged right atrium and right ventricle.
ECG	Broad P waves in standard leads; broad negative phase of diphasic P in V$_1$. If pulmonary hypertension is present, tall peaked P waves, right axis deviation, or right ventricular hypertrophy appears.	Left axis deviation or frank left ventricular hypertrophy. P waves broad, tall, or notched in standard leads. Broad negative phase of diphasic P in V$_1$.	Left ventricular hypertrophy.	Left ventricular hypertrophy.	Tall, peaked P waves. Possible right ventricular hypertrophy.	Right axis usual.

(continued)

TABLE 8–30. VALVULAR HEART DISEASE: DIAGNOSTIC EVALUATION. *(CONTINUED)*

	Mitral Stenosis	Mitral Regurgitation	Aortic Stenosis	Aortic Regurgitation	Tricuspid Stenosis	Tricuspid Regurgitation
			Echocardiography			
Two-dimensional echocardiography	Thickened, immobile mitral valve with anterior and posterior leaflets moving together. "Hockey stick" shape to opened anterior leaflet in rheumatic mitral stenosis. Annular calcium with thin leaflets in calcific mitral stenosis. LA enlargement, normal to small left ventricle. Orifice can be traced to approximate mitral valve orifice area.	Thickened mitral valve in rheumatic disease; mitral valve prolapse; flail leaflet or vegetations may be seen. Dilated left ventricle in volume overload. Operate for left ventricular end-systolic dimension >4.5 cm.	Dense persistent echoes from the aortic valve with poor leaflet excursion. Left ventricular hypertrophy late in the disease. Bicuspid valve in younger patients.	Abnormal aortic valve or dilated aortic root. Diastolic vibrations of the anterior leaflet of the mitral valve and septum. In acute aortic insufficiency, premature closure of the mitral valve before the QRS. When severe, dilated left ventricle with normal or decreased contractility. Operate when left ventricular end-systolic dimension >5.0 cm.	In rheumatic disease, tricuspid valve thickening, decreased early diastolic filling slope of the tricuspid valve. In carcinoid, leaflets fixed, but no significant thickening.	Enlarged right ventricle with paradoxical septal motion. Tricuspid valve often pulled open by displaced chordae.

Continuous and color flow Doppler and TEE	Prolonged pressure half-time across mitral valve allows estimation of gradient. MVA estimated from pressure half-time. Indirect evidence of pulmonary hypertension by noting elevated right ventricular systolic pressure measured from the tricuspid regurgitation jet.	Regurgitant flow mapped into LA. Use of PISA helps assess MR severity. TEE important in prosthetic mitral valve regurgitation.	increased transvalvular flow velocity; severe AS when peak jet >4 m/sec (64 mm Hg). Valve area estimate using continuity equation is poorly reproducible.	Demonstrates regurgitation and qualitatively estimates severity based on percentage of left ventricular outflow filled with jet and distance jet penetrates into left ventricle. TEE important in aortic valve endocarditis to exclude abscess. Mitral inflow pattern describes diastolic dysfunction.	Prolonged pressure half-time across tricuspid valve can be used to estimate mean gradient. Severe tricuspid stenosis present when mean gradient >5 mm Hg.	Regurgitant flow mapped into right atrium and venae cavae. Right ventricular systolic pressure estimated by tricuspid regurgitation jet velocity.

A_2 = aortic second sound; AS = aortic stenosis; ICS = intercostal space; LA = left atrial; MCL = midclavicular line; MR = mitral regurgitation; MVA = measured valve area; P_2 = pulmonary second sound; $PISA$ = proximal isovelocity surface area; PMI = point of maximal impulse; S_1 = first heart sound; S_2 = second heart sound; S_4 = fourth heart sound; SVC = superior vena cava; TEE = transesophageal echocardiography; V_1 = chest ECG lead 1.

Reproduced with permission, from McPhee SJ, Papadakis MA, Rabow MW (editors). Current Medical Diagnosis & Treatment 2012, 51st ed. McGraw-Hill, 2012.

TABLE 8-31. WHITE BLOOD CELLS: INTERPRETATION OF WHITE CELL COUNT AND DIFFERENTIAL.[1]

Cells	Range (10^3/mcL)	Increased in	Decreased in
WBC count (total)	4.0–11.0	Infection, hematologic and lymphoid malignancies.	Decreased production (aplastic anemia, folate or B_{12} deficiency, drugs [eg, ethanol, chloramphenicol]); decreased life span (sepsis, hypersplenism, drugs).
Neutrophils	1.8–6.8	Infection (bacterial or early viral), acute stress, acute and chronic inflammation, tumors, drugs (eg, G-CSF), diabetic ketoacidosis, leukemia (rare).	Aplastic anemia, drug-induced neutropenia, chemotherapy, folate or B_{12} deficiency, myelodysplasia, marrow infiltration, cyclic neutropenia, autoimmune or isoimmune neutropenia, Felty syndrome, hypersplenism, sepsis, viral marrow suppression, myelokathexis, congenital (eg, Kostmann syndrome), bone marrow failure syndromes.
Lymphocytes	0.9–2.9	Viral infection (especially infectious mononucleosis, pertussis), thyrotoxicosis, adrenal insufficiency, lymphoid leukemia/lymphoma, chronic infection, drug and allergic reactions, autoimmune diseases.	Immune deficiency syndromes (eg, HIV), idiopathic, drugs.
Monocytes	0.1–0.6	Inflammation, infection, malignancy, tuberculosis, myeloproliferative disorders (eg, CMML).	Depleted in overwhelming bacterial infection, hairy cell leukemia.
Eosinophils	0.0–0.4	Allergic states, asthma, drug sensitivity reactions, skin disorders, parasitic and certain fungal infections, Churg-Strauss syndrome, polyarteritis nodosa, response to malignancy (eg, Hodgkin disease, T-cell lymphoma, adenocarcinoma), eosinophilic pneumonia, hypereosinophilic syndrome, leukemia (eg, chronic eosinophilic leukemia), myeloid or lymphoid neoplasm with abnormality of PDGF receptor (alpha or beta) or FGF receptor, mastocytosis.	Acute and chronic inflammation, stress, drugs (corticosteroids).

| Basophils | 0.0–0.1 | Hypersensitivity reactions, drugs, myeloproliferative disorders (eg, CML), basophilic or mast cell variant of acute or chronic leukemia, inflammatory reaction, certain infections, hypothyroidism. | Not applicable. |

[1]In the automated differential, white cells are classified as neutrophils, monocytes, lymphocytes, eosinophils or basophils based on its size and surface/internal characteristics (eg, granularity, peroxidase). Different instruments use different methodologies for the differential.

The reproducibility of 100-cell manual differentials is notoriously poor. Review of blood smears is useful to visually identify abnormal cells (eg, immature granulocytes, toxic changes, dysplastic cells, blasts, nucleated RBCs, etc).

CML = chronic myeloid leukemia; **CMML** = chronic myelomonocytic leukemia.

9

Diagnostic Algorithms

Chuanyi Mark Lu, MD, Stephen J. McPhee, MD, Diana Nicoll, MD, PhD, MPA, and Michael Pignone, MD, MPH

HOW TO USE THIS SECTION

This section shows how diagnostic tests can be used in differential diagnosis and difficult diagnostic challenges. Material is presented in algorithmic forms, and contents are listed in alphabetical order by condition.

Abbreviations used throughout this section include the following: N = Normal; ↑ = Increased or high; ↓ = Decreased or low.

Each algorithm uses the following conventions:

SUSPECTED DIAGNOSIS/CLINICAL SITUATION

↓

Diagnostic test

↙ ↘

Test abnormal   Test normal

↓ ↓

Diagnosis   *Diagnosis*

↓

Treatment

Contents (Figures)   *Pages*

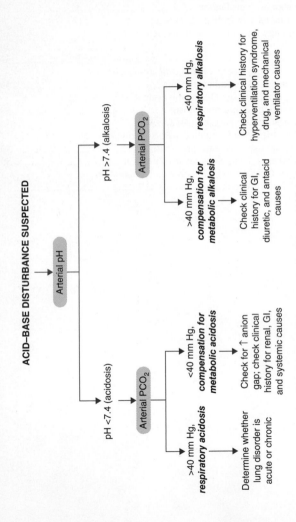

Figure 9–1. ACID–BASE DISTURBANCES: Diagnostic approach. **GI** = *gastrointestinal.*

ACID–BASE DISTURBANCE SUSPECTED

Arterial pH

pH <7.4 (acidosis)

Arterial PCO_2

>40 mm Hg, *respiratory acidosis*

Determine whether lung disorder is acute or chronic

<40 mm Hg, *compensation for metabolic acidosis*

Check for ↑ anion gap; check clinical history for renal, GI, and systemic causes

pH >7.4 (alkalosis)

Arterial PCO_2

>40 mm Hg, *compensation for metabolic alkalosis*

Check clinical history for GI, diuretic, and antacid causes

<40 mm Hg, *respiratory alkalosis*

Check clinical history for hyperventilation syndrome, drug, and mechanical ventilator causes

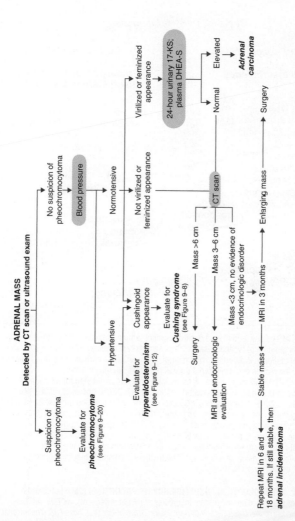

Figure 9-2. ADRENAL MASS: Diagnostic evaluation. **CT** = computed tomography; **DHEA-S** = dehydroepiandrosterone sulfate; **17-KS** = 17-ketosteroids; **MRI** = magnetic resonance imaging.

ADRENOCORTICAL INSUFFICIENCY SUSPECTED

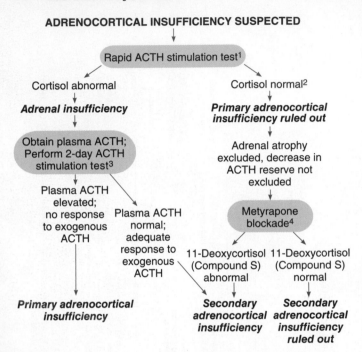

[1]In the rapid ACTH stimulation test, a baseline cortisol sample is obtained; Cosyntropin, 1–25 mcg, is given IM or IV; and plasma cortisol samples are obtained 30 or 60 minutes later.
[2]The normal response is a cortisol increment of >7 mcg/dL. If a cortisol level of >20 mcg/dL is obtained, the response is considered normal regardless of the increment.
[3]Administer ACTH, 250 mcg IV every 8 hours, as a continuous infusion for 48 hours, and measure daily urinary 17-hydroxycorticosteroids (17-OHCS) or free cortisol excretion and plasma cortisol. Urinary 17-OHCS excretion of >27 mg during the first 24 hours and >47 mg during the second 24 hours is normal. Plasma cortisol >20 mcg/dL at 30 or 60 minutes after infusion is begun and >25 mcg/dL 6–8 hours later is normal.
[4]Metyrapone blockade is performed by giving 2–2.5 g metyrapone orally at 12 midnight. Draw cortisol and 11-deoxycortisol levels at 8 AM. 11-Deoxycortisol level <7 mcg/dL indicates secondary adrenal insufficiency (as long as there is adequate blockade of cortisol synthesis [cortisol level <10 mcg/dL]).

Figure 9–3. ADRENOCORTICAL INSUFFICIENCY (HYPOCORTISOLISM): Laboratory evaluation of suspected adrenocortical insufficiency (hypocortisolism). ***ACTH*** = adrenocorticotropic hormone. (*Modified, with permission, from Miller WL, Tyrrell JB. The adrenal cortex. In: Endocrinology and Metabolism, 3rd ed. Felig P, Baxter JD, Frohman LA [editors]. McGraw-Hill, 1995.*)

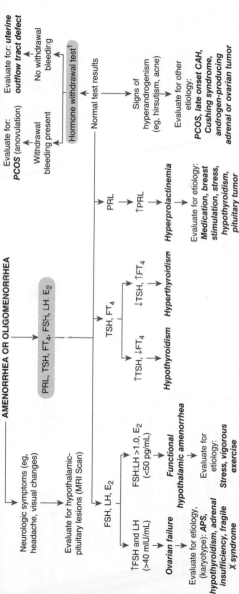

AMENORRHEA OR OLIGOMENORRHEA

PRL, TSH, FT₄, FSH, LH E₂

Neurologic symptoms (eg, headache, visual changes)

Evaluate for hypothalamic-pituitary lesions (MRI Scan)

FSH, LH, E₂

↑FSH and LH (>40 mIU/mL)

Ovarian failure

Evaluate for etiology, (karyotype): *APS, hypothyroidism, adrenal insufficiency, fragile X syndrome*

FSH:LH >1.0, E₂ (<50 pg/mL)

Functional hypothalamic amenorrhea

Evaluate for etiology: *Stress, vigorous exercise*

TSH, FT₄

↑TSH, ↓FT₄

Hypothyroidism

↓TSH, ↑FT₄

Hyperthyroidism

PRL

↑PRL

Hyperprolactinemia

Evaluate for etiology: *Medication, breast stimulation, stress, hypothyroidism, pituitary tumor*

Normal test results

Hormone withdrawal test[1]

Withdrawal bleeding present

Evaluate for: *PCOS* (anovulation)

No withdrawal bleeding

Evaluate for: *uterine outflow tract defect*

Signs of hyperandrogenism (eg, hirsutism, acne)

Evaluate for other etiology: *PCOS, late onset CAH, Cushing syndrome, androgen-producing adrenal or ovarian tumor*

---

[1]Give medroxyprogesterone 5–10 mg orally daily for 5 days. If withdrawal bleeding ensues, endogenous estrogen is adequate (eg, anovulation is occurring).

Figure 9–4. AMENORRHEA OR OLIGOMENORRHEA: Diagnostic laboratory evaluation for amenorrhea or oligomenorrhea. Primary amenorrhea is defined as the failure of menses to appear by age 16. Secondary amenorrhea is defined as occurring in women who have secondary sexual characteristics, have experienced menarche, and are presenting with consistently absent menses (more than 3 consecutive months). Oligomenorrhea is defined as scanty menses, or menses occurring at intervals of >35 days with only 4–9 menstrual periods in 1 year. Pregnancy must be ruled out before pursuing the testing outlined in the algorithm. *APS* = autoimmune polyglandular syndrome; *CAH* = congenital adrenal hyperplasia; *E₂* = estradiol; *FSH* = follicle-stimulating hormone; *FT₄* = free thyroxine; *LH* = luteinizing hormone; *MRI* = magnetic resonance imaging; *PCOS* = polycystic ovarian syndrome; *PRL* = prolactin; *TSH* = thyroid-stimulating hormone. (Modified, with permission, from Gardner DG, Shoback D [editors]: Greenspan's Basic & Clinical Endocrinology, 9th ed. Copyright © 2011 by The McGraw-Hill Companies, Inc.)

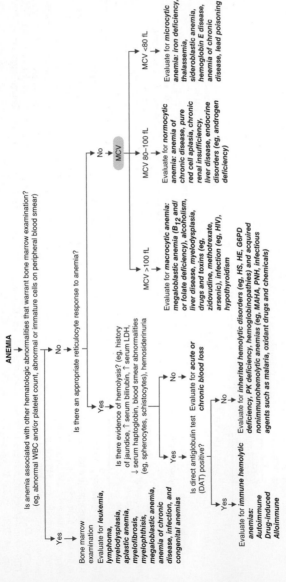

Figure 9–5. ANEMIA: General considerations and initial evaluation. The initial evaluation of anemia should include complete blood cell count, reticulocyte count and review of peripheral blood smear. *G6PD* = glucose-6-phosphate dehydrogenase; *HE* = hereditary elliptocytosis; *HS* = hereditary spherocytosis; *LDH* = lactate dehydrogenase; *MAHA* = microangiopathic hemolytic anemia; *MCV* = mean corpuscular volume; *PK* = pyruvate kinase; *PNH* = paroxysmal nocturnal hemoglobinuria.

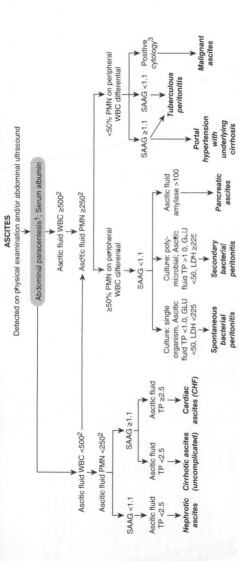

ASCITES
Detected on physical examination and/or abdominal ultrasound

Abdominal paracentesis[1]; Serum albumin

Ascitic fluid WBC <500[2]

   Ascitic fluid PMN <250[2]

      SAAG <1.1 — Ascitic fluid TP <2.5 → ***Nephrotic ascites***

      SAAG ≥1.1 — Ascitic fluid TP <2.5 → ***Cirrhotic ascites (uncomplicated)***

          — Ascitic fluid TP ≥2.5 → ***Cardiac ascites (CHF)***

Ascitic fluid WBC ≥500[2]

   Ascitic fluid PMN ≥250[2]

≥50% PMN on peripheral WBC differential

  SAAG <1.1

   Culture: single organism, Ascitic fluid TP <1.0, GLU <50, LDH <225 → ***Spontaneous bacterial peritonitis***

   Culture: poly-microbial; Ascitic fluid TP >1.0, GLU <50, LDH ≥225 → ***Secondary bacterial peritonitis***

   Ascitic fluid amylase >100 → ***Pancreatic ascites***

<50% PMN on peripheral WBC differential

  SAAG ≥1.1 → ***Portal hypertension with underlying cirrhosis***

  SAAG <1.1 → ***Tuberculous peritonitis***

    Positive cytology[3] → ***Malignant ascites***

[1]Note the gross appearance of fluid (crystal clear, transparent or cloudy yellow, bloody, milky, or dark brown), and send ascitic fluid for cell count and differential, total protein, albumin, glucose, LDH, amylase, Gram stain, AFB stain, bacterial and other cultures and cytology as indicated. Also send triglyceride for milky fluid, bilirubin for dark-brown fluid. (See Table 8–5.)
[2]For bloody fluid, subtract 1 WBC per 750 RBC and subtract 1 PMN per 250 RBC (cells/mm³).
[3]Malignant cells present.

Figure 9–6. ASCITES: Diagnostic evaluation. ***CHF*** = congestive heart failure; ***GLU*** = glucose (mg/dL); ***LDH*** = lactate dehydrogenase (IU/L); ***PMN*** = polymorphonuclear neutrophil (cells/mm³); ***RBC*** = red blood cell count (cells/mm³); ***SAAG*** = serum-ascites albumin gradient (g/dL); ***TP*** = total protein (g/dL); ***WBC*** = white blood cell count (cells/mm³). (Modified, with permission, from Feldman M, Friedman LS, Brandt LJ [editors]: Sleisenger and Fordtran's Gastrointestinal and Liver Disease: Pathophysiology, Diagnosis, Management. 9th ed. Saunders, 2010.)

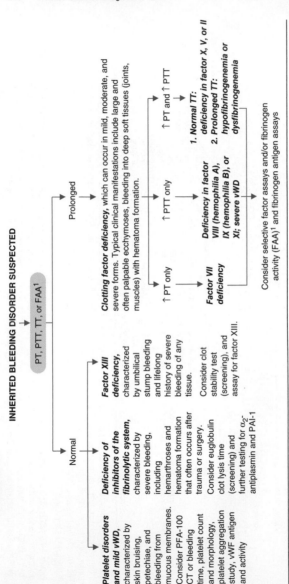

INHERITED BLEEDING DISORDER SUSPECTED

PT, PTT, TT, or FAA[1]

Normal

Prolonged

Platelet disorders and mild vWD, characterized by skin bruising, petechiae, and bleeding from mucous membranes. Consider PFA-100 CT or bleeding time, platelet count and morphology, platelet aggregation study, vWF antigen and activity.

Deficiency of inhibitors of the fibrinolytic system, characterized by severe bleeding, including hemarthroses and hematoma formation that often occurs after trauma or surgery. Consider euglobulin clot lysis time (screening) and further testing for α₂-antiplasmin and PAI-1.

Factor XIII deficiency, characterized by umbilical stump bleeding and lifelong history of severe bleeding of any tissue. Consider clot stability test (screening), and assay for factor XIII.

Clotting factor deficiency, which can occur in mild, moderate, and severe forms. Typical clinical manifestations include large and often palpable ecchymoses, bleeding into deep soft tissues (joints, muscles) with hematoma formation.

↑ PT only → *Factor VII deficiency*

↑ PTT only → *Deficiency in factor VIII (hemophilia A), IX (hemophilia B), or XI; severe vWD*

↑ PT and ↑ PTT →
1. *Normal TT: deficiency in factor X, V, or II*
2. *Prolonged TT: hypofibrinogenemia or dysfibrinogenemia*

Consider selective factor assays and/or fibrinogen activity (FAA)[1] and fibrinogen antigen assays

---

[1] *FAA (fibrinogen activity assay)* is now routinely available in clinical laboratories and has largely replaced the need for TT for evaluation of fibrinogen activity (function).

Figure 9–7. **BLEEDING DISORDERS, INHERITED:** Evaluation of suspected inherited bleeding disorders. *PAI-1* = plasminogen activator inhibitor 1; *PFA-100 CT* = platelet function analyzer-100 closure time; *PT* = prothrombin time; *PTT* = partial thromboplastin time; *TT* = thrombin time; *vWD* = von Willebrand disease; *vWF* = von Willebrand factor.

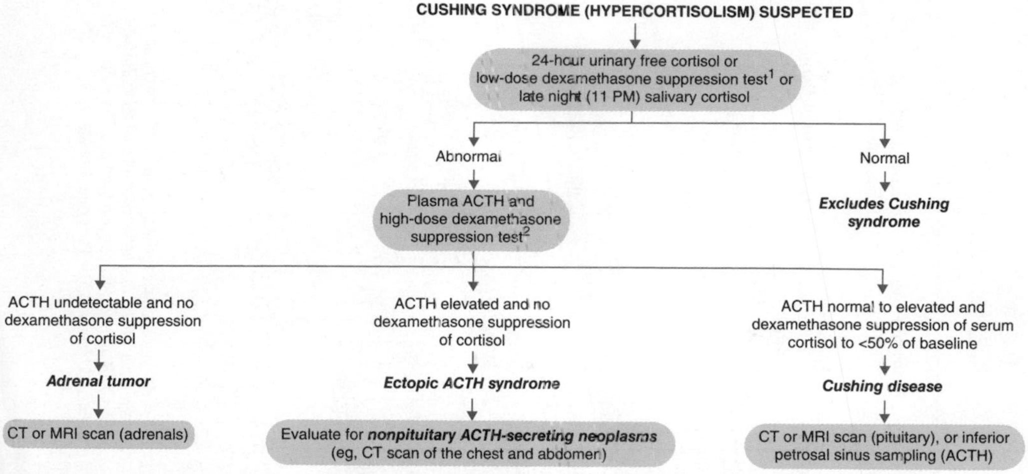
CUSHING SYNDROME (HYPERCORTISOLISM) SUSPECTED
24-hour urinary free cortisol or low-dose dexamethasone suppression test[1] or late night (11 PM) salivary cortisol
Abnormal
Normal
Plasma ACTH and high-dose dexamethasone suppression test[2]
Excludes Cushing syndrome
ACTH undetectable and no dexamethasone suppression of cortisol
Adrenal tumor
CT or MRI scan (adrenals)
ACTH elevated and no dexamethasone suppression of cortisol
Ectopic ACTH syndrome
Evaluate for nonpituitary ACTH-secreting neoplasms (eg, CT scan of the chest and abdomen)
ACTH normal to elevated and dexamethasone suppression of serum cortisol to <50% of baseline
Cushing disease
CT or MRI scan (pituitary), or inferior petrosal sinus sampling (ACTH)

[1]Low dose: Give 1 mg dexamethasone at 11 PM; draw serum cortisol at 8 AM. Normally, AM cortisol is <1.8 mcg/dL (50 nmol/L).
[2]High dose: Give 8 mg dexamethasone at 11 PM; draw serum cortisol at 8 AM or collect 24-hour urinary free cortisol. Normally, AM cortisol is <5 mcg/dL (<135 nmol/L) or 24-hour urinary free cortisol is <20 mcg.

Figure 9–8. CUSHING SYNDROME (HYPERCORTISOLISM): Diagnostic evaluation of suspected Cushing syndrome (hypercortisolism). ***ACTH*** = *adrenocorticotropic hormone;* ***CT*** = *computed tomography;* ***HPLC*** = *high-performance liquid chromatography;* ***MRI*** = *magnetic resonance imaging.*

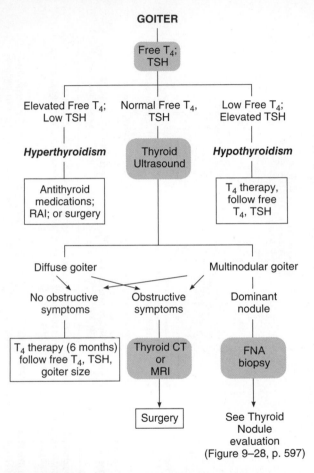

Figure 9–9. GOITER: Diagnostic evaluation and management strategy. **CT** = computed tomography; **FNA** = fine-needle aspiration; **MRI** = magnetic resonance imaging; **RAI** = radioactive iodine; **T₄** = L-thyroxine. **TSH** = thyroid-stimulating hormone. (Modified, with permission, from Goldman L, Bennett JC [editors]. Cecil's Textbook of Medicine, 22nd edition. Saunders, 2004.)

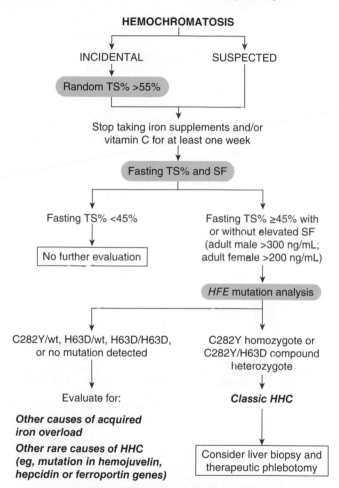

Figure 9–10. HEMOCHROMATOSIS: Diagnostic evaluation of suspected hemochromatosis. **HHC** = hereditary hemochromatosis. **SF** = serum ferritin; **TS%** = transferrin-iron saturation percentage (serum iron/total iron binding capacity × 100%).

HIRSUTISM

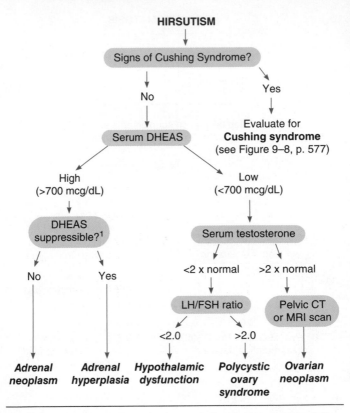

---

[1]DHEAS < 170 mcg/dL after dexamethasone 0.5 mg orally every 6 hours for 5 days, with DHEAS repeated on the fifth day.

Figure 9–11. HIRSUTISM: Evaluation of hirsutism in females. Exceptions occur that do not fit this algorithm. **CT** = computed tomography; **DHEAS** = dehydroepiandrosterone sulfate; **FSH** = follicle-stimulating hormone; **LH** = luteinizing hormone. (Reproduced, with permission, from Fitzgerald PA [editor]. Handbook of Clinical Endocrinology, 2nd edition. Originally published by Appleton & Lange. Copyright © 1992 by the McGraw-Hill Companies, Inc.)

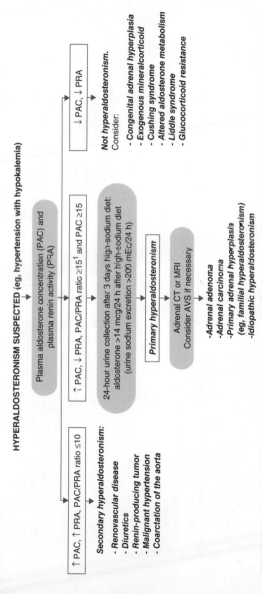

HYPERALDOSTERONISM SUSPECTED (eg, hypertension with hypokalemia)

Plasma aldosterone concentration (PAC) and plasma renin activity (PRA)

↑ PAC, ↑ PRA, PAC/PRA ratio ≤10

Secondary hyperaldosteronism:
- Renovascular disease
- Diuretics
- Renin-producing tumor
- Malignant hypertension
- Coarctation of the aorta

↑ PAC, ↓ PRA, PAC/PRA ratio ≥15[1] and PAC ≥15

24-hour urine collection after 3 days high-sodium diet: aldosterone >14 mcg/24 h after high-sodium diet (urine sodium excretion >200 mEq/24 h)

Primary hyperaldosteronism

Adrenal CT or MRI
Consider AVS if necessary

- *Adrenal adenoma*
- *Adrenal carcinoma*
- *Primary adrenal hyperplasia (eg, familial hyperaldosteronism)*
- *Idiopathic hyperaldosteronism*

↓ PAC, ↓ PRA

Not hyperaldosteronism. Consider:
- Congenital adrenal hyperplasia
- Exogenous mineralcorticoid
- Cushing syndrome
- Altered aldosterone metabolism
- Liddle syndrome
- Glucocorticoid resistance

[1]The cutoff for a "high" PAC/PRA ratio is laboratory-dependent and, more specifically, PRA assay-dependent, and therefore an increased PAC is required for the diagnosis.

Figure 9–12. HYPERALDOSTERONISM: Laboratory evaluation of suspected hyperaldosteronism. *AVS* = adrenal venous sampling; *CT* = computed tomography; *MRI* = magnetic resonance imaging; *PAC* = plasma aldosterone concentration (ng/dL); *PRA* = plasma renin activity (ng/mL/hr); *PAC/PRA ratio* = plasma aldosterone concentration to plasma renin activity ratio.

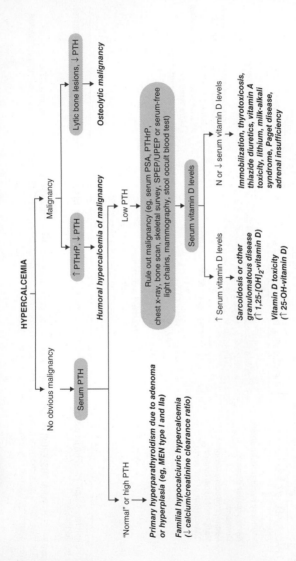

Figure 9–13. HYPERCALCEMIA: Diagnostic approach to hypercalcemia. **PTH** = parathyroid hormone (measured by intact PTH assay); **PTHrP** = PTH related protein; **PSA** = prostate specific antigen; **SPEP** = serum protein electrophoresis; **UPEP** = urine protein electrophoresis; ↑ = increase; ↓ = decrease.

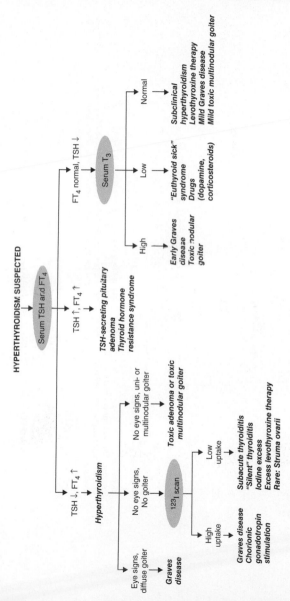

Figure 9–14. HYPERTHYROIDISM: Laboratory evaluation. **FT₄** = free thyroxine; **T₃** = 3,5,3'-triiodothyronine; **TSH** = thyroid-stimulating hormone. (Modified with permission from Gardner DG, Shoback D [editors]. Greenspan's Basic & Clinical Endocrinology, 9th edition. Originally published by Appleton & Lange. Copyright © 2011 by the McGraw-Hill Companies, Inc.)

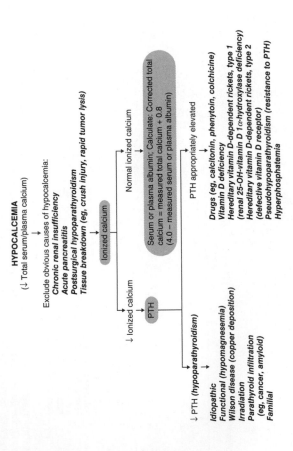

Figure 9–15. HYPOCALCEMIA: Diagnostic approach to hypocalcemia. *PTH = parathyroid hormone.*

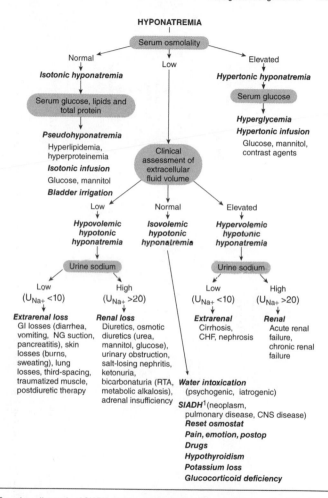

HYPONATREMIA

Serum osmolality

Normal → **Isotonic hyponatremia**

Serum glucose, lipids and total protein

Pseudohyponatremia
Hyperlipidemia, hyperproteinemia
Isotonic infusion
Glucose, mannitol
Bladder irrigation

Low → Clinical assessment of extracellular fluid volume

Elevated → **Hypertonic hyponatremia**

Serum glucose

Hyperglycemia
Hypertonic infusion
Glucose, mannitol, contrast agents

Low → **Hypovolemic hypotonic hyponatremia**

Urine sodium

Low (U$_{Na+}$ <10) → **Extrarenal loss**
GI losses (diarrhea, vomiting, NG suction, pancreatitis), skin losses (burns, sweating), lung losses, third-spacing, traumatized muscle, postdiuretic therapy

High (U$_{Na+}$ >20) → **Renal loss**
Diuretics, osmotic diuretics (urea, mannitol, glucose), urinary obstruction, salt-losing nephritis, ketonuria, bicarbonaturia (RTA, metabolic alkalosis), adrenal insufficiency

Normal → **Isovolemic hypotonic hyponatremia**

Water intoxication (psychogenic, iatrogenic)
SIADH[1] (neoplasm, pulmonary disease, CNS disease)
Reset osmostat
Pain, emotion, postop
Drugs
Hypothyroidism
Potassium loss
Glucocorticoid deficiency

Elevated → **Hypervolemic hypotonic hyponatremia**

Urine sodium

Low (U$_{Na+}$ <10) → **Extrarenal**
Cirrhosis, CHF, nephrosis

High (U$_{Na+}$ >20) → **Renal**
Acute renal failure, chronic renal failure

[1]To make a diagnosis of SIADH, must exclude hypothyroidism and glucocorticoid insufficiency first.

Figure 9–16. HYPONATREMIA: Evaluation of hyponatremia. ***CHF*** = *congestive heart failure;* ***CNS*** = *central nervous system;* ***GI*** = *gastrointestinal;* ***NG*** = *nasogastric;* ***RTA*** = *renal tubular acidosis;* ***SIADH*** = *syndrome of inappropriate antidiuretic hormone;* ***U***$_{Na+}$ = *urinary sodium (mg/dL).* (*Adapted, with permission, from Narins RG et al. Diagnostic strategies of fluid, electrolyte, and acid-base homeostasis.* Am J Med *1982;72:496.* [PMID: 7036739])

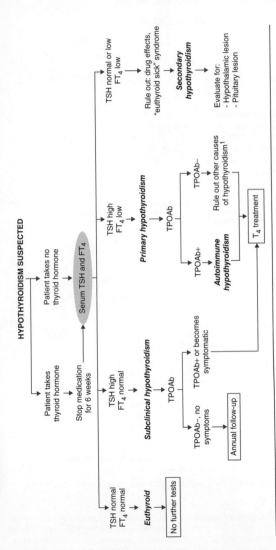

Figure 9–17. HYPOTHYROIDISM: Diagnostic approach. *FT₄* = free thyroxine; *TPOAb+* = thyroid peroxidase antibodies positive; *TPOAb−* = thyroid peroxidase antibodies negative; *TSH* = thyroid-stimulating hormone.

[1]Other causes of hypothyroidism include iatrogenic (eg, irradiation, thyroidectomy), drugs (eg, lithium, antithyroid drugs), congenital, iodine deficiency, and infiltrative disorders involving thyroid gland.

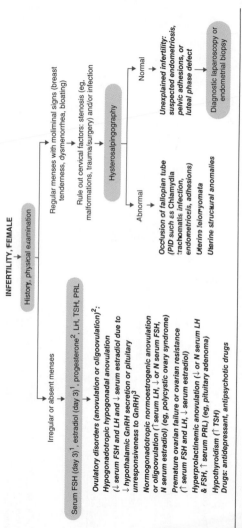

INFERTILITY, FEMALE

History, physical examination

Irregular or absent menses

Serum FSH (day 3)[1], estradiol (day 3)[1], progesterone[2], LH, TSH, PRL

Ovulatory disorders (anovulation or oligoovulation)[2]:

Hypogonadotropic hypogonadal anovulation (↓ serum FSH and LH and ↓ serum estradiol due to ↓ hypothalamic GnRH secretion or pituitary unresponsiveness to GnRH)[3]

Normogonadotropic normoestrogenic anovulation or oligoovulation (↑ serum LH, ↓ or N serum FSH, N serum estradiol) (eg, polycystic ovary syndrome)

Premature ovarian failure or ovarian resistance (↑ serum FSH and LH, ↓ serum estradiol)

Hyperprolactinemic anovulation (↓ or N serum LH & FSH, ↑ serum PRL) (eg, pituitary adenoma)

Hypothyroidism (↑ TSH)

Drugs: antidepressant, antipsychotic drugs

Regular menses with molimina signs (breast tenderness, dysmenorrhea, bloating)

Rule out cervical factors: stenosis (eg, malformations, trauma/surgery) and/or infection

Hysterosalpingography

Abnormal

Occlusion of fallopian tube (PID such as Chlamydia trachomatis infection, endometriosis, adhesions)

Uterine leiomyomata

Uterine structural anomalies

Normal

Unexplained infertility: suspected endometriosis, pelvic adhesions, or luteal phase defect

Diagnostic laparoscopy or endometrial biopsy

[1]Day 1 is the first day of full menstrual flow.

[2]A mid-luteal phase serum progesterone level <3 ng/mL suggests anovulation.

[3]Hypogonadotropic hypogonadal anovulation (hypothalamic-pituitary amenorrhea) can be caused by Kallman syndrome, Sheehan syndrome, empty sella syndrome, autoimmune diseases (eg, lymphocytic hypophysitis), tumors/trauma/radiation of the hypothalamic or pituitary area, stress, eating disorders, and intense exercise.

Figure 9-18. INFERTILITY, FEMALE: Evaluation of female infertility. *FSH* = follicle-stimulating hormone; *GnRH* = gonadotropin-releasing hormone; *LH* = luteinizing hormone; *PID* = pelvic inflammatory disease; *PRL* = prolactin; *TSH* = thyroid stimulating hormone.

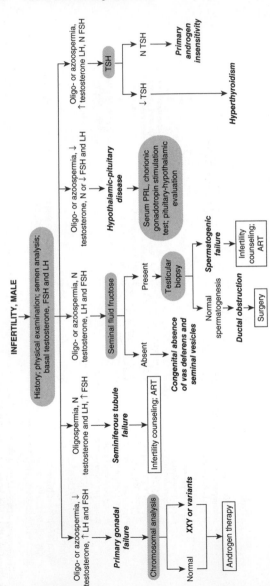

Figure 9–19. INFERTILITY, MALE: Evaluation of male factor infertility. **ART** = assisted reproductive technologies; **FSH** = follicle-stimulating hormone; **LH** = Luteinizing hormones; **PRL** = prolactin; **TSH** = thyroid-stimulating hormone. (Adapted, with permission, from Gardner DG, Shoback D [editors]. Greenspan's Basic and Clinical Endocrinology, 9th edition. McGraw-Hill, 2011.)

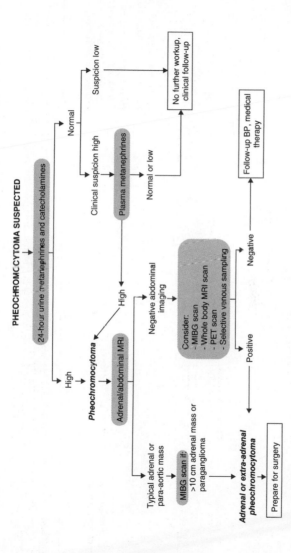

Figure 9–20. PHEOCHROMOCYTOMA: Evaluation and localization of a possible pheochromocytoma. Clinical suspicion is triggered by paroxysmal symptoms (especially hypertension); hypertension that is intermittent, unusually labile, or resistant to treatment; family history of pheochromocytoma or associated conditions; or an incidentally discovered adrenal mass. *BP = blood pressure; **MIBG** = ^{131}I- or ^{123}I-labeled metaiodobenzylguanidine; **MRI** = magnetic resonance imaging; **PET** = positron emission tomography.*

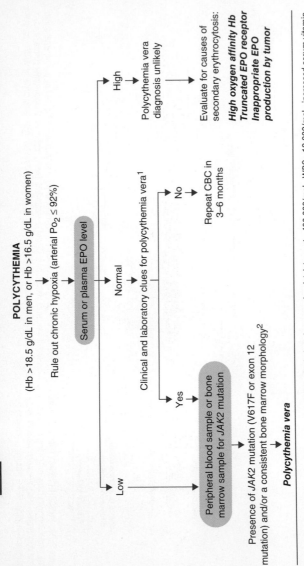

POLYCYTHEMIA
(Hb >18.5 g/dL in men, or Hb >16.5 g/dL in women)

Rule out chronic hypoxia (arterial Po₂ ≤ 92%)

Serum or plasma EPO level

Low → Peripheral blood sample or bone marrow sample for *JAK2* mutation

Presence of *JAK2* mutation (V617F or exon 12 mutation) and/or a consistent bone marrow morphology[2]

Polycythemia vera

Normal → Clinical and laboratory clues for polycythemia vera[1]

Yes → Peripheral blood sample or bone marrow sample for *JAK2* mutation

No → Repeat CBC in 3–6 months

High → Polycythemia vera diagnosis unlikely → Evaluate for causes of secondary erythrocytosis:
High oxygen affinity Hb
Truncated EPO receptor
Inappropriate EPO production by tumor

[1]Clinical and laboratory clues for polycythemia vera include splenomegaly, platelet count >400,000/mcL, WBC >12,000/mcL, increased serum vitamin B₁₂ or vitamin B₁₂ binding capacity, and no history of familial erythrocytosis.

[2]*JAK2*ᵛ⁶¹⁷ᶠ mutation has been found to be present in >95% of patients with polycythemia vera; mutation in exon 12 of *JAK2* has also been reported. Bone marrow biopsy shows panmyelosis with prominent erythroid and megakaryocytic proliferation.

Figure 9–21. POLYCYTHEMIA: Diagnostic evaluation. *CBC* = complete blood cell count; *EPO* = erythropoietin; *Hb* = hemoglobin; *JAK2* = Janus kinase 2 gene.

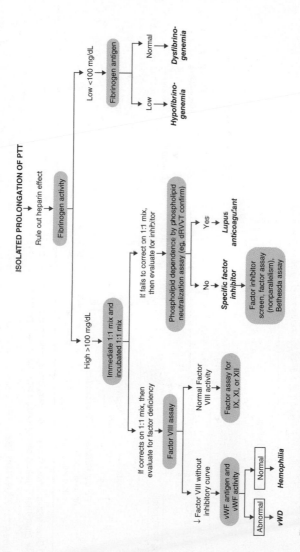

Figure 9–22. ISOLATED PROLONGATION OF PTT: Laboratory evaluation. **dRVVT** = dilute Russell viper venom time; **PTT** = activated partial thromboplastin time; **vWF** = von Willebrand factor; **vWD** = von Willebrand disease.

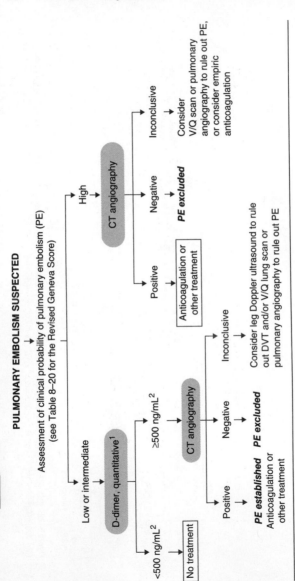

PULMONARY EMBOLISM SUSPECTED

Assessment of clinical probability of pulmonary embolism (PE)
(see Table 8–20 for the Revised Geneva Score)

[1]D-Dimer testing is typically used in the emergency department to rule out PE.
[2]The cutoff value is method-dependent (eg, 500 ng/mL is the cutoff for the ELISA-based D-dimer assay).

Figure 9–23. PULMONARY EMBOLISM: Diagnostic strategy for patients with suspected pulmonary embolism. **CT** = *computed tomography;* **DVT** = *deep venous thrombosis;* **PE** = *pulmonary embolism;* **V/Q scan** = *ventilation-perfusion scan.* (Modified from Le Gal G et al. Prediction of pulmonary embolism in the emergency department: the revised Geneva score. Ann Intern Med 2006;144:165. [PMID: 16461960])

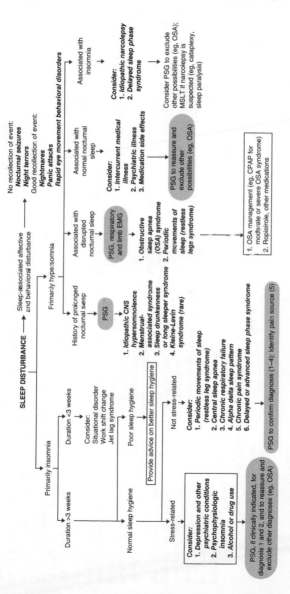

Figure 9–24. SLEEP DISTURBANCE: Diagnostic evaluation. Poor sleep hygiene refers to products or behaviors that can interfere with sleep, such as caffeine, alcohol, and tobacco, intense exercise in the evening, and irregular sleeping schedule. ***CNS*** = central nervous system; ***CPAP*** = continuous positive airway pressure; ***EMG*** = electromyogram; ***MSLTs*** = multiple sleep latency tests (note: patient must be off antidepressants and stimulants to undergo an MSLT); ***PSG*** = polysomnography.

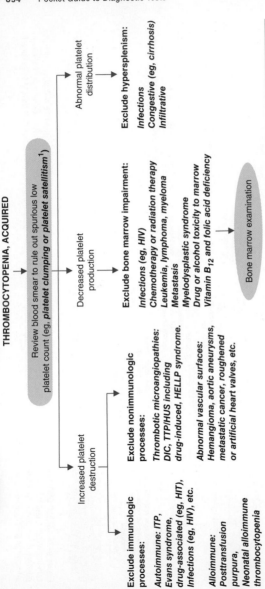

THROMBOCYTOPENIA, ACQUIRED

Review blood smear to rule out spurious low
platelet count (eg, *platelet clumping or platelet satellitism*[1])

Increased platelet destruction

Exclude immunologic processes:

Autoimmune: ITP,
Evans syndrome,
drug-associated (eg, HIT),
Infections (eg, HIV), etc.

Alloimmune:
Posttransfusion
purpura,
Neonatal alloimmune
thrombocytopenia

Exclude nonimmunologic processes:

Thrombotic microangiopathies:
DIC, TTP/HUS including
drug-induced, HELLP syndrome.

Abnormal vascular surfaces:
Hemangioma, aortic aneurysms,
metastatic cancer, roughened
or artificial heart valves, etc.

Decreased platelet production

Exclude bone marrow impairment:

Infections (eg, HIV)
Chemotherapy or radiation therapy
Leukemia, lymphoma, myeloma
Metastasis
Myelodysplastic syndrome
Drug or alcohol toxicity to marrow
Vitamin B_{12} and folic acid deficiency

Bone marrow examination

Abnormal platelet distribution

Exclude hypersplenism:

Infections
Congestive (eg, cirrhosis)
Infiltrative

[1]Platelet satellitism, a rare peripheral blood finding, is adherence of 4 or more platelets to the surface of a neutrophil or monocyte. Similar to platelet clumping, it is an *in vitro* phenomenon often seen in EDTA-anticoagulated (lavender tube) whole blood. It may cause false thrombocytopenia with automated cell counters.

Figure 9–25. ACQUIRED THROMBOCYTOPENIA: Diagnostic approach to acquired thrombocytopenia. **DIC** = *disseminated intravascular coagulation;* **HELLP syndrome** = *hemolytic anemia, elevated liver enzymes, and low platelet count;* **HIT** = *heparin-induced thrombocytopenia;* **HIV** = *human immunodeficiency virus;* **HUS** = *hemolytic uremic syndrome;* **ITP** = *idiopathic thrombocytopenic purpura;* **TTP** = *thrombotic thrombocytopenic purpura.*

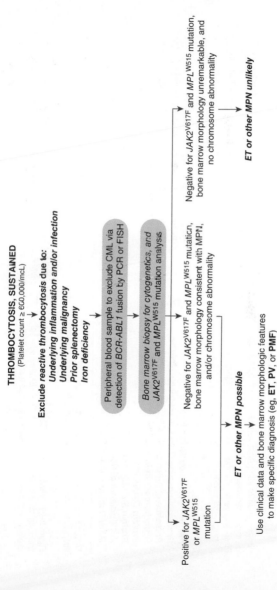

THROMBOCYTOSIS, SUSTAINED
(Platelet count ≥ 600,000/mcL)

Exclude reactive thrombocytosis due to:
  Underlying inflammation and/or infection
  Underlying malignancy
  Prior splenectomy
  Iron deficiency

Peripheral blood sample to exclude CML via detection of *BCR-ABL1* fusion by PCR or FISH

Bone marrow biopsy for cytogenetics, and $JAK2^{V617F}$ and MPL^{W515} mutation analysis

Positive for $JAK2^{V617F}$ or MPL^{W515} mutation

ET or other MPN possible

Use clinical data and bone marrow morphologic features to make specific diagnosis (eg, **ET**, **PV**, or **PMF**)

Negative for $JAK2^{V617F}$ and MPL^{W515} mutation, bone marrow morphology consistent with MPN, and/or chromosome abnormality

Negative for $JAK2^{V617F}$ and MPL^{W515} mutation, bone marrow morphology unremarkable, and no chromosome abnormality

ET or other MPN unlikely

Figure 9–26. THROMBOCYTOSIS: Diagnostic evaluation of sustained thrombocytosis. **CML** = chronic myeloid leukemia; **ET** = essential thrombocythemia; **FISH** = fluorescence in-situ hybridization; **JAK2** = Janus kinase 2 gene; **MPL** = myeloproliferative leukemia gene; **MPN** = myeloproliferative neoplasms; **PCR** = polymerase chain reaction; **PMF** = primary myelofibrosis; **PV** = polycythemia vera.

VENUS THROMBOSIS, ESTABLISHED

Exclude acquired thrombosis (eg, malignancy, orthopedic surgery, trauma, immobilization, CHF, CMPD, nephrotic syndrome, hyperviscosity, PNH[1])

If none present, and:

First episode of idiopathic venous thrombosis at age <50 years OR
History of recurrent thrombotic episodes OR
First-degree relative(s) with documented thromboembolism at age <50 years

Evaluate for:

Factor V Leiden mutation by PCR
Prothrombin gene G20210A mutation by PCR
Presence of lupus anticoagulant (eg, dRVVT)
Hyperhomocysteinemia
Protein C deficiency
Protein S deficiency
Antithrombin deficiency
MTHFR mutation by PCR

First episodes of idiopathic venous thromboembolism at age ≥50 years and
Negative family history of thromboembolism

Evaluate for:

Factor V Leiden mutation by PCR
Prothrombin gene G20210A mutation by PCR
Presence of lupus anticoagulant (eg, dRVVT)
Hyperhomocysteinemia

[1]Thrombosis occurs in 40–45% of patients with PNH, often at unusual sites, including hepatic veins (Budd-Chiari syndrome), other intra-abdominal veins (portal, splenic, splanchnic), cerebral sinuses, and dermal veins.

Figure 9–27. VENUS THROMBOSIS: Evaluation for possible hypercoagulability (thrombophilia) causing venous thrombosis. **CHF** = congestive heart failure; **CMPD** = chronic myeloproliferative disorder; **dRVVT** = dilute Russell viper venom clotting time; **MTHFR** = methylene tetrahydrofolate reductase; **PCR** = polymerase chain reaction; **PNH** = paroxysmal nocturnal hemoglobinuria.

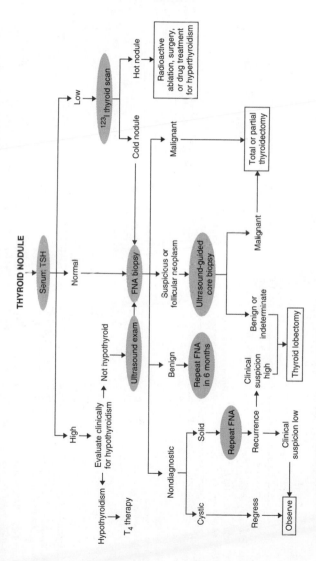

Figure 9-28. THYROID NODULE: Diagnostic evaluation. *FNA* = fine-needle aspiration, *TSH* = thyroid-stimulating hormone. (Modified, with permission, from Burch HB. Evaluation and management of the solid thyroid nodule. Endocrinol Metab Clin North Am 1995;24:663.)

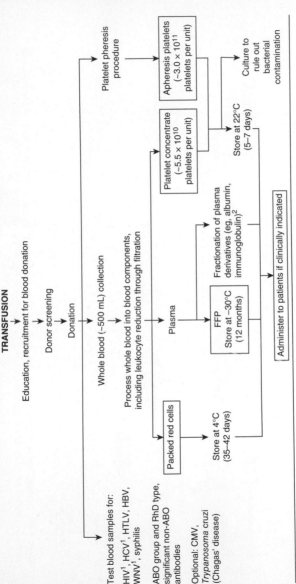

Figure 9–29. TRANSFUSION: Blood donation and preparation of blood components. ***CMV*** = *cytomegalovirus;* ***FFP*** = *fresh frozen plasma;* ***HBV*** = *hepatitis B virus;* ***HCV*** = *hepatitis C virus;* ***HIV*** = *human immunodeficiency virus;* ***HTLV*** = *human T-cell leukemia virus;* ***WNV*** = *West Nile virus.*

[1]Nucleic acid testing (NAT) should be included for HIV, HCV, and WNV screening.

[2]Plasma derivatives are also prepared through plasmapheresis.

10

Nomograms and Reference Material

Michael Pignone, MD, MPH, Stephen J. McPhee, MD,
Diana Nicoll, MD, PhD, MPA, and Chuanyi Mark Lu, MD

HOW TO USE THIS SECTION

This section contains useful nomograms and reference material. Material is
presented in alphabetical order by subject.

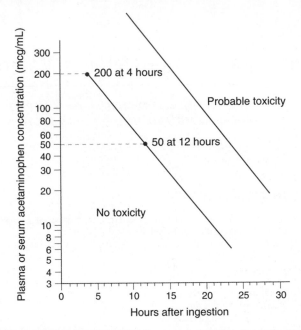

Figure 10–1. ACETAMINOPHEN TOXICITY: Nomogram for prediction of acetaminophen hepatotoxicity following acute overdosage. The upper line defines serum acetaminophen concentrations known to be associated with hepatotoxicity; the lower line defines serum levels 25% lower than those expected to cause hepatotoxicity. To give a margin for error, the lower line should be used as a guide to treatment. (*Modified and reproduced, with permission, from Rumack BH, Matthew H. Acetaminophen poisoning and toxicity.* Pediatrics *1975;55:871. Reproduced by permission of Pediatrics. Copyright© 1975.*)

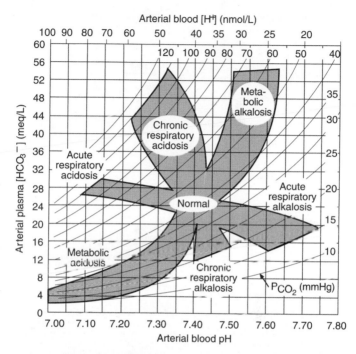

Figure 10–2. ACID–BASE NOMOGRAM: Shown are the 95% confidence limits of the normal respiratory and metabolic compensations for primary acid–base disturbances. (*Reproduced, with permission, from Brenner BM, Rector FC [editors]. Brenner & Rector's the Kidney, 8th ed. Saunders/Elsevier, 2008.*)

Extrinsic pathway　　　　　　　**Intrinsic pathway**

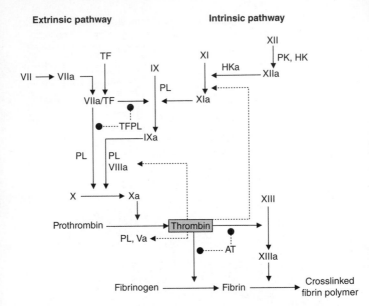

Figure 10–3. THE COAGULATION CASCADE: Schematic representation of the coagulation pathways. The central precipitating event is considered to involve tissue factor (TF), which under physiologic conditions, is not exposed to the blood. With vascular or endothelial cell injury, TF acts together with Factor VIIa and phospholipids (PL) to convert Factor IX to IXa and Factor X to Xa. The "intrinsic pathway" includes "contact" activation of Factor XI by XIIa-activated high molecular-weight kininogen complex (XIIa-HKa). Factor XIa converts Factor IX to IXa, which, in turn, converts Factor X to Xa, in concert with Factor VIIIa and PL. Factor Xa is the active ingredient of the "prothrombinase" complex, which includes Factor Va and PL, and converts prothrombin to thrombin (TH). TH cleaves fibrinopeptides from fibrinogen, allowing the resultant fibrin monomers to polymerize, and converts Factor XIII to XIIIa, which cross-links the fibrin clot. TH also accelerates and augments the process (in dashed lines) by activating Factor V and VIII, but continued proteolytic action also dampens the process by activating protein C, which degrades Factor Va and VIIIa. TH activation of Factor XI to XIa is a proposed pathway. There are natural plasma inhibitors of the cascade: tissue factor pathway inhibitor (TFPI) blocks VIIa/TF and thus inactivates the "extrinsic pathway" after the clotting process is initiated; antithrombin (AT) blocks IXa, and Xa, and thrombin. Arrows = active enzymes; dashed lines with arrows = positive feedback reactions, which are considered important to maintain the process after the "extrinsic pathway" is shut down by TFPI; dashed lines with solid dots = inhibitory effects; *PK* = *prekallikrein*. Note that the contact system (PK, HK, and XII) actually contributes to fibrinolysis and bradykinin formation in vivo, and its role in initiation of the intrinsic pathway in vivo is questionable.

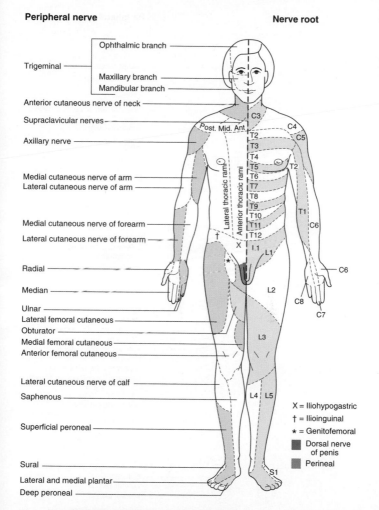

Figure 10–4. DERMATOME CHART: Cutaneous innervation. The segmental or radicular (root) distribution is shown on the right side of the body, and the peripheral nerve distribution on the left side. **Above:** anterior view; **next page:** posterior view. (*Reproduced, with permission, from Simon R et al [editors]. Clinical Neurology, 7th ed., McGraw-Hill, 2009.*)

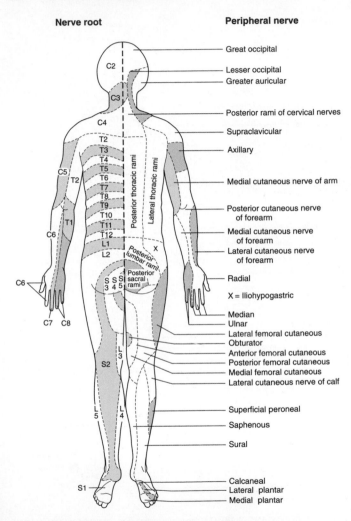

Figure 10–4. *(Continued)*

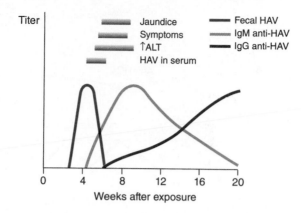

Figure 10–5. HEPATITIS A: Usual pattern of serologic changes in hepatitis A. **ALT** = *alanine aminotransferase;* **Anti-HAV** = *hepatitis A virus antibody;* **HAV** = *hepatitis A virus;* **IgM** = *immunoglobulin M;* **IgG** = *immunoglobulin G. (Reproduced, with permission, from Koff RS: Acute viral hepatitis. In:* Handbook of Liver Disease. *Friedman LS, Keeffe EB [editors], 2nd ed.* © *Elsevier, 2004.)*

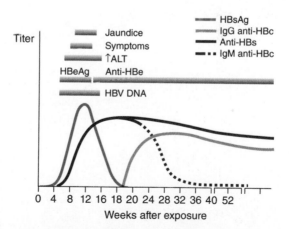

Figure 10–6. HEPATITIS B: Usual pattern of serologic changes in hepatitis B. **ALT** = *alanine aminotransferase;* **Anti-HBc** = *hepatitis B core antibody;* **Anti-HBe** = *antibody to hepatitis B e antigen;* **Anti-HBs** = *hepatitis B surface antibody;* **HBeAg** = *hepatitis B e antigen;* **HBsAg** = *hepatitis B surface antigen;* **HBV** = *hepatitis B virus;* **HBV DNA** = *Hepatitis B viral DNA;* **IgG** = *immunoglobulin G;* **IgM** = *immunoglobulin M. (Reproduced, with permission, from Koff RS: Acute viral hepatitis. In:* Handbook of Liver Disease. *Friedman LS, Keeffe EB [editors], 2nd ed.* © *Elsevier, 2004.)*

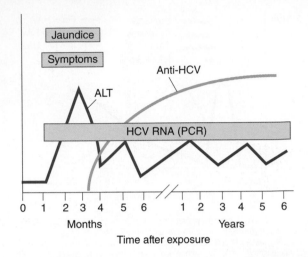

Figure 10–7. HEPATITIS C: The typical course of chronic hepatitis C. **ALT** = *alanine amino-transferase.* **Anti-HCV** = *antibody to hepatitis C virus by enzyme immunoassay;* **HCV RNA [PCR]** = *hepatitis C viral RNA by polymerase chain reaction.* (*Reproduced, with permission, from McPhee SJ, Papadakis MA, Rabow MW [editors].* Current Medical Diagnosis & Treatment 2012. *McGraw-Hill, 2012.*)

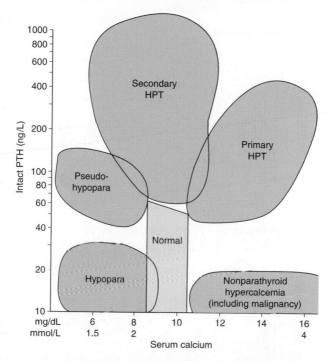

Figure 10–8. PARATHYROID HORMONE AND CALCIUM NOMOGRAM. Relation between
serum intact parathyroid hormone (PTH) and serum calcium levels in patients with hypo-
parathyroidism, pseudohypoparathyroidism, nonparathyroid hypercalcemia, primary
hyperparathyroidism, and secondary hyperparathyroidism. ***HPT*** = *hyperparathyroidism.*
(*Used with permission from Gordon Strewler, MD.*)
Note: A recent study suggests that a multivariate model that adds clinical and demographic
information may perform better than the nomogram alone. (*See O'Neill SS et al. Multivariate
analysis of clinical, demographic, and laboratory data for classification of disorders of
calcium homeostasis. Am J Clin Pathol 2011;135:100. [PMID: 21173131]*)

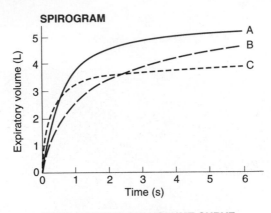

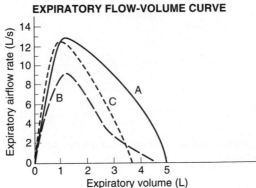

Figure 10–9. PULMONARY FUNCTION TESTS: SPIROMETRY. Representative spirograms (upper panel) and expiratory flow-volume curves (lower panel) for normal (A), obstructive (B), and restrictive (C) patterns. (*Reproduced, with permission, from Tierney LM Jr, McPhee SJ, Papadakis MA [editors]. Current Medical Diagnosis & Treatment 2005, 44th ed.* McGraw-Hill, 2005.)

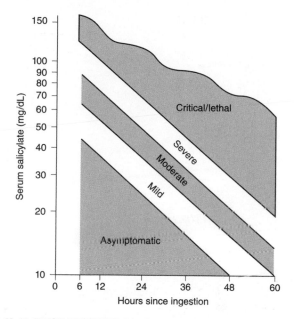

Figure 10–10. SALICYLATE TOXICITY: Nomogram for determining severity of salicylate intoxication after acute ingestion of non–enteric-coated aspirin preparation. (*Modified and reproduced, with permission, from Done AK. Significance of measurements of salicylate in blood in cases of acute ingestion. Pediatrics 1960;26:800. Reproduced by permission of* Pediatrics. *Copyright © 1960.*)

Index

NOTE: A *t* following a page number indicates tabular material, and an *f* following a page number indicates a figure.